The Health Collection
provided by
Genesis Health Services
Foundation

GASPING FOR AIR

GASPING
FOR AIR

How Breathing Is Killing Us and What We Can Do about It

Kevin Glynn, MD

ROWMAN & LITTLEFIELD
Lanham • Boulder • New York • London

Published by Rowman & Littlefield
A wholly owned subsidiary of The Rowman & Littlefield Publishing Group, Inc.
4501 Forbes Boulevard, Suite 200, Lanham, Maryland 20706
www.rowman.com

Unit A, Whitacre Mews, 26-34 Stannary Street, London SE11 4AB, United Kingdom

British Library Cataloguing in Publication Information Available

Library of Congress Cataloging-in-Publication Data

Names: Glynn, Kevin, 1936– author.
Title: Gasping for air : how breathing is killing us and what we can do about
    it / Kevin Glynn, M.D.
Description: Lanham : Rowman & Littlefield, [2017] | Includes bibliographical
    references and index.
Identifiers: LCCN 2016057285 (print) | LCCN 2017013096 (ebook) | ISBN
    9781442246249 (electronic) | ISBN 9781442246232 (cloth : alk. paper)
Subjects: LCSH: Respiratory organs—Diseases. | Respiratory
    organs—Diseases—Treatment.
Classification: LCC RC736 (ebook) | LCC RC736 .G59 2017 (print) | DDC
    616.2—dc23
LC record available at https://lccn.loc.gov/2016057285

♾™ The paper used in this publication meets the minimum requirements of
American National Standard for Information Sciences—Permanence of Paper
for Printed Library Materials, ANSI/NISO Z39.48-1992.

Printed in the United States of America

To Patty:
You take my breath away

"The Lord God formed the man from the dust of the ground and breathed into his nostrils the breath of life, and the man became a living being."[1]

—Genesis 2:4

CONTENTS

TIMELINE

How Breathing Kills	Year	What We Can Do about It
	1543	Andreas Vesalius publishes *On the Fabric of the Human Body*
	1628	William Harvey demonstrates circulation of blood
John Bunyan labels consumption (tuberculosis) "captain of the men of death"	1680	
	1700	Bernardino Ramazzini publishes treatise on occupational diseases
	1774	Joseph Priestley discovers oxygen
	1796	Edward Jenner performs first cowpox vaccination (against smallpox)

How Breathing Kills	Year	What We Can Do about It
	1797	Giovanni Venturi demonstrates jet effect of forcing liquid through a small orifice
	1819	René Laennec describes the pathology of emphysema
Charles Dickens pens *Pickwick Papers*, in which he describes respiratory failure in obesity	1836	
	1856	Rudolph Virchow connects venous blood clots and pulmonary emboli
Henry Salter describes clinical features of asthma	1860	
	1874	Germany passes compulsory vaccination law
James Bonsack invents cigarette rolling machine	1880	Workable infant incubator invented Louis Pasteur and George Sternberg discover pneumococcus
	1882	Robert Koch discovers tuberculosis bacillus
	1885	Edward Trudeau opens tuberculosis sanatorium at Saranac Lake, NY
First description of coccidioidal fungus infection	1892	
First polio outbreak in the United States	1894	
William Osler notes pneumonia has replaced tuberculosis as "captain of the men of death"	1901	

How Breathing Kills	Year	What We Can Do about It
Pierre and Marie Curie isolate radium	1902	
Iroquois Theater fire in Chicago kills 600 people	1903	
	1904	Founding of National Association for Prevention and Treatment of Tuberculosis
	1907	Christmas Seals launched
	1908	US Congress passes first federal workers' compensation law
First case of sickle-cell disease in the United States described	1910	
Great Influenza kills 35 million	1918	
	1921	BCG vaccine against tuberculosis first administered
	1926	Alvan Barach invents first workable oxygen tent
	1929	Philip Drinker invents iron lung
J. M. Campbell describes farmers' lung	1932	
	1933	Evarts Graham performs first successful pneumonectomy for lung cancer
Hawk's Nest silicosis disaster kills 400 workers	1936	
Dorothy Andersen describes clinical picture of cystic fibrosis	1938	Jonas Salk and Thomas Francis develop first influenza vaccine
	1939	Karl Link and Harold Campbell isolate anticoagulant dicumarol

How Breathing Kills	Year	What We Can Do about It
	1942	First civilian use of penicillin
Los Angeles "gas" attack begins war on smog	1943	
	1944	Selman Waksman and Albert Schatz discover streptomycin active against tuberculosis
Donora, PA, air pollution catastrophe	1948	Bennett valve used to assist ventilation in polio patients
Ernst Wynder and Evarts Graham report tobacco a possible factor in lung cancer	1949	Public Health Service Act establishes NIH as research arm of federal government
	1950	Edward Kendall and Philip Hench win Nobel Prize for discovering adrenal steroids
Killer fog hits London Global polio epidemic	1952	Isoniazid revolutionizes treatment of tuberculosis Henrik Ibsen in Denmark uses positive-pressure ventilation to treat polio victims
Golfer Ben Hogan sustains massive pulmonary emboli after auto accident Hyaline membrane disease described as cause of respiratory distress of newborns	1953	Virginia Apgar describes scoring system to predict survival of newborns
	1955	Salk vaccine against polio released
	1959	Mary Ellen Avery and Jere Mead connect respiratory distress of newborns with lack of surfactant Amphotericin B antifungal introduced

How Breathing Kills	Year	What We Can Do about It
	1965	Linde liquid oxygen reservoir introduced Henri Gastaut notices a connection between breathing and airway obstruction
	1966	Kimishige Ishizaka and Gunnar Johansson describe immunoglobulin E role in allergies
	1967	Fluconazole, first oral antifungal agent, released
	1968	Puritan–Bennett introduces MA-1 ventilator
	1969	Thomas Petty shows oxygen keeps COPD patients out of hospital
	1973	American Lung Association adopts current name
Philadelphia outbreak of Legionnaires' disease	1976	California establishes Air Quality Management District Karen Ann Quinlan withdrawn from ventilator support after court order
	1977	First pneumococcal vaccine licensed
Indiana outbreak of histoplasmosis	1978	
	1980	Colin Sullivan in Australia describes CPAP to treat sleep apnea
Bhopal disaster in India kills thousands	1981	
	1982	Albert Jonsen and Mark Siegler publish first edition of *Clinical Ethics*

How Breathing Kills	Year	What We Can Do about It
	1989	Gene that causes cystic fibrosis recognized
New Mexico hantavirus outbreak	**1993**	
	1995	Actor Christopher Reeve injures spinal cord and is kept alive on ventilator
FDA releases OxyContin; opioid epidemic starts	**1996**	
Discovery of atmospheric brown cloud	**1999**	
9/11 attack in New York, DC, and Pennsylvania	**2001**	
SARS epidemic Hon Lik invents e-cigarette	**2003**	
	2004	ADAM$_{33}$ gene discovered in asthmatics
	2005	Sildenafil approved to treat primary pulmonary arterial hypertension
MERS-CoV epidemic Colorado and Washington become first states to legalize recreational marijuana	**2012**	FDA releases ivacaftor to treat cystic fibrosis Anne Glover coins term *age of biology* to describe twenty-first century
Jahi McMath declared brain dead after sleep apnea surgery tragedy	**2013**	

How Breathing Kills	Year	What We Can Do about It
	2014	FDA approves nivolumab Immunotherapy for non-small-cell lung cancer begins Sublingual oral therapy for allergic asthma approved Pirfenidone approved in United States for treatment of pulmonary fibrosis
	2015	FDA approves oral anticoagulant dabigatran

AUTHOR'S NOTE

Thirty-six million Americans live with respiratory impairment. Three hundred thousand of them will die this year: 140,000 from chronic pulmonary diseases and 160,000 from lung cancer. Worldwide, over six million people will die this year from respiratory diseases like pneumonia, COPD, and tuberculosis. Only cancer and cardiovascular diseases are responsible for more fatalities in the developed world.[1]

In January 2011, I read *The Emperor of All Maladies: A Biography of Cancer*. It was interesting and informative, and I thought, "Someone should do the same thing for breathing disorders." *Emperor* became a best-seller and later won a Pulitzer Prize. It was clear the public was interested in this approach to medical subjects, so in 2012, I began writing *Gasping for Air*.

This is a story of breathing, of the life-giving rhythm that fuels everything we do. So automatic and unconscious we take it for granted—until we can't breathe. Then we choke and gasp and succumb. If we stop breathing, within five minutes our brains begin to die.

Gasping for Air is part history, part biography, and part science. It is about science but is not a scientific book. It contains stories of personal experiences but is not a memoir. It tackles these questions: What forces threaten to suffocate us? How do we fight back? How must we adjust? Ancient diseases lurk in the atmosphere to asphyxiate the unlucky or ill-defended, while society invents new toxins with the potential to suffocate us. But nature has supplied us with weapons to defend ourselves: ingenuity, perseverance, and adaptability. Yet the question remains: Do we know how to use them?

Writing history and biography is straightforward. Published books and articles are ready resources. Telling stories of personal experiences is more difficult. Memory is imperfect, and time has passed since events occurred. Records have been destroyed. People have died or can't be interviewed. Patients' privacy demands respect. So, I have used false names to camouflage identities and have altered details to protect privacy or fill in gaps caused by incomplete recall. In dialogue, where I cannot remember the exact words, I have crafted language that reflects what I know of the context of the conversation and what the speaker most likely would have said. Otherwise, these stories describe events that really happened.

INTRODUCTION

"When you take away their breath, they die and return to the dust."

—Psalm 104:29[1]

My first visit to the hospital emergency room remains vivid in my mind seventy years later. I awoke in the middle of the night, coughing and wheezing. I sat on the edge of the bed and felt my chest muscles straining to move air in and out, my lungs so tight I thought I would suffocate. My mother heard me and came into my bedroom. Her furrowed brow showed her concern. "Let me get you a drink of water," she said. "Maybe it will help the coughing."

Soon my father joined her, his face also tense with worry. After they called the doctor, Dad said, "Put on your jacket over your pajamas. We're going to the hospital."

I grew up fighting asthma. By the time I reached third grade, I realized I was different from most of the kids in the neighborhood. They rarely went to the doctor, but for me, office visits and house calls were standard events. Whenever I got a cold, it went to my chest, and I coughed and wheezed and became short of breath. Every month I missed at least a couple of school days due to difficulty breathing. I swallowed medicines that made me vomit, inhaled sprays that made me cough, and endured shots that left my arms and rear end swollen for days. Sometimes I felt like a medical guinea pig.

My classmates went home the same day after having their tonsils removed. I was hospitalized afterward because of my breathing difficulties. I remember the day after tonsil surgery, lying in a near-empty pediatric ward, listening to radio news about a military attack in France that had the nurses chattering among themselves. The date was June 7, 1944. I've often thought, while the GIs were fighting on the beaches of Normandy, I was fighting to breathe.

Athletics really highlighted the difference between me and my friends. When I ran, I wheezed. Later, when I became a physician, I realized that exercise-induced bronchospasm is common in asthma. Ice skating was the worst. I became so choked up I sometimes couldn't walk home and had to wait in the warming hut until the attack subsided or someone would offer me a ride. Later, I learned that inhaling cold dry air so regularly provokes wheezing in asthmatics it is used as a diagnostic test.

In eighth grade, I tried out for the school football team. After two days with my face in the grassy dirt, learning the three-point stance, how to block, and how to make a clean tackle, I went home and wheezed for the next three days. When I missed practice the entire next week, I realized this wasn't going to work and abandoned football.

As time went on, I resigned myself to episodes of gasping for air as part of life, unaware of how the disease was defining my personality. In high school, I came to accept I was not going to become the star of any athletic team, no matter how much I dreamed of it. But the days at home, hardly able to get from the bed to the bathroom, gave me time to read and think. There had to be a place in the world for me. When I was eighteen, I decided I wanted to go to medical school. I achieved my ambition and eventually chose to specialize in respiratory diseases because I felt I understood patients with difficulty breathing. We shared a common bond.

I practiced pulmonary medicine for thirty-three years in San Diego, including twenty-two years as medical director of respiratory care at Scripps Mercy Hospital. During that time, the field of respiratory medicine exploded. Between 1940, when the first certificates were awarded, until 1970, the year after I became certified, the American Board of Internal Medicine granted a total of 346 diplomas in pulmonary disease. By the end of 2016, the board had certified a total of more than 17,000 pulmonary specialists.[2]

I watched chronic lung diseases increase in prevalence, tuberculosis decline and then come back, asthma treatment become a growth industry, and smoking-related diseases like lung cancer and COPD burgeon. Mechanical ventilators went from plastic boxes with a few valves to complicated marvels of microprocessor technology. I had a ringside seat to the advances in respiratory care during the last half-century and used them to help patients.

With a surface area the size of a tennis court, the lungs invite invasion by bacteria, chemicals, and infinitesimally small shreds of dusts, such as asbestos. The air we breathe continues to be both a source of life and a threat to it. One-eighth of the US population has chronic respiratory diseases. Twenty-four million people live with asthma; 12 million suffer from COPD and other chronic lung diseases; and 10 million have sleep apnea.[3] Respiratory diseases are the third-most frequent cause of death in the United States and fourth-most common worldwide.[4]

Epidemic respiratory infections circle the globe and are only a plane ride away. Stop to take a picture of a camel in Saudi Arabia, and you may be exposed to the MERS virus, which causes pneumonia with respiratory failure and is fatal in a third of cases. Shop at your local grocery store or ride the bus during the winter months, and you may encounter influenza. The CDC estimates that as many as 50,000 deaths occur annually due to influenza-induced pneumonia and respiratory failure.

Atmospheric toxins assault our ability to breathe. Visit Beijing, and observe residents wearing face masks on smoggy days.[5] Travel to New Delhi, and breathe six times the amount of particulate dust the World Health Organization considers safe. The WHO estimates seven million people die prematurely each year worldwide from inhaling contaminated air.[6]

Americans breathe our share of toxins as well. Despite leading the way in efforts to reduce smog, Los Angeles residents inhale the most ozone of all the cities in the country, and children who live in the most contaminated regions of the city have lower pulmonary function than their counterparts in cleaner areas.[7] Fresno, in California's Central Valley, enjoys the unenviable status of having the highest concentration of atmospheric dust in the United States.[8]

But we aid our attackers. Refusing to vaccinate leads to epidemics; burning fossil fuel produces air pollution; smoking tobacco causes lung cancer. As the once-popular cartoon character Pogo Possum commented, "We have met the enemy, and he is us."

Are we destined collectively to choke to death? By no means. Morbidity figures cause concern, but medical advances offer hope. Respiratory medicine is a dynamic and expanding area of research and treatment. A few decades ago, we could only offer those with bronchitis and emphysema advice to stop smoking and take antibiotics for infection and steroids for acute flare-ups. Now patients benefit from inhaling new drugs that reduce inflammation and open their airways.

Lung cancer is declining in the United States (but is on the rise worldwide). Results of treatment have been disappointing, though immunotherapy may change that. At present, only one-sixth of patients survive five years, but PET scans and genetic labeling techniques foresee the time when we will diagnose lung cancer soon enough to treat it effectively. These advances are only the beginning. Our understanding of immunology grows year by year, and genomics is still in its infancy. Bioelectronics is exploding. Who knows where the future will take us?

Gasping for Air tells the stories of the men and women who fight to help us breathe. Many are physicians and scientists, but many are engineers, entrepreneurs, and teachers as well. Plus, patients themselves, by their courage and resourcefulness, inspire the rest of us.

Recognizable medical weapons include oxygen and ventilators, antibiotics and vaccines. But education is also a powerful tool. Public service campaigns to promote immunization have wiped out smallpox, nearly eradicated polio, and reduced the impact of measles and whooping cough. Antismoking TV commercials show COPD and lung cancer patients emaciated and tethered to oxygen. The victims gasp their regrets for not having kicked the habit sooner. The images are shocking, but the CDC estimates they have helped 100,000 people to give up tobacco.[9]

Yet, medicine and science have limits. High-tech respiratory care creates ethical dilemmas. Who should be placed on a ventilator? How long should it be continued when there is no progress? What about the millions of people around the world dying because they don't have access to effective medicines for tuberculosis? Or those forced to work in jobs that suffocate them? Or to live near toxic waste dumps? Surely, we owe them help as well.

It's been a lifetime since that first terrifying night when my father rushed me to the hospital emergency room, but I still remember it. We drove north along the "outer drive," a local name for Chicago's Lake Shore Drive. The windows of my Dad's Dodge coupe were foggy with mist except where the windshield wiper blades etched half-circles of clear vision. The lights of the other cars were blurred, and in spite of my difficulty breathing, I remember being surprised at the traffic. At that age, I considered any time after ten o'clock the middle of the night. We were headed to the hospital. Was it going to hurt? Could they help me to breathe? The answers were unknown, and I was scared.

We arrived at Presbyterian Hospital, with its white tiled walls and floors and the odor of carbolic acid, a disinfectant used in those days. A doctor, probably an intern, examined me. My breathing came harder and harder, and my wheezing decreased. The doctor must have been worried too, because he told my father, "He needs a shot of adrenaline right away."

I didn't know he meant that I wasn't even moving enough air in and out to create a wheeze and that I could die. He injected a needle into my arm. My heart pounded and my hands shook. I began to sweat. I know now these were characteristic effects of adrenaline. In a few minutes my breathing relaxed.

After a while, the jitteriness subsided, and I didn't breathe normally, but I could more easily move air in and out. Adrenaline saved my life.

Since then, medicine has advanced in leaps to help those with breathing disorders, and I'm grateful for the chance I've had to participate. Two of my children and two grandchildren also have asthma. I'm happy to say their treatment works better than mine two generations ago, and they lead full and active lives.

Respiratory medicine, like all medicine, is full of ironies. Economic growth results in air pollution; global travel spreads infections; and technologic advances produce toxins and carcinogens. For nearly four decades, I practiced on the front lines of pulmonary medicine. I saw patients live and die, get well, get sicker. The story that follows is as much about those patients as it is about the scientists and physicians working to help them. I'm often asked if I'm optimistic about the future. I've seen such tremendous progress in a short time. I've seen the once-condemned run marathons. I've seen the miraculous become ordinary. Yes, I'm optimistic. Medicine can do much—but it must be humble enough to recognize its limits. So, I remind myself of the admonition of Paracelsus five centuries ago: "The art of healing comes from nature, not from the physician."[10]

I
WORLDWIDE PLAGUES

1

THE DISEASE THAT
MEDICINE NEVER CURED

"The captain of all these men of death that came against him to take him away, was the Consumption, for it was that that brought him down to the grave."

—John Bunyan[1]

"A disease which medicine never cured, wealth never warded off . . . which sometimes moves in giant strides, and sometimes at a tardy sluggish pace, but slow or quick, is ever sure and certain."

—Charles Dickens[2]

In April 2014, I enjoyed the privilege of attending an "Evening with Paul Farmer" in San Diego. Farmer is a professor at Harvard Medical School and founder of Partners in Health (PIH), a global organization to bring the benefits of modern science to those in greatest need, the poorest and most overlooked. Tall and thin, with wire-framed glasses, Farmer looked professorial but talked rapidly and emphatically, like an evangelist. Skilled in riposte, he answered questions with a wit as quick as any talk-show host.

Radiating energy as he spoke, he informed us he had just flown in from Russia, stopped in San Francisco, was leaving San Diego for Boston the next morning, and then was on to Haiti. His message was compelling. We in developed countries have the responsibility to help the world's poor fight the diseases that are killing them—and at the top of the list is tuberculosis, especially drug-resistant tuberculosis.

Farmer was born in Massachusetts in 1959 but grew up in Florida in a family of eight who lived wherever Farmer's father found work.[3] When money was short, the Farmer children pitched in to help, and one summer in Brooksville, north of Tampa, Paul Farmer picked fruit alongside migrant laborers from Haiti. Helping Haitians was to become his life work.

Farmer received a scholarship to Duke University, where he studied medical anthropology. He spent time in Haiti, learned to speak Creole, and took in the island's history and culture. He moved on to Harvard Medical School and graduated in 1990 with both an MD and a PhD, the latter in anthropology. He remained in Boston for residency training and during this time launched a program in the inner city to combat rising rates of HIV and tuberculosis. While he did this, he also commuted back and forth between Massachusetts and Haiti every few months.

In Haiti, Farmer helped to establish a community health project called Zanmi Lasante (Creole for "Partners in Health") that served a poverty-stricken rural area of 150,000 people where tuberculosis was a major challenge. Under Farmer's guidance, the project achieved success rates that rivaled results from the best clinics in the United States but for a fraction of the cost.

That evening in San Diego, Farmer told us how Partners in Health improved the lives of the poor. Treating tuberculosis was a major component of the initiative. Its success depended on creating an organized system of community health clinics staffed by locals. These gained the trust of the people and dealt with common obstacles, like procuring scarce medicines. Farmer was optimistic. He could show this approach worked worldwide, and he challenged us in the audience to help.

My reaction to listening to Farmer was that he wants more than to treat the sick. He seeks to change how the developed world sees care for the poor. He wants to open our eyes about what is possible. In this context, tuberculosis is more than a disease that kills millions of people every year; it is a symbol of poverty and despair that we have the resources to treat if we have the will.

Tuberculosis is the archetypical respiratory disorder, though difficulty breathing comes late in the course of the disease. The lungs are the usual site of entry and the organs most affected with tuberculosis. Infection begins when a contagious patient coughs. The force of the exhalation catapults microscopic droplets of fluid containing tuberculosis bacilli into the atmosphere. These droplets dry out but remain airborne for several hours, and if inhaled by a susceptible individual, bacilli begin multiplying in that person's lungs.

The newly infected person may run a slight fever or cough or feel tired or may not realize anything is wrong. As immunity develops, most people control the infection, but a few unlucky ones experience a spread through the lungs or to other organs. Fever, weight loss, cough with sputum production, and profound fatigue follow.

For the rest of the infected person's life, tuberculosis bacilli remain in the lungs. Thirteen million Americans are in this category. For many, the only footprint of the infection is a scar in the lung. If the person's immune resistance later drops, from alcoholism, poor nutrition, diabetes, cancer, or HIV, tuberculosis organisms begin to multiply, reproducing every twenty-four hours, liquefying lung tissue, invading blood vessels, and sucking away the victim's life. A person with advanced disease coughs up blood, becomes short of breath, weakens, and dies. This late stage may last months or be over in a day. Unpredictability is a distinguishing characteristic of the tuberculosis bacillus.

Tuberculosis has attacked humans since the beginning of history. Bone fragments from 8000 BCE show changes consistent with the disease. Egyptian and Incan mummies demonstrate tuberculous lesions in the spine. Historians of science feel that tuberculosis has been an intimate companion of humans since our species began, aggressive during times of deprivation, in check during good times, but never absent.[4] The disease kills the most susceptible individuals and sickens those who are resistant but doesn't prevent them from surviving. Those who are highly resistant show no sign of disease but forever retain microscopic nests of organisms hidden amid scar tissue in the lungs.

Tuberculosis has a place in history and literature as the most-feared plague of the ages; a metaphor for a slow and lingering death; an insidious, implacable thief of life.[5] The disease has occurred in waves over millennia. We are now in the late stage of an epidemic that likely began in sixteenth-century England and spread to the rest of Europe during the Industrial Revolution, when people moved to cities and crowded together in squalid conditions.

If we trace the history of tuberculosis over the centuries, we can recognize different threads in the tapestry. Before 1860, the pattern was one of multiple forms of treatment, mostly ineffective (not surprising for a disease that has killed nearly a billion people since the human species began). In addition, treatments were based mostly on ignorance and superstition.

Clovis, a fifth-century king of the Franks, was said to be able to cure scrofula, tuberculosis of the glands in the neck, by touching the afflicted person. King Edward I of England was reported to have touched 533 sick people in one month, and in what may be the record for hands-on medicine, in 1660, Charles II of England is said to have touched 6,000 people in one month. If the monarch merely put his chain of office over the head of the afflicted person, the "royal touch" was supposedly able to effect cure.[6]

Other approaches we today would classify as quackery included drinking potions of garlic mixed with dog fat and inhaling smoke from burning cow

dung. Vomiting was felt to exercise the chest muscles, and so physicians prescribed ocean voyages, both for the sea air and to induce seasickness. René
Laennec, inventor of the stethoscope, noticed that tuberculosis seemed less
prevalent near the ocean and so suggested patients place seaweed under their
beds.

Many methods contradicted each other. Some experts recommended exercise; others, rest. Some urged patients to be outside to breathe fresh air,
while others favored staying inside in an airtight room wrapped in a feather
blanket near a hot stove. When physicians recommend many treatments, it's
a sign that none work. It's also a sign of the desperation felt by both patients
and doctors.

In the mid-nineteenth century, George Bodington, a British country doctor,
founded a small nursing home to provide a calm restful environment where
tuberculosis patients could breathe fresh air.[7] This was the forerunner of the
sanatorium, a hospital to treat a specific disease, tuberculosis. Unfortunately,
the medical establishment disputed his theories, and Bodington abandoned
his studies of tuberculosis to concentrate on treating the mentally ill.

But Bodington's ideas did not die. Hermann Brehmer, a university student
from Silesia, then an eastern province of Prussia, contracted tuberculosis, and
his doctor recommended he move to a healthier climate.[8] Brehmer went to
the Himalayas, and while there, he improved. He returned home and decided
to enter medical school. After graduating in 1854, Brehmer opened a tuberculosis sanatorium in Gorbersdorf, Germany. He located it in a wooded area,
where patients breathed fresh air, ate well, and enjoyed the smell of the pine
trees while they recuperated. Brehmer's sanatorium and a similar one in Da-
vos, Switzerland, provided inspiration for the fictitious sanatorium depicted in
Thomas Mann's *The Magic Mountain.*

Edward L. Trudeau founded the first tuberculosis sanatorium in the United
States. Born in New York City in 1848, Trudeau considered a career in the
navy, but when his older brother Frank contracted tuberculosis, Edward gave
up his naval appointment to take care of him. The disease progressed rapidly,
and Frank died three months after becoming ill. This tragedy changed Edward's life. He decided to become a physician.[9] He graduated from Columbia
University College of Physicians and Surgeons in 1871 and started a medical
practice in New York City. He married and had a child. Then, a few months
later, he noticed he was tiring easily, was running a fever, and had swollen
lymph glands in his neck. Like his brother, he had tuberculosis.[10] Demoral-
ized by the diagnosis, Trudeau resigned himself to dying.

Trudeau loved the woods of upper New York, and if he was to die, he
wanted to die there. At the suggestion of friends, he moved to a rustic camp
in the Adirondack Mountains near Saranac Lake.[11] Like other young people

of his era facing death from tuberculosis, he was so weak and emaciated he had to be carried into the hut he later dubbed the "little red house," where he was to reside. He expected to go quickly, but with rest and time, he began to improve. He gained strength and became able to exercise outdoors.[12] Trudeau brought his family to live with him at the camp and in 1876, after four years there, decided to stay in Saranac Lake and open a medical practice.

Convinced that the healthy climate, rest, good diet, and therapeutic exercise were responsible for his getting better, Trudeau became an advocate of the "rest cure" for tuberculosis. Soon he concentrated his practice on the white plague, and in 1885, he officially founded the Adirondack Cottage Sanatorium, dedicated to treating tuberculosis patients by prolonged rest and being outdoors.[13]

Trudeau required his guests (i.e., patients) to follow a strict program of diet and exercise. They received three meals every day and a glass of milk every four hours. Plus, they were to spend as much time as possible outside, sitting or lying in bed on an open-air porch in all seasons and in all types of weather. Trudeau took in patients regardless of their ability to pay, which meant both natives and immigrants. He covered the costs of care for those without funds by soliciting donations from wealthy friends in New York City. Soon doctors all over the country began to refer patients for treatment at his sanatorium, and Trudeau became a leader in American tuberculosis medicine.[14] In 1904, he was one of the founders of the National Society for the Prevention and Treatment of Tuberculosis, forerunner of today's American Lung Association.

If we trace the history of tuberculosis during the sanatorium era, from the 1860s until the 1950s, we see additional threads in the tapestry: the discovery of the cause of the disease, preoccupation with rest as a cure, incarceration of those infected, invasive and sometimes mutilating procedures, and the isolation and hopelessness that shrouded patients.

While the sanatorium movement grew, researchers looked for medicines to alleviate the effects of tuberculosis, but without knowledge of its cause, they were searching in the dark. However, in 1882, Robert Koch, a German medical scientist, presented a paper before the Physiological Society of Germany in Berlin entitled *Die Tuberculose* ("On Tuberculosis").[15] By means of a specific method of staining, Koch demonstrated bacteria in diseased organs of tuberculosis patients. In cheesy masses from the lungs of human sufferers, he not only found the organisms, but he was also able to inject them into guinea pigs and cause tuberculosis in those animals. Science finally knew what caused tuberculosis. Would it then be possible to find a cure?

Recognizing the cause of tuberculosis and being able to make a specific diagnosis were breakthroughs, but effective treatment was sixty years away. Rest, fresh air, and healthy food remained the foundation of therapy until the mid-twentieth century.

During the heyday of the sanatorium, adventurous physicians and surgeons sought ways to augment the benefits of rest, diet, and fresh air for tuberculosis patients. Many appear bizarre or barbaric today and hardly suggest progress. But they made more sense than garlic and dog fat or seaweed under the pillow—treatments from earlier times. That they endured for fifty years indicates how desperate patients and physicians were to control the disease.

British physician James Carson injected air into the pleural space, which caused the lung to collapse.[16] The theory was that shrinking the diseased segment of lung tissue permitted it to rest and thus to heal. Surgeons inserted Lucite spheres, like miniature ping-pong balls, inside the chest to collapse the upper lobes of the lungs. Paraffin bricks served the same purpose in some cases. The goal was to put the lung at rest.

Surgeons also performed thoracoplasty. This involved fracturing the upper ribs, removing portions of them, and then pushing the remaining rib segments down to collapse the underlying lung. The procedure was often performed in stages, which meant multiple operations, until the rib cage was virtually flattened and the underlying lung was like a pancake. It was deforming, disfiguring, and produced a compensatory spine tilt that made exercise difficult. It also eventually led to heart failure and death.

Sanatorium care likely helped patients, though the exact reason is difficult to pinpoint. Probably it was a combination of rest, a good diet, and a quiet environment. But the patients, their families, and society paid a price.[17] Taking the cure worked fine for the wealthy, but confining the breadwinners of households for months and years left working-class families destitute. In addition, many people were remanded by court order to local sanatoriums. During the peak years of the sanatorium movement, 1890 to 1950, children considered at risk for tuberculosis were taken from their families and treated in institutions known as preventoriums. These were a combination hospital, school, and sanatorium, in which children were confined in an attempt to keep them from getting sick from tuberculosis.[18]

We in the twenty-first century have difficulty grasping the fear that cloaked tuberculosis patients, their families, and the public throughout history. It meant ostracism and an inexorable, painful descent to invalidism and death. The tuberculosis hospital was a different world: isolated, often in a rural area, with its own procedures and staff. Young people would be admitted, start to cough up blood, and the next day be dead from pulmonary hemorrhage.

In his autobiography, Edward Trudeau described his reaction to being told his diagnosis:

> I think I know something of the feelings of the man at the bar who is told he is to be hanged on a given date, for in those days pulmonary consumption was

considered as absolutely fatal. . . . I felt stunned. It seemed to me the world had suddenly grown dark. The sun was shining and the street was filled with the rush and noise of traffic but to me the world had lost every vestige of brightness. I had consumption—that most fatal of diseases! Had I not seen all its horrors in my brother's case? It meant death and I had never thought of death before![19]

Corwin Hinshaw, a twentieth-century pioneer in the treatment of tuberculosis, described conditions in American sanatoria during the 1940s and '50s:

The majority of patients were in the age group 20–35 years. The basic remedy was "bed rest" in its most stringent form: Twenty-four hours flat. Meals were spooned to each patient by registered nurses, bed baths and the universal bedpans were imposed on these youngsters who looked and felt normal but who had shadows—even small shadows—on their chest X-ray films.

All this in an effort to halt the persistent and almost inevitable trend for such small lesions to advance and destroy the patient. The average patient spent more than a full year in bed, many others much more. Careers were abandoned, marriage was discouraged, and pregnancy virtually forbidden. Stress in any form and to any degree must be avoided.[20]

Even when effective therapy became available, former tuberculosis patients lived with frightening flashbacks from their sanatorium days. Anxiety and concern haunted them for the rest of their lives. During my early years in practice, nearly every week, an ex-tuberculosis patient would telephone our office, petrified because of coughing up a speck of blood or running a fever. Our policy was to see them as quickly as possible and to take a chest X-ray. Most of the time it was not serious, usually bronchitis arising in an area where the lung was scarred, but to these patients, fever or blood-spitting brought on terror. They had seen fellow sanatorium patients cough up blood and the next day die from pulmonary hemorrhage.

From the time of Koch's discovery of the tuberculosis bacillus in 1882, scientists labored to find a drug or vaccine that worked against the disease. Building on the early twentieth-century successes in creating vaccines, researchers applied their knowledge to tuberculosis. In 1908, Albert Calmette and Camille Guerin, working at the Institut Pasteur de Lille in France, discovered a strain of tuberculosis bacilli that had lost its virulence. From this strain, they made a vaccine, called Bacillus-Calmette-Guerin, or BCG, that has been used ever since in parts of Europe and in developing countries with a high prevalence of tuberculosis. BCG never became widely accepted in the United States because it makes the tuberculin skin test become positive, thus destroying the value of the skin test as a case-finding tool.

The early decades of the twentieth century were disappointing and frustrating for those in the laboratory struggling to find weapons against the white plague. Then, in 1943, Selman Waksman discovered streptomycin, and the antibiotic age arrived for tuberculosis. This revolutionized treatment forever and announced the end of the sanatorium era. It also presaged the problem we face today: drug resistance.

Selman Waksman was born in 1888 in what is now the Ukraine. He came to the United States in 1910 and six years later became an American citizen.[21] After graduation from Rutgers University, he enrolled in graduate school at the University of California, Berkeley, where he performed research on soil bacteria. Waksman received a PhD in biochemistry in 1918, after which he returned to Rutgers to continue his investigations.[22] Following the discovery of penicillin, scientists everywhere were interested in finding other drugs with similar properties, and soil microbiology was an important area of study.

Albert Schatz, a graduate student working under Waksman, isolated a substance from a bacterial family called *Actinomycetes* that was effective against the tuberculosis bacillus. Waksman and Schatz called it streptomycin and patented their method of extracting it. Waksman sent samples of the drug to Corwin Hinshaw at the Mayo Clinic, who verified that streptomycin worked against tuberculosis in guinea pigs. The pharmaceutical company Merck produced the drug for human use, and Waksman received royalties of $2.3 million, most of which he turned over to Rutgers to establish an institute of microbiology. In 1952, Waksman won the Nobel Prize for medicine for discovering streptomycin.

Soon other drugs followed: PAS in 1948 and, in 1952, isonicotinic acid hydrazide, or INH. INH had dramatic effects in tuberculosis: Fever disappeared in a few days, and contagiousness subsided in two weeks. This was a remarkable achievement.[23] These three drugs, INH, streptomycin, and PAS, called triple-drug therapy, arrested disease in more than 96 percent of patients within two years. Failures usually resulted from intolerance to medications or not adhering to the prescribed schedule. And patients could be treated in general hospitals or outpatient clinics. Thus, by the late 1950s, the sanatorium era came to an end. In 1954, Trudeau's cottages at Saranac Lake shut down.

However, the history of tuberculosis is one of progress and optimism, followed by setbacks and disappointment. Antituberculosis drugs had side effects. Streptomycin caused dizziness and permanent hearing loss. Vernon Wyborney, my associate, received streptomycin injections when he contracted tuberculosis as an intern in the 1940s. It caused such difficulty in hearing he eventually could not hear what patients were saying and was forced to retire. PAS caused severe gastrointestinal upset that made it intolerable for many patients. INH caused a painful neuropathy and occasionally liver damage. No progress occurred without an accompanying price.

Also, no matter what medical science achieved, the wily bacillus figured a way to thwart it. Tuberculosis is truly a consummate parasite, sapping energy from its victims to nourish itself while permitting them to continue living but in a diminished, walking-dead state. Within a short time after the discovery of streptomycin, tuberculosis patients taking the drug developed resistance and relapsed. Physicians fought back by using several drugs simultaneously to attack the bacillus in different parts of its metabolism. Their goal was to arrest the disease but avoid drug resistance.

Imagine a million bacilli in a patient's lung. Say that 1 percent were resistant to streptomycin. That meant 10,000 organisms would survive treatment with streptomycin and continue to multiply. In tuberculosis, that was enough to cause relapse in a year or two. Those residual organisms led to death within three years for almost 20 percent of patients.[24]

Suppose therapy consisted of two drugs administered together. If streptomycin could eradicate 99 percent of the organisms and drug number 2 suppressed 90 percent of the remainder, that would mean out of a million bacilli, only one hundred would remain that were resistant to both drugs. Unfortunately, those one hundred bacilli would continue to multiply, and a percentage of patients would relapse. So, it was essential to use a broad enough drug combination to knock out virtually all the organisms in affected areas of the lungs and trust that the patient's own defenses could finish the job.

Resistance developed mainly in two ways: One was when patients took a single drug at a time. Another was when patients took medicines intermittently. Skipping doses or stopping and restarting temporarily suppressed the bacteria but didn't fully eradicate them. Relapse of disease soon followed.

Drug resistance was a gnawing threat to control of the disease. When I was on the medical chest staff at Milwaukee County General Hospital in the late 1960s, we had responsibility for the tuberculosis service. The unfortunate patients with drug-resistant disease needed to take as many as five different drugs for months or sometimes a year to have any hope for successful treatment. Each medicine had its own set of side effects, often serious themselves. Dizziness, seizures, hallucinations, vomiting, muscle weakness, liver toxicity, and kidney impairment were constant problems among the drug-resistant patients on the tuberculosis ward.

Meanwhile the pattern of advances followed by setbacks continued. With triple therapy, tuberculosis prevalence declined to the point that, in the 1960s, experts even talked about eradicating what Charles Dickens had called a "disease that medicine never cured." But these were dreams.

Tuberculosis did not disappear. If we trace the history of the disease since 1960, we discern still more threads in the tapestry. Those at the margins of society continued as carriers. HIV disease complicated both diagnosis and treatment. Immigrants brought tuberculosis to the United States from the developing world. And with immigration came multidrug resistance, the current threat articulated by Paul Farmer in his writings and lectures.

By the 1960s, though antituberculosis drugs worked, public health physicians grappled with how to reach those who most needed treatment. Alcoholics, homeless people, the elderly, and immigrants remained tuberculosis repositories. Authorities tried to corral them to screen for active disease. Cities mandated that jails have X-ray facilities, and when the police arrested vagrants for loitering or petty theft, they performed chest X-rays and frequently found active tuberculosis. A prisoner showing evidence of tuberculosis would be confined in the hospital by court order until pronounced no longer contagious.

In Milwaukee, when patients were admitted to the tuberculosis service from the jail, someone from the medical staff (usually me, lowest on the totem pole) had to go to court and testify the individual was a threat to the public health. The judge ordered the inmate to remain hospitalized for however long it took to achieve control, which could be as long as two years. This worked for the jail population, but what about those on the street? They also had tuberculosis. How could they be reached?

Francis Curry was director of public health in San Francisco. In 1958, he opened a clinic in the Tenderloin (San Francisco's skid row), where he enticed alcoholics to be skin-tested for tuberculosis by giving them cards that sent them to the head of the food line. He ran satellite clinics throughout the high-incidence areas of the city and opened them at hours convenient for patients.

Knowing that the best medicines available would not work unless taken, Curry assigned public health nurses to administer antituberculosis medications either at the clinic or in the place where the patients lived. These were the forerunners of what is today a cornerstone of tuberculosis treatment: neighborhood clinics and direct-observation therapy, or DOT. Studies in Hong Kong; India; and Denver, Colorado, showed this method worked better than trusting patients to take medicines on their own. It was labor-intensive but successful.

But progress was again followed by setback. Even while Curry was pioneering patient-centered therapy, two other susceptible groups emerged to challenge public health experts: the elderly and AIDS patients—the elderly because immunity wanes with age and AIDS because HIV attacks lymphocytes, the white blood cells intimately involved in immunity to tuberculosis.

With HIV, even recognizing tuberculosis became difficult. The disease could look like heart failure, blood clots, pneumonia, or cancer. It could be in the upper, lower, or middle lung fields. Physicians had to discount every-thing they knew about the radiographic signs of tuberculosis when consulting on HIV patients. Fortunately, this obstacle was temporary. When effective antiviral therapy for HIV became available, treatment of coexisting tuberculosis became easier and worked better. The battle goes on, but prospects are brighter than they were twenty years ago.

Standard treatment today involves administering four drugs simultaneously by direct observation: INH, rifampin, ethambutal, and pyrazinamide. After two months, ethambutal and pyrazinamide can be stopped and the other two continued an additional four months. This schedule achieves control in 95 percent of cases. Six months sounds like a long time, but a generation ago, treatment lasted eighteen to twenty-four months, and a generation before that, treatment could require several years in a sanatorium.

Immigrants have always been a major source of tuberculosis. Those from Asia, Africa, and Latin America bring with them a high incidence of drug resistance. Since 1997, the fraction of US-born tuberculosis patients with resistance to antituberculosis drugs has hovered at one case per hundred thousand persons.[25] But the proportion of foreign-born patients with drug-resistant disease is higher and has been increasing. In San Diego County, more than a third of tuberculosis cases have a cross-border connection.[26] People live in Mexico and cross the border to work in San Diego or live in San Diego and work in Mexico. Because drug resistance in Baja California is four times more frequent than in San Diego, tuberculosis threatens people on both sides of the border.

In the last twenty years, more than 50 million patients have been treated for tuberculosis worldwide, and an estimated 22 million deaths have been prevented.[27] Yet millions of patients become infected every year and go untreated. In 2014, the most recent year for which statistics are available, 9.6 million people around the world acquired the disease, and 1.5 million died.[28] These 9.6 million are the ones Paul Farmer wants to reach.

When Farmer confronted drug-resistant tuberculosis in Haiti, he sought a model on how to deal with the challenge. In the late 1980s, New York City faced an outbreak of drug-resistant tuberculosis. The Department of Public Health used rapid lab tests to identify which of the dozen available antituberculosis agents could eradicate drug-resistant organisms and administered these via direct observation. This approach was costly, but it worked. Farmer set up similar procedures in Haiti and achieved nearly as good outcomes. Furthermore, he employed the same strategy in Peru and Russia, where multidrug-resistant tuberculosis was reaching epidemic levels. Farmer showed, even in poor areas of the world, it's possible to achieve results in treating tuberculosis almost as good as in wealthy countries.[29]

Farmer is a physician, academician, and medical missionary. He's also a prophet, circumnavigating the globe, preaching that wealthy countries can learn from experiences in poorer nations. Millions of migrants from poverty-stricken countries continue to flood into the developed world. Many come illegally and so hide from the authorities. Many have tuberculosis. Farmer urges citizens of well-to-do nations to join the battle against tuberculosis for both altruistic and selfish reasons. Helping people in developing countries to receive effective treatment will improve their health and reduce immigrant-related tuberculosis in affluent countries.

The biggest challenge the developed world faces today in controlling tuberculosis is to remember: to remember how recently the white plague was a terrifying killer in our country, to remember the poor and disenfranchised who perpetuate the disease, to remember the public health measures that control spread, to remember that setbacks follow advances.

Refugees come to America today just like in the time of Trudeau: poor, dispossessed, often sick, and seeking a better life. With them comes tuberculosis. But today we possess powerful weapons in our battle: X-rays and blood tests that can tell whether a person has been infected and effective medicines with additional new drugs in development. Yet the adversary is notoriously resilient. We should never become smug. History reminds us that, in the struggle against tuberculosis, progress and setbacks are the pattern. Trailblazers like Trudeau, Koch, Waksman, Curry, and Farmer have shown that to break that pattern will require vigilance, dedication, and persistence.

2

CAPTAINS OF THE MEN OF DEATH

"In the Mortality Bills, pneumonia is an easy second to tuberculosis; indeed in many cities the death rate is now higher, and it has become, to use the phrase of Bunyan, the captain of the men of death."

—William Osler[1]

I spent the winter of 1962–1963 as a medical resident at the Ann Arbor VA Hospital across the Huron River from the University of Michigan Medical Center. Two months on the pulmonary service kindled my interest in respiratory diseases, but the sleepless nights and stress as admitting resident nearly squelched that attraction. It seemed, whenever I was on call, a beleaguered emergency room doctor someplace in southern Michigan or northern Indiana or Ohio would phone: "I have a gentleman with pneumonia here. He's a veteran, and I'm sending him to Ann Arbor. I know you'll take good care of him. Thanks. Good-bye." (Medicare didn't yet exist, and many retirees had no hospital insurance.)

Several hours later, usually after midnight, an ambulance would arrive and discharge into our admitting ward an elderly man, unable to muster the strength to give a history, coughing, straining the muscles in his neck to breathe, sweating, ashen gray, his heart pounding, with wheezes and rattling sounds in his lungs so loud they echoed through the stethoscope into the examining room. The chest X-ray would show lungs whited out by infection and fluid. I would slap an oxygen mask over his face, take cultures of blood, suction mucus from his throat, admit him to the ward, and start antibiotics. Sometimes we had to put a tube into the trachea and begin mechanical ventilation.

Night after night, the scenario repeated itself until the hospital was so full there were no empty beds, but the patients were too sick to be moved elsewhere. Most of them didn't have only pneumonia. They had pneumonia plus heart failure or COPD or liver cirrhosis or diabetes. Many went into shock, sustained cardiac arrest, and died. It became a morbid joke among the residents. Being the admitting doctor at the VA in the winter was like finding customers for the undertaker. It was grim work, and many questioned whether we wanted to do it the rest of our lives.

Pneumonia acquired in a community setting can result from dozens of different viruses and bacteria. But the single species that is the most frequent cause of lower respiratory tract infections is the pneumococcus. At the turn of the twentieth century, William Osler labeled it "captain of the men of death" and yet also the "friend of the aged."

Pneumococci are bacteria. Differing from influenza, tuberculosis, or many of the other lethal respiratory infectious agents, they illustrate a sobering fact of biology: Organisms that normally live inside us can break out and kill us. Pneumococci ordinarily reside in the noses and throats of humans, where they dwell quietly until the person's resistance changes. Should the unlucky individual lose consciousness, drink too much alcohol, or suffer loss of immune capacity, these indolent microbes migrate into the lungs, where they furiously attack, overwhelming natural defenses, entering the bloodstream, chewing up tissue, spreading to the nervous system, and leading to shock and death, especially among infants and the elderly.

Each year, 500,000 cases of pneumococcal pneumonia occur in the United States.[2] Untreated, the mortality rate hovers at 35 percent, though antibiotics cut that in half. Pneumococcal infections occur mostly in the winter months, thought to be related to coexisting viral infections reducing resistance.

Fatal complications of pneumococcus, like bloodstream infection and meningitis, usually occur during the first or second week of infection. Once the crisis passes, the majority of victims recover over a period of several weeks, though some remain weak and fatigued for several months. Not all recover. Pleural effusion, accumulation of fluid in the space between the lung and chest wall, occurs a third of the time and can deteriorate into empyema, a collection of pus inside the chest. The latter requires prompt surgical drainage, or it is lethal.

Osler called pneumonia the "most widespread and most fatal of all acute diseases" and described the typical symptoms, which are the same today: abrupt onset with chills, headache, and muscle pains, followed by a painful cough and difficulty breathing. He described a typical patient as flushed, with rapid respirations and spiking fevers. Sputum was thick and often rusty in color. Osler called it "lung fever."[3]

In 1910, pneumonia caused 13 percent of recorded deaths in the United States.[4] By 1999, that fraction fell to less than 5 percent in a much larger overall population. Better medical care, better nutrition, and an improved standard of living all contributed to that drop. But bacterial pneumonia, exemplified by pneumococcus, remains a major threat to breathing a century after Osler's time.

In 1875, as bacteriology was emerging as a new branch of biology, Edwin Klebs, a German scientist, reported seeing bacteria in the lungs of patients with pneumonia. But Klebs didn't follow through on the observation and so lost his chance to discover one of the most important causes of disease and death in all of history. Six years later, George Sternberg in the United States and Louis Pasteur in France, working independently, were more persistent and so more fortunate.

Sternberg was a US Army surgeon. In the 1870s, he spent his spare time learning about the new science of bacteriology, and in 1880, this effort paid off. Sternberg performed experiments in which he injected his own saliva under the skin of rabbits. The animals developed fever and weakness, followed within forty-eight hours by shock and death. Perplexed by the "virulent properties" of his own saliva, he repeated the experiment with water—no result— and "putrid" wine—also no result. Next, he injected saliva from ten other individuals, patients and colleagues, without effect. What was in Sternberg's saliva but not in that of most other people that killed rabbits?

Meanwhile, 5,000 miles away in Paris, Louis Pasteur performed a similar experiment. For some reason lost in the lore of science, Pasteur injected saliva from an infant who had died of rabies into rabbits and observed results similar to those of Sternberg. Perhaps he focused on saliva because, in the terminal phases of rabies, victims salivate profusely. Pasteur also recovered small organisms that he called *microbe septicemique de salive* from the infected rabbits.[5] Pasteur published his results three months before Sternberg, and so by scientific etiquette, he is credited with being the discoverer of these comma-shaped rabbit killers. Acknowledging this, Sternberg called the organisms *Micrococcus pasteuri*.[6] Neither of the two scientists realized they had identified the organism that was the most common bacterial cause of pneumonia throughout the world, to be named later *Streptococcus pneumoniae*.

The saliva of Sternberg and the rabid child killed rabbits because Sternberg and the child both carried pneumococci. Most children are exposed to pneumococci by the time they learn to walk, and nearly half retain the organisms in their throats. As they grow up, pneumococci usually disappear, so that only 10 percent of adults are carriers. Pneumococci are transmitted from one person to another by close contact, but paradoxically, carriers are not contagious. Children's day care centers, college dormitories, and military recruit barracks are notorious sources of transmission, likely related to the closeness involved, but patients recovering from pneumococcal pneumonia do not ordinarily require isolation.

Treatment of pneumococcal infection has passed through two phases: preantibiotics and postantibiotics. In the early twentieth century, Osler recommended rest, fluids, and nutrition, supporting the patient until nature heals. Osler was dubious about the value of adding oxygen, which was just becoming available in his era, to alleviate the cyanosis, or blueness of the skin that frequently accompanies pneumonia. He commented that, whenever he was asked to consult on a case of pneumonia and saw an oxygen bottle at the bedside, he knew the prognosis was grave. Yet, today, oxygen and cool mist to wet the dry, inflamed airways are important adjuncts in managing severe cases of pneumonia in hospitalized patients.

Antibiotics did not exist in Osler's time, but he mentioned a promising innovation undergoing trial in the early twentieth century, administration of antibody-containing serum from a patient who had immunity to the disease. (Serum is the fluid portion of blood that separates from red and white blood cells when blood clots.) Medical science calls this passive immunization to distinguish it from vaccination, or active immunization, which means stimulating the patient's own system to make antibodies.

Pneumococci possess antigens, substances that the body recognizes as foreign, in their thick outside layer, or capsule. Humans and other animals acquire protective immunity by making antibodies to these capsular antigens. Antibodies are complex compounds that bind to antigens and assist white blood cells to destroy invading microorganisms.

Bacteria that have the same antigens are said to belong to the same strain. In the early twentieth century, four known strains of pneumococci existed. Serum from a patient or an animal (rabbits and horses were frequent sources of serum) immune to one group of antigens wouldn't work on a patient with a different strain because the antibodies wouldn't bind to different antigens. So, matching serum antibodies to specific pneumococcal strains was necessary. It was complicated and tedious, but serum treatment worked and improved survival rates in pneumonia.

The prevalence of pneumonia and its lethality made investigators search for a vaccine even before antiserum became popular. In 1886, gold was discovered in South Africa.[7] This created a huge demand for laborers to dig out the precious substance from underground veins of ore. Mine owners imported workers from rural areas, and in the crowded conditions, these men came down with pneumococcal pneumonia with such frequency the success of

African gold mining was in danger. Pneumonia mortality rates were so high the British government threatened to close down the mines. To combat this threat, in 1911, officials retained the services of Sir Almoth Wright, a British scientist known for earlier work on a typhoid vaccine.

Wright recommended inoculating the miners with a vaccine made of ground-up pneumococcal cells. Wright must have been aware of the different pneumococcal strains. But he conducted vaccine trials on 50,000 miners, ignoring which antigens the vaccine contained, so Wright's vaccine depended on luck to work. When he reported the vaccine was effective, a major segment of the scientific community was skeptical of his conclusions.

The controversy became worse when F. Spencer Lister, a Wright protégé, vaccinated workers in one mine and used workers from a different mine as controls to confirm Wright's observations. Unfortunately, Lister neglected to take into account that pneumococcal attack rates vary among different groups in different locations. It was like vaccinating people in Los Angeles and comparing their pneumonia rates with New Yorkers. Doubts about Lister's studies reinforced disbelief in Wright's work. Wright and Lister were on the right track, but poorly designed trials rendered their results unreliable. The march of science is full of false starts and detours like this.

Vaccine research continued, however, both in Europe and in the United States. In 1930, scientists at the Rockefeller Institute discovered complex sugars, called polysaccharides, in the pneumococcal capsule. These were not proteins, like most antigens, but nevertheless were recognized by the body as foreign. This was a big step forward, but creating an effective pneumococcal vaccine was still years in the future.

Because vaccines are biological compounds made from cells of living organisms, developing and testing them is more complex than testing drugs, like antibiotics or pain relievers, which are chemicals and whose behavior is relatively predictable. During the 1930s and '40s, scientists produced vaccines against tetanus, whooping cough, typhoid, cholera, and plague and antitoxin against diphtheria. These bacteria contained few enough antigens that vaccine neutralized most strains of each species. Pneumococci, in contrast, produced over ninety different types of polysaccharide (though we know now that most human infections are due to twenty of them). So, progress in pneumococcal vaccine was slow, and it was not until 1977 that a vaccine against pneumococcus was finally licensed in the United States.

Pneumococcal vaccine remains complicated. Currently two types exist. The first is made from polysaccharide. It contains twenty-three different antigens that protect against more than 90 percent of the strains that affect humans. However, children under the age of two are unable to mount a full immune response to the twenty-three-antigen vaccine, so the pharmaceutical companies created a vaccine that splices a carrier protein to the polysaccharide, thus making it more potent. The protein-polysaccharide conjugate covers the thirteen most prevalent strains and is used to immunize infants and toddlers. After they pass the age of two, children can then be revaccinated with the full twenty-three-strain mixture.

Pneumococcal vaccines were administered at first to infants, pregnant women, the elderly, and those working in health care—those most at risk. Then diabetics and HIV-infected individuals were added. Since 2013, the vaccine is recommended for everyone. But pneumococcal vaccine is only 60 percent effective, not surprising if one realizes it is the most complex of all the immunizations administered to humans. Furthermore, experience is too recent to be sure how long immunity lasts. Current studies suggest at least five years, so some authorities recommend revaccination after five to ten years.

Science invented vaccines decades before it discovered antibiotics. Sulfa drugs, synthesized in the 1930s, produced good results in pneumonia. However, the popularity of antiserum delayed sulfa's acceptance by the medical establishment, showing how ingrained habits can resist even a revolutionary improvement.

By the 1940s, penicillin proved much better than sulfa and supplanted it as the treatment of choice for bacterial pneumonia. Initially, military personnel had priority for the wonder drug, but after World War II, penicillin became available for civilian use. It transformed the treatment of all infections but particularly bacterial pneumonia. Between 1930 and 1950, mortality rates from pneumococcal bloodstream infections, the most lethal complication of pneumonia, dropped by half.

But nearly from the beginning, scientists saw a problem looming: antibiotic resistance. As physicians prescribed antibiotics for common colds, which are caused by viruses and thus not helped by antibiotics, populations of bacteria resistant to antibiotics were able to survive in the patient's tissues. Combining penicillin with other antibiotics, such as streptomycin, attempted to hit the attacking organisms in several places. Researchers called it a "one-two punch." To illustrate, penicillin blocks bacteria from making their outer protective wall, while streptomycin inhibits synthesis of proteins inside the bacterial cell. This strategy helped combat resistance but didn't eliminate it.

In the 1950s and '60s, pharmaceutical companies churned out new antibiotics nearly every year. These were chemically different from penicillin, possessing action against many species, and were called broad-spectrum. Some attacked penicillin-resistant strains of pneumococci, which everyone hoped would turn the tide against drug resistance. This hope would prove naïve and premature.

Studies soon showed prompt treatment of pneumonia produced greater success, and so physicians came under pressure to start antibiotics within hours of diagnosis. This meant they had to make an educated guess as to possible causes and initiate treatment immediately. Today, initial treatment of pneumonia is either a broad-spectrum antibiotic or a combination of several antibiotics. When cultures become available a day or two later, the antibiotics used can be narrowed to focus on the specific organisms causing infection.

One percent of the US population develops pneumonia each year—three million people. But pneumonia is a heterogeneous diagnosis. Viruses and organisms between viruses and bacteria, called mycoplasma, also cause lung infections. Among bacterial causes, in nearly half, pneumococci are the culprit.[8] But dozens of other species can invade the lungs, and each of these follows a different course, responds differently to antibiotics, and has different degrees of contagiousness. Successful treatment depends on knowing the bug, the drug, and the patient.

Nancy, the young woman to be described in the chapter on influenza, suffered from staphylococcal pneumonia in the wake of influenza. Staph pneumonia is less prevalent than pneumococcal but is responsible for 10 percent of bacterial pneumonia cases seen in a typical hospital and is near the top of the list of infections sending patients to the intensive care unit. Staphylococci, like pneumococci, live in the nose and throat and on the skin. They spread via direct contact. From a tiny pimple on the skin, they may invade the bloodstream and produce multiple abscesses in the lung, making them one of the most frightening types of respiratory infection.

Other species, like *Klebsiella* and *Hemophilus*, live in the gastrointestinal tract. However, if body defenses deteriorate, any of these can invade the lungs and produce pneumonia, septicemia, and death.[9] Add viruses and mycoplasma to the mix, and it becomes easy to see why pneumonia is such a complex medical problem. Sometimes, in our medical zeal to eradicate diseases, we overlook that pneumonia may be one of nature's ways of softening death. A friend of mine was diagnosed with inoperable pancreatic cancer two years ago. He was weak, without appetite, and dwindling away. Then he had a heart attack and developed pneumonia. His wife courageously decided to stop treatment, and he died within a couple of days. Afterward she told me the pneumonia was a blessing. It spared him dying slowly and miserably from cancer of the pancreas.

This is not a new idea. William Osler was the most prominent physician in the world during the early twentieth century. In his lifetime and for a century afterward, he has been a model of the thoughtful inquiry, equanimity under stress, and respect for the human side of medicine to which all good physicians aspire. One Osler adage, often forgotten today, was "Pneumonia may well be called the friend of the aged. Taken off by it in an acute, short, not often painful illness, the old man escapes those cold gradations of decay so distressing to himself and to his friends."[10]

In another irony of medical history, Osler joked that the pneumococcus would someday carry him off. Maybe he knew he was a carrier. In the summer of 1919, while preparing to celebrate his seventieth birthday, he contracted a cold accompanied by chills. He said, "Friday night my Pneumococcus struck, and I had a high fever and have been in bed ever since."[11] Osler did not die immediately; he survived the acute illness. But through the fall of 1919, he languished, unable to shake off pneumococcal complications. As the infection slowly destroyed his lungs, the consummate physician made notes of his own illness.

As recorded by his biographer Harvey Cushing, Osler sent the notes with letters to his professional friends as though he were in charge of care for some patient in whose welfare he knew they were interested. "No fever since the 16th, but the cough persists and an occasional paroxysm—bouts as bad as senile whooping cough," read one quote.

The nights were the worst, preventing him from sleeping, so that he was administered "morphia," the term at that time for morphine, to permit him some rest. Then fluid collected in his chest. His physicians drained the pleural space and found pus, an ominous sign indicating an underlying lung abscess. On December 29, 1919, pneumonia finally killed the renowned physician. The dean of Christ Church, Oxford, eulogized Osler at his funeral: "He achieved many honors and many dignities, but the proudest of all was his unwritten title, 'the young man's friend.'"[12]

Earlier, Osler had urged his colleagues, "Keep an open mind toward pneumonia. Our grandchildren will be interested and are likely to have as many differences of opinion regarding treatment as we have."[13] A century later, this has turned out to be true, perhaps in a different way from how Osler intended. New causes of pneumonia continually emerge. Many species, bacteria, viruses, fungi, and exotic organisms, carried by travelers from all over the globe, attack. Malignancies and autoimmune diseases weaken resistance. The invaders become resistant to drugs. Despite our arsenal of antibiotics and antivirals, lower respiratory tract infections remain the fourth-most prevalent cause of death in the world.[14] Osler's advice about keeping an open mind toward pneumonia remains relevant a century after his death.

3

THEY STACKED CASKETS
IN THE HALLS

"But the most terrifying aspect of the epidemic was the piling up of bodies. Undertakers, themselves sick, were overwhelmed. They had no place to put bodies. Gravediggers either were sick or refused to bury influenza victims . . . they stacked caskets in halls, in their living quarters."

—John M. Barry[1]

I first met Nancy on a chilly January evening in 1975. I was choosing books to read to the children before they went to bed when the phone rang. The doctor in the emergency department wanted me to take care of a female patient being admitted to the intensive care unit with pneumonia. I apologized to the kids, kissed my wife, told her I wasn't sure when I'd be home, and headed for the hospital. As I drove along the freeway, I asked myself questions as I usually did. How old was she? I had forgotten to inquire. How was her breathing? As adrenaline kicked in, I felt the hyperalert state that always accompanied an urgent problem in the ICU.

To save time, I stopped by the emergency department first in hopes of catching a look at her chest X-ray before it went over to the radiology department for official reading. Her left lung looked like a snowstorm had hit it, and the right one was almost entirely whited out as well. This meant both lungs were inflamed, swollen, and boggy with fluid, the picture of bilateral pneumonia. I wasted no time in hightailing it to the ICU.

The unit becomes quiet in the evening. Visitors go home, and procedures like X-rays and cardiac catheterizations are finished for the day unless an emergency arises. The nurses turn down the lights to help patients sleep. The only sounds are the clicks and whooshes of ventilator valves opening and clos-ing. At the nursing station, technicians watch screens that display electrocar-diograms, blood pressures, oxygen levels, and other vital signs. Nurses silently glide from bed to bed checking to be sure patients are OK. Charts in hand, respiratory therapists record the numbers that show mechanical ventilators are doing their job. The atmosphere is quiet, but everyone is on alert.

In Nancy's room that night, the staff was ready for action. Her nurse was at the bedside. The respiratory therapist had parked a ventilator near the foot of her bed. Perhaps the emergency department staff had instructed them to be ready to intubate her. I quickly looked over her record—thirty-three years old; married; one son, age six; no history of serious illness. Part-time job with an accounting firm.

When I introduced myself, she was so drowsy she couldn't even respond. She gasped inaudibly through the oxygen mask, her lips and tongue dry, un-able to make a sound. Her pulse was 140, and her respiratory rate was 30, both twice normal. Her skin was moist and ashen, her hair wet with sweat and plastered down in soggy twists. The muscles in her neck tensed as she tried to breathe. I put a stethoscope on her chest and heard the crackling sounds of inflammation, like someone crushing cellophane inside her lungs. She would have a respiratory arrest in the next hour unless we intervened. I took her hand and said, "We're going to take care of you. It'll be all right."

I instructed the nurse and respiratory therapist to bring the crash cart to the bedside and asked how to reach her husband. "He's outside," came the reply.

Nancy's husband sat in the little anteroom outside the unit. He was in his early thirties, with sandy brown hair and glasses. He wore a sport coat and tie. I learned he had come home from work to take her to the hospital. His eyes were set in a grimace that suggested confusion as much as anxiety. He leaned forward when I asked him how she got sick. "She was fine until a week ago," he explained. "Then she got the flu and it really wiped her out. She went to the doctor the day before yesterday, but he said he couldn't see anything serious and told her she'd be okay in a few days."

I nodded. "Then what?"

"This afternoon she called me at work and said she felt terrible. Said she couldn't breathe. Asked me to take her to the hospital."

"No past history of any medical problems? Not a smoker? No recent travel? Not taking any drugs or medicines?" I checked off the points in my mind, and he told me all were negative. She had been in good health before this hit her.

I looked at him. "She has a bad pneumonia. I think it started with influenza. There may be a secondary bacterial infection in addition. That happens fre-quently. I'm going to cover her with antibiotics, but most important, she needs a ventilator to help her breathe." He nodded, his face fixed, and I continued,

"It'll require a tube in her windpipe. It'll be uncomfortable for her and she won't be able to talk, but I'm afraid we have to do it if we hope to save her."

Influenza typically comes on suddenly; causes fever, muscle aches, cough, and sore throat; and lasts seven to ten days. Infected individuals shed virus particles in tiny droplets they cough or sneeze out during the first three days up to two weeks after becoming infected. This is the time when flu passes from one person to another.

The illness has appeared under different names through the centuries, called "grippe," "sweating sickness," and "epidemic catarrh" at various times. The British name was "knock-me-down" fever, while in the colonies it was the "jolly rant." The term *influenza* comes from an old Italian folk word for "influence or visitation" because people thought epidemics resulted from the stars visiting pestilence on them. "Influenza di Fredo," the influence of the cold, was applied originally to scarlet fever, but by the mid-eighteenth century, *influenza* came to refer to what we today call the flu.[2]

Like many infections, influenza spreads to humans from animals. Birds and swine are the reservoirs for the virus, and humans pick it up by contact with chickens, ducks, and hogs. Seasonal flu affects millions during the winter months, and 200,000 people are hospitalized every year in the United States because of complications of the disease. Of these, 35,000 die from pneumonia or underlying chronic lung and heart diseases.[3]

The virus is a crafty, resourceful adversary and worldwide a major respiratory problem. Its power comes from its ability to assume multiple identities. Viruses have proteins on their surface called antigens that permit them to infect host animals and plants. Influenza depends on two antigens to carry its attack. They are known as hemagglutinins and neuraminidases, H and N in shorthand. More than fifteen types of H and nine of N exist, so investigators label specific strains of virus by where and when they first appeared and their H/N type. For example, the vaccine recommended for the winter of 2015–2016 seeks to protect against three strains of virus. It contains as its two main ingredients antigens from influenza virus A/California 2009 H1N1 and A/Switzerland 2013 H3N2.[4]

The influenza virus also mutates frequently. This means its surface antigens change constantly, a process referred to as antigen drift. The host is unable to develop lasting immunity because, with each mutation, the virus looks slightly different to the immune system. Imagine a terrorist who is a master of disguise. Each time he strikes, he changes clothes, wears a different wig, or grows a beard. Thus, he keeps the defense systems off balance. Antigen drift occurs every few years and leads to epidemics, with increases in hospitalizations and deaths. No matter how hard researchers try, they can't keep up with this sneaky enemy.

Seasonal influenza usually starts in birds in Asia and, as humans become infected, spreads to the western hemisphere. That is why every year virologists and public health experts review influenza cases from Asia and make an educated guess as to which strains to recommend to vaccine manufacturers for the following winter. Antiviral drugs can reduce the duration of symptoms and help infected patients return to work sooner, but because it can't be wiped out in the millions of wild birds in the world, vaccination is the main hope for controlling influenza in humans.

Periodically, antigen drift becomes so extreme the surface of the influenza virus is completely unrecognizable to host defenses. Called antigen shift, this is a situation in which no one has immunity. This is how pandemics occur; the terrorist actually changes identity, resulting in infections that spread like wildfire through the entire world population. Recent pandemics occurred in 1957, 1968, 1977, 1997, and 2009. None of these, however, caused even a fraction of the deaths or provoked a fraction of the terror that the 1918–1919 Spanish flu produced. It was the worst infectious catastrophe in human history.

Nineteen-eighteen was a sad year. The Great War, the war to end all wars, smoldered on. Five million soldiers lay dead. The western world was weary of the struggle and the carnage.[5] Then nature launched its own attack on humanity. In March, influenza erupted at a US Army camp in Kansas. It was a frightening illness that quickly spread to other military camps and into the civilian population. As troops debarked to Europe, they carried it to Britain, France, and Germany. Authorities in these war-torn countries tried to keep the public from becoming frightened and so downplayed its importance. Only the Spanish, who were neutral in the war and whose king was reportedly infected, were willing to acknowledge its presence, which is why the world called it Spanish flu.[6] It was horrific. Many victims died within a few hours of developing symptoms. They collapsed on sidewalks and in streetcars. Whole families were wiped out. Physicians and nurses became infected and died as well.

Hundreds of thousands of people fell ill, and a quarter of them died. The public panicked. People began to conjure images of the Black Death, the name given to the infamous bubonic plague that ravaged Europe in the fourteenth century. From 1918 through 1919, nearly half of all deaths in the United States resulted from influenza and the associated pneumonia it triggered in unlucky victims. Public health experts estimated that 675,000 more people died in this country than would have absent the flu epidemic. Considering that the US population in 1918 was approximately 105 million and now is 315 million, 2 million extra deaths would be a comparable casualty rate today.

Experts weren't even sure of the cause. At first, they suspected bacteria and cultured many kinds of organisms from the lungs of victims but couldn't show for sure any of them were the culprits. Scientists worked frantically to develop antiserum or some immunizing technique, but all failed. They didn't even know the killer was a virus, not a bacterium. It was not until 1931 that swine virus was shown to be the agent that caused the great influenza pandemic of 1918.[7]

In 2005, investigators at the CDC reconstructed the virus that caused the great influenza.[8] They found the gene sequences resemble those of viruses that exist today in birds and swine and cautioned that a recurrence of such a severe pandemic, while unlikely, is possible. The 1918 strain contained surface antigens H1 and N1, and so epidemiologists have worried this antigen combination may spawn a particularly potent strain, but so far, global disaster has not occurred.

For individual patients like Nancy, however, statistics matter little, and this can be even more frightening. Nancy wasn't immunized against influenza in 1975. She was young and in good health. Yet within a week she was on the verge of dying.

Influenza vaccines vary in effectiveness from year to year. This has made some experts dubious about their value in reducing mortality rates in the general population.[9] But many patients who die from influenza succumb to secondary pneumonia or heart failure, and death certificates are misleading. The CDC recommends vaccination annually for everyone over six months old, especially health care workers and those most susceptible: the elderly; pregnant women; and those with diabetes, heart diseases, and lung diseases.

Most hospitals in the United States now require all staff who have patient contact to be vaccinated during the months when influenza occurs or to wear a mask while around patients if they refuse. Protection depends on good respiratory care and standard public health measures of isolation and personal hygiene.

Influenza challenges even the most experienced physicians. Traditionally, we think of infants and the elderly, those at the extremes of life, as the most vulnerable. Or those already affected with diseases that weaken the heart and lungs, like coronary heart disease and COPD. Or immunologically weakened patients, such as cancer patients on chemotherapy, diabetics, and pregnant mothers. Yet, recent epidemics have targeted adolescents and young adults, which is why public health authorities have extended recommendations for immunization to include all segments of the population.

In the ICU that January night, when I told Nancy's husband she needed a machine to breathe for her, the color drained from his face. He spoke quietly, "What are her chances?"

"Too early to know. She's young and healthy, so I'd say the odds are in her favor. But this is very serious."

He stared at the wall. I was used to these moments when patients or family ponder difficult situations. Even so, I felt the awkward silence, and after a few minutes I asked, "You and she have a son, right? Any other family here in San Diego?"

"One boy. He's with his grandparents now."

"Come with me to her bedside. It will help her if she can see you," I said. "And it will help you to see her." He held her hand while I explained to Nancy what we needed to do. She was able to give a little nod, and I looked at her husband. "Would you wait outside while we set up the ventilator?" Fortunately, an obstetrical anesthesiologist was in the hospital that evening, and I enlisted his help to sedate her and pass the endotracheal tube, after which we attached the machine that was going to do the work of breathing for Nancy for the next few days or weeks.

Bacteria called staphylococci grew from her secretions, and based on the history of a viral illness the week before, I felt sure Nancy had postinfluenza staphylococcal pneumonia, the disease that killed 20 million people during the great flu pandemic of 1918–1919 and continues to kill thousands of people every winter in the United States.[10] Measurement of serum antibodies three weeks later returned positive for influenza, confirming the diagnosis, but this was not known at the start.

Nancy spent ten days on the mechanical ventilator and six weeks in the hospital. Despite big-gun antibiotics and heroic respiratory care, her right upper lobe liquefied and turned into a balloon-like cavity that replaced part of her lung and then slowly shrunk down into scar tissue. But she survived. Today she is able to live a normal life as long as she doesn't overstress herself. However, she still gets short of breath with heavy exertion, is susceptible to respiratory infections, and has to be diligent about keeping her immunizations up to date. She is one patient in whom I had no qualms about prescribing antibiotics for a cold.

Influenza reveals the vulnerability of our respiratory system. Six hundred times an hour, 14,000 times a day, humans inhale to stay alive. Viruses need cells to parasitize, and air offers an easy way to travel from host to host. We humans are often no more than accidental way stations in natural cycles that include birds and swine as viral hosts.

We can't eradicate the natural reservoirs of influenza, so how are we to defend ourselves against these constantly mutating coils of RNA? Surely technical advances like intensive respiratory care and mechanical ventilators save countless lives among the very sick. But, as they have for over a century, isolation, quarantine, and good hygiene remain the bedrock of our collective defenses against influenza as well as the other airborne viruses that cause pneumonia and respiratory death. Modern techniques augment but don't replace these age-old public health measures.

Influenza is only one of many infectious agents that threaten breathing. Some, like tuberculosis, are ancient, while other viruses, like SARS and MERS, are so new they have barely received names. Whether old or new, their behavior and natural history are mysterious, and this makes them all the more frightening and all the more challenging.

4

THE MAN IN THE IRON LUNG

"Life ultimately means taking the responsibility to find the right answer to its problems and to fulfill the tasks which it constantly sets for each individual."

—Victor Frankl[1]

When I was growing up, polio was the most frightening of the epidemic diseases that threatened us. Adults talked about the Spanish flu and its terrors, but that seemed remote. We were all vaccinated against smallpox. TB was a vague ghost about which we knew little. But polio was right there, and every summer it brought fear to the neighborhood. The disease was said to come from contaminated water, especially swimming pools. My parents were so concerned that during August and September we weren't allowed even to swim in Lake Michigan. Each summer, several kids would get the disease, and in every elementary school were students who walked with braces or crutches, their withered legs unable to bear weight. But paralysis of the breathing muscles was the most terrifying complication of polio, carrying the risk of suffocation and the specter of being in an iron lung, maybe forever.

In the early 1950s, I was lucky enough to make frequent trips from Chicago to South Bend, Indiana, to watch Notre Dame football. A friend's father had season tickets and was always willing to take a couple of us along. We walked up Notre Dame Avenue, pulled along with the noisy, joyful crowd, excitement mounting, as ahead we saw, like a shrine, the famous golden dome of the administration building. We bought tickets outside the stadium, confident we would have a good view wherever we sat. Notre Dame Stadium did not have a track around the field, so spectators were close to the action.

This was the era of Frank Leahy, and every year Notre Dame fielded one of the top teams in the country. Whether nature gave us crisp sunny days or black clouds that poured cold rain, we enjoyed enthusiasm matched nowhere else. When the band struck up "Cheer, cheer for Old Notre Dame" and the students roared in one great voice, "Onward to victory," accompanied by the women from St. Mary's College, with their green sweaters, pleated skirts, and white bobby socks, a shiver went up my spine.

But it was not all fun and thrills. From the tunnel at the north end of the stadium, where some of the nation's best athletes had just jogged onto the field, a bus would back into an area near the corner of the end zone, and an attendant would open its back doors. Out would come a six-foot-long cylinder on wheels, like a giant tin can, with a man's head protruding from its end. It was Fred Snite Jr., the "man in the iron lung." Snite was well-known in Chicago. A Notre Dame graduate, he had contracted polio in 1936 at the age of twenty-six and was paralyzed afterward. He traveled from Chicago to South Bend for all home games in a bus specially fitted to accommodate him.

As I sat in the stands, I couldn't stop staring at the iron lung. Snite watched the games through a mirror, his every breath dependent on the motor that changed the pressure inside the cylinder and allowed his lungs to expand. I admired his courage and perseverance but cringed to think about his predicament. How did he manage bathing or going to the bathroom? How did he survive, day after day, year after year, inside that thing?

Though vaccination has wiped out the disease in most of the world, polio will quickly return if immunization levels wane. Most young parents and most young physicians have never seen a case of polio. This is a blessing but carries the risk of complacency. One hundred million new humans are born every year around the world, and they are all vulnerable until vaccinated.

Polio occurs in waves. The first recorded polio outbreak in the United States was in Vermont in 1894, and a major epidemic struck New York in the summer of 1916. Six thousand people lost their lives, and 27,000 were left with various types of paralysis.[2] The city was in a panic. No one knew how it spread. Dr. Haven Emerson, professor of public health at Columbia University and health commissioner of New York City, quarantined families with members affected by polio in an effort to check its contagiousness.

The majority of patients who got polio didn't even realize it. Any germ could cause fever and weakness. About a quarter of polio patients had some form of muscle paralysis, and of those, a small subgroup, fewer than 5 percent, lost their ability to breathe, which was nearly universally fatal. Because most polio fatalities were due to respiratory paralysis, the disease stimulated the development of machines to assist breathing, precursors of the mechanical ventilators that are now mainstays in operating rooms and intensive care units. Contrivances existed to aid breathing, but they weren't effective. Then in 1929 came the first workable treatment for the respiratory muscle paralysis that killed polio victims: the iron lung.[3] To us eighty years later, it may seem like an arcane device of doubtful interest. But in the era before the advent of polio vaccine, when thousands of children contracted the disease every year, it was revolutionary.

Philip Drinker and Jack Emerson were scions of prominent families, both highly intelligent but of entirely different temperaments. Pictures show Drinker to be handsome, formally dressed, and reserved, while Emerson appears informal, smiling, and tieless. Drinker was born in 1894 in Haverford, Pennsylvania, son of the president of Lehigh University. He graduated from Princeton in 1915 and in 1917 earned a degree in chemical engineering from Lehigh. He moved to Boston, where he joined the faculty of Harvard University and in 1923 became an instructor in the newly created School of Public Health.

In 1926, executives of the Consolidated Gas Company of New York became concerned about the number of workers who were victims of electric shock or gas and smoke inhalation.[4] They sought help from Dr. Cecil Drinker, Philip's brother, who was professor of physiology at Harvard. At that time, Philip Drinker was working with Louis A. Shaw, studying respiration in cats. For their experiments, they devised an airtight iron box into which they could place an anesthetized cat, with its head exposed by means of a tight-fitting rubber collar in one end. A hand-operated pump connected to the box allowed them to suck out air, which caused the pressure inside the box to fall and made the cat inhale. When air was pumped back in, the animal exhaled.

Using this apparatus, they could keep cats alive for extended periods of time, and it occurred to Philip Drinker that a larger version of the box might be helpful to humans who couldn't breathe. He and Shaw constructed an adult-sized model, which he called a respirator, powered by an electric motor attached to a vacuum cleaner mechanism.

Cecil Drinker enthusiastically informed the gas company about his brother's invention, and by 1929, the first operational version was ready. The gas company donated it to Bellevue Hospital, and it was put into use almost immediately when a young woman unconscious from a drug overdose was brought to the hospital. She survived, which led a newspaper reporter to dub the respirator the iron lung. Later that year, Philip Drinker and his associate, pediatrician Charles McKhann, reported in the *Journal of the American Medical Association* the successful clinical use of the respirator in polio, and demand skyrocketed.[5]

Drinker and Shaw secured patents on the device and licensed its manufacture to the Warren E. Collins Company. Philip Drinker's son, an engineer himself, later said the success of the respirator was due to the availability of electricity, which allowed the device to be powered by motors that could operate continuously for long periods of time, and involvement by engineers in all stages of development. However, the Drinker-Shaw respirator had drawbacks. It was heavy, full of complicated fittings, expensive, and hot inside. Nevertheless, it revolutionized the treatment of respiratory paralysis due to polio and was used successfully to treat tetanus, diphtheria, poisonings, and drug overdoses, as well. By 1931, there were hundreds of Drinker respirators in use throughout the country.

John Haven Emerson, known as Jack, was born in 1906, the son of Dr. Haven Emerson, the same New York City public health commissioner during the 1916 polio epidemic.[6] The family was descended from William Emerson, brother of Ralph Waldo Emerson. Upper-class New Englanders, they were a scholarly, erudite clan of Brahmins who traditionally attended either Harvard or Radcliffe. But Jack was different. He was not much of a student and liked tinkering with machines better than attending classes. He never graduated from high school. In 1928, Jack moved to Boston, where his brother, who was at Harvard, got him a job sweeping floors in the physics lab. There he learned how to repair and maintain instruments used in research.

He borrowed $1,600 from his mother and bought the equipment for a small machine shop, which he located in a warehouse near Harvard Square. The office was described as dusty and cluttered with papers. Emerson himself answered the telephone. The shop was a model of ordered activity, where Harvard students who worked there would shout for Jack when they needed help.[7] In 1929, Emerson designed an oxygen tent for James Wilson, a pediatrician at Boston Children's Hospital.[8] As Emerson himself described it, because Wilson needed a way to cool the oxygen-rich air inside the tent, he bought a milk pail at Sears Roebuck and filled it with ice. He attached a motor to it, which was supposed to blow mist from the ice to the interior of the oxygen tent. But the combination of salt, water, and oxygen rusted the tinny metal, and the resulting leaks made the apparatus unworkable. So, Emerson made him a copper bucket, and the oxygen tent became functional.

Wilson showed Emerson the Drinker respirator and asked if he had any ideas on how to improve it. Emerson looked at it, thought about it, and said he felt having two motors was unduly complicated. He constructed a box with a piece of leather from a car seat as its top. Turning the box on its side he moved the leather sheet inward and outward to change the pressure in the box. Emerson gave the prototype to Wilson to show to Drinker, but Drinker rejected it, saying, "That won't work. We thought of that."[9]

Emerson discussed Drinker's reaction with his father in New York. The elder Emerson wrote to his son, saying, "We're heading for a bad epidemic of polio this year. If you're ever going to try that idea of yours, now's the time to do it." (According to Jack Emerson, this was in 1930 or 1931.)[10]

Emerson crossed the Charles River to the Robertson Boiler Works in Boston and, without any drawings or formal plans, told them, "Make me a round tank, about so big, well, twenty-eight inches maybe in diameter, and put some legs on it. We'll take it from there."[11] Within two weeks he constructed a simplified respirator. He took it to New York and presented it to his father, who suggested on his way back to Boston that Jack also show it to the doctors at the Chapin Hospital in Providence, which was the regional contagious disease hospital for Rhode Island. When Jack arrived in Providence, he found the Rhode Islanders had four patients on Drinker respirators and another patient in need of support, a young priest with severe respiratory paralysis who was expected to die that night. Emerson put the priest-patient into his respirator, and it worked perfectly. It ran for six months, the patient lived, and Emerson decided he would make more respirators. (The original Emerson machine, called Old No. 1, is now in the Smithsonian Institution in Washington.)

Emerson asked Robertson to make five more tanks, one of which he planned to exhibit at an equipment show of the American Hospital Association to be held in Toronto in 1931. Drinker learned of this and visited Emerson in his shop in Cambridge. He told Emerson that he had patents, and if Emerson continued making respirators, he would put him out of business. Emerson was angry because he felt his modifications had created a quieter, more reliable, and less expensive iron lung and that life-saving devices should be shared, not hoarded.

With his cousin and associate David Garrison, Emerson drove to Toronto, carrying one of the machines in the backseat of a Dodge touring car with its top down. According to Garrison, the headrest of the iron lung protruded so far it knocked over several street signs as they went through Albany, New York. The two entrepreneurs made it to Toronto and set up their iron lung among the exhibits. Emerson's iron lung sold for $1,000, a little more than half of what a Drinker cost, plus it was simpler and quieter. It was such a hit that representatives from Massachusetts General Hospital, a teaching institution of Harvard Medical School, ordered one on the spot.

Drinker was indignant. He was a Harvard professor. Who was this upstart to intrude on his domain? He reported the impertinence to Dean Edsel of Harvard, who persuaded Emerson not to advertise for six months, during which time the Collins Company came out with a new model incorporating several of Emerson's features.[12] The story of the conflict between the professor and the mechanic went viral by 1931 standards. *Time* magazine reported that Harvard's retiring president, A. Lawrence Lowell, tried to stop Jack Emerson from making ventilators. "I will like hell!" Emerson responded and strode out of the presidential mansion.[13] Drinker and Collins sued Emerson for infringing on their patents.

Emerson received added support from several members of the Harvard Medical School faculty when it was disclosed that Drinker was receiving royalties on every respirator sold by Collins. (Drinker allegedly got $300 on each $1,500 respirator.) Emerson claimed that $1,500 for a Drinker machine was robbery, and while he was selling similar machines for $1,000, he could lower the price even further if he had enough orders to build them in quantity. As the suit got nastier, the Harvard Corporation pinned up a notice in both the Medical School and School of Public Health that read,

> No member of either of these schools should take out for his own profit, or make any profit on, a patent upon any invention or discovery that affects the health of individuals or the public. If, to protect the public against misuse of the invention or discovery, it is necessary to control it by means of a patent, that should be applied for in such a name and under such conditions as the Corporation may determine.[14]

Mammals breathe by contracting respiratory muscles to enlarge the chest cavity. This lowers the pressure in the lungs below that of the atmosphere so that air rushes in. When the breathing muscles relax, the chest becomes smaller, and air leaves the lungs. Aware of this, inventors of machines to assist breathing sought to mimic nature to the extent possible. Emerson based his defense on showing that negative-pressure breathing machines existed long before Drinker and Shaw invented theirs. While Drinker had made important improvements, his ideas were not original.

Emerson searched the archives of the US Patent Office and reviewed the medical literature on negative-pressure body-encasing respirators. He compiled a historical list of the various contraptions invented, some of which were ingenious, some so impractical they bordered on crazy, and few of which had any success. Using these examples of early negative-pressure respirators, Emerson won the lawsuit. He rubbed salt in the Harvard wound when he credited the library at Massachusetts General Hospital with being the resource that permitted him to prevail. Several of Drinker's patents were disallowed, and Emerson continued making and selling iron lungs.

Meanwhile, polio remained the frightening disease I remember from my childhood, and iron lungs were cornerstones in treatment. They are now archaic emblems of another era but then were technological marvels. James Wilson, the pediatrician who asked Jack Emerson to look over the Drinker iron lung, started a respirator room at Boston Children's Hospital, in which several patients could be treated simultaneously. Caring for respirator patients was difficult and required expertise not readily available in small communities. The iron lungs worked well enough that many polio patients survived, but some required assisted ventilation for weeks; months; or, like Fred Snite Jr., for the rest of their lives. In truth, physicians weren't even sure whether prolonged inability to breathe was a sign of lingering polio effect or whether patients' breathing muscles had simply become weak from disuse.

Wilson said, "Of all the experiences the physician must undergo, none can be more distressing than to watch respiratory paralysis in a child with poliomyelitis."[15] He was convinced respirator centers offered patients the best chance of survival. With the support of President Franklin D. Roosevelt, himself a polio survivor, the National Foundation for Infantile Paralysis (which later became the March of Dimes) promoted using iron lungs for long-term care. The March of Dimes funded thirteen new centers at academic medical centers across the country. In 1944, Wilson became chair of the Department of Pediatrics at the University of Michigan, where he was a key organizer of the center there, which was the third in the nation.

Soon many hospitals had respirator wards like the ones Wilson envisioned. However, even the proponents of iron lungs realized that they were a stopgap measure. They did not treat the infection itself but, like rehabilitative exercises and leg casts, only ameliorated the impact of polio. However, iron lungs helped patients with poisonings, drug overdoses, and chest injuries, so they had other applications besides polio.

But the role of the iron lung in respiratory distress soon came to an end. A polio vaccine was on the horizon. It had been known since 1908 that polio was caused by a virus, but it took until 1949 before John Enders, Thomas Weller, and Frederick Robbins at Boston Children's Hospital were able to culture quantities of the virus large enough for study.[16] For this breakthrough, they received the Nobel Prize in medicine and physiology in 1954. Their work made it possible for Jonas Salk at the University of Pittsburgh to develop a killed-cell vaccine in 1955 and for Albert Sabin at the University of Cincinnati to follow with a live vaccine in 1961. Widespread vaccination caused a marked decrease in polio cases in the developed world after 1955 and, with that, less need for iron lungs. Before the polio vaccine became available, more than 15,000 cases of paralysis occurred each year in the United States. Following the introduction of the vaccine, the number of cases fell rapidly to less than one hundred in the 1960s and fewer than ten in the 1970s.[17] Polio has almost been eradicated worldwide because of vaccination. In 2016, only thirty-nine cases of polio of any kind were reported globally, confined to Pakistan, Afghanistan, and Nigeria.[18]

In the early 1950s, there were thousands of Drinker and Emerson iron lungs in use in the United States. By 1959, the number dropped to 1,200 and, by 2004, to fewer than 50.[19] Emerson stopped manufacturing iron lungs in 1970 and parts for them in 1974. Respironics, which acquired Emerson's company, continued repairing them and replacing parts until 2004. Today, there are fewer than twenty-five patients throughout the United States sleeping in iron lungs, some having spent more than fifty years dependent on them.[20]

Jack Emerson continued making ventilators but became interested in other projects. During World War II, he devised valves for high-altitude flight and underwater breathing. In 1942, he developed a resuscitator for victims of asphyxiation. In 1949, in collaboration with the Anesthesia Department at Harvard Medical School, he invented a device to assist breathing during anesthesia. And so, his connections with Harvard continued, in spite of the earlier conflict over the iron lung. Emerson later said, "All the things I've done have been because doctors have come to me with something they were trying to do. We didn't set out and say, 'Now we're going to get into this field and make this.' It's because of what doctors asked me for. That's the way my business is run."[21]

Emerson acquired over twenty patents for various devices he designed and in 1979 was awarded the Chadwick Medal by the American Thoracic Society, the first nonphysician to be honored in this way. He moved to Arlington, Massachusetts, and worked into his late eighties, attending trade shows and tinkering with instruments. One of his inventions is still used today, the Cough-Assist, a device to help clear secretions in patients with cystic fibrosis. Emerson died in 1997.

Despite being in the iron lung, Fred Snite Jr. led a full life. His family had a winter home in Florida, and he traveled there. In time, he became able to use a portable chest respirator he called Junior that permitted him to come out of the iron lung for several hours each day. He visited the famous shrine in Lourdes, France, though he experienced no miraculous cure from that pilgrimage. In 1939, Snite married and over the next six years fathered three daughters. He became a serious bridge player and participated in tournaments from inside his respirator. Gifted with a positive spirit and friendly personality, he made radio, and later television, broadcasts on behalf of the March of Dimes, becoming an inspiration for polio sufferers everywhere. He also remained a dedicated Notre Dame fan. In 1956, his attendant, Leonard Hawkins, wrote a book in which he praised Snite as an "example of courage every one of us hopes he'll have when his own hour of trial arrives."[22] Frederick Snite Jr. died in 1954 of cor pulmonale, heart failure due to chronic respiratory insufficiency.

But the iron lung became obsolete for another reason. Subatmospheric pressure worked for situations where the lungs were normal, like patients suffocating from neurological or muscular weakness, as in polio or drug overdoses. But the tank respirator wasn't powerful enough to inflate lungs inflamed with pneumonia or boggy with edema fluid. Medical science soon learned a better way to support breathing in these patients. It was called intermittent positive-pressure ventilation. More on this later.

5

PRODUCTS OF PARASITIC BEINGS

"All infections, of whatever type, with no exceptions, are products of parasitic beings; that is, by living organisms that enter in other living organisms, in which they find nourishment, that is, food that suits them, here they hatch, grow and reproduce themselves."

—Agostino Bassi[1]

"Remember how much you do not know."

—William Osler[2]

The warmest part of the year occurs later in the southwest than in the rest of the United States. Even after the equinox, when the oak leaves have begun to turn brown and football dominates the sports pages, the belatedly rising sun, as if to give the earth one last roasting as it moves south, marches across the sky, unimpeded by clouds, and sucks the last molecules of water out of the already-parched ground. Cooling winds from the west stand still, allow the atmosphere to reach baking temperatures, then swirl up from the east, becoming the infamous "devil winds" or "Santa Anas" that fuel brush and forest fires. And on those dessicating fall days, amid the choking dust, valley fever stalks the land.

The disease, coccidioidomycosis, or Coccy for short, is caused by inhaling a fungus, called *Coccidioides immitis/posadasii*, that lives in the arid soil. It can manifest itself as no more than a bad case of flu or as a relentless killer that eats into nearly every organ in the body. Though the organism was recognized as early as 1892, medical science knew little about its behavior until decades later. For the first quarter of the twentieth century, physicians thought it was universally fatal and that valley fever was something else. Then in 1929, one of those peculiar chance events that keep popping up in science occurred and changed everything.

Harold Chope was a twenty-six-year-old Stanford University medical student examining a culture of *Cocci* in the microbiology lab when he inadvertently breathed on the plate, causing a cloud of spores to rise into the air.[3] Nine days later, Chope developed chest pain, cough, and blood-streaked sputum. A chest X-ray showed pneumonia in the right lung. Everyone thought he would die; this was the dreaded Coccy. University officials were distraught. They were responsible for the safety of students and felt the least they could do was to make him as comfortable as possible. So they put him into a private hospital room and procured a radio for him, a major perk in those days. Sputum samples grew *Cocci*, confirming the fatal diagnosis. Newspapers and nationally circulated magazines wrote up the story, portraying Chope as a young investigator about to become a martyr to science.

But Chope didn't die. A month later, he developed red bumps on his extremities, an allergic reaction known as erythema nodosum, and slowly began to improve. After three months, he was healed and returned to his medical school classes. The students and faculty at Stanford were overjoyed that he had been spared. (Chope was likely happy, too.) And from Chope's experience, the scientists acquired an important insight: Acute pulmonary Coccy developed between one and two weeks after exposure and was not always fatal.

After Chope graduated, another Stanford medical student, Charles Smith, came onboard in the microbiology lab. Soon after, Smith developed a respiratory illness with chest pain and pleurisy. He worried he might have tuberculosis, but sputum tests were negative. Like Chope, Smith had acquired acute Coccy in the lab but didn't recognize it. Insight number 2: Coccy could mimic tuberculosis.

Smith decided to stay on in the lab and study the mysterious fungus. He probably didn't know it then, but he was embarking on what would become his life's work, and his investigations would unlock many of the secrets of Coccy and profoundly influence medicine's view of the disease for years to come.

In 1934, Dr. Myrnie Gifford, yet another Stanford medical graduate working in the Kern County Health Department in California's Central Valley, while reviewing records of patients with Coccy, noted that, of fifteen cases, three had erythema nodosum. The syndrome of cough, chest pain, fever, pneumonia, and erythema nodosum was already well-known in Kern County under the names valley fever, desert fever, and San Joaquin fever. Gifford mentioned this to her mentor, Ernest Dickson, in whose laboratory Chope had worked, and he reminded her that Chope also had erythema nodosum.

After this, Gifford began to skin-test all patients in Kern County who developed valley fever for *Cocci*. They were universally positive. The fungus had been cultured from soil on a ranch near Delano, so the health department knew it grew in the area. Gifford also noted that the majority of valley fever patients had a history of dust exposure, strengthening the association. Insight number 3: San Joaquin Valley fever was actually acute Coccy. While rarely fatal, it was an important disease, affecting thousands of people in California and Arizona every year, necessitating hospitalization for many and confusing doctors who thought they were seeing tuberculosis or lung cancer.

In 1937, Smith undertook study of the natural history of Coccy in the San Joaquin Valley. He obtained the addresses of all newly diagnosed valley fever cases from the Kern and Tulare Health Departments and visited the patients' homes, skin-testing them for *Cocci*. He found half were recently arrived migrant workers, farmers from the midwest who had left the dust bowl to seek a better life in California. By repeated skin testing of these workers, Smith showed that the *Cocci* skin tests turn positive around two weeks after the onset of symptoms.

Smith heard from local doctors that a patient almost never had a second case of valley fever. He then became certain that a positive skin test reaction indicated protection from reinfection. He also wondered how long the skin test remained positive after a patient had Coccy and persuaded Chope to be skin-tested. Chope had had no further exposure to *Cocci* in the years after he left the lab. The skin test produced a large blistered red area on Chope's arm that sloughed the skin, leaving him with a permanent scar. Needless to say, Chope refused further skin tests.[4] Insight number 4: The skin test remained positive indefinitely, likely throughout one's lifetime, and was a sign of immunity.

Smith also became convinced that the disease was not contagious. He found no clustering of cases in people who worked together, and bed partners of patients rarely became infected unless they also had dust exposure. However, he came to appreciate its infectiousness. Eighteen people working in his department developed the disease with no exposure except to laboratory cultures. Because of this, Smith was said to hire only individuals known to have a positive response to the *Cocci* skin test to work in the lab, as they were immune to the disease.[5]

While Smith was conducting epidemiologic studies in various areas of California, the world was being drawn into global conflict, and Coccy became important to the war effort. During World War II the US Army decided to train aviators at fields in central California and Arizona. The terrain was flat, skies were often cloudless, and winters were mild enough to permit year-round flying. Smith, among others, warned about the risk of Coccy for newcomers, but the military leaders felt that the geographic advantages outweighed the medical danger. They did, however, agree not to train ground troops in regions known to be endemic for the fungus. Smith was able to extend his Coccy studies on these recruits and confirmed the disease affected those newly arrived the most. Of the 100,000 trainees, 25,000 became skin-test-positive during their first year in the valley.[6] He also observed that the disease disseminated throughout the body ten times more frequently in blacks than in whites.[7]

Wartime policies provided more opportunities for Smith to study Coccy when German, Italian, and Japanese prisoners were housed on military reservations in the southwestern United States. Many of these had tuberculosis, and authorities were concerned they would get Coccy as well. No evidence accrued that Coccy aggravated tuberculosis, but the military moved those patients to other parts of the country in order to avoid criticism about violating the Geneva Conventions regarding humane treatment of prisoners of war.[8]

Smith also observed Japanese Americans interned at camps in areas endemic for *Cocci* in California and Arizona and concluded they had approximately the same susceptibility to infection as Caucasians, though possibly more tendency to disseminate.[9] Perhaps those discriminated against in one of America's saddest policies were able to gain some reassurance from these studies.

Smith's observations made public health authorities aware of another type of discrimination. Public health regulations required placing anyone with a chest X-ray consistent with tuberculosis into a sanatorium. Many of those individuals showed no sign of tuberculosis bacilli in their sputum. They were later found to have a positive *Cocci* skin test. To make matters worse, some had been admitted without really having tuberculosis but acquired it after residing in a sanatorium for several months. How many lives were needlessly disrupted by these policies? These tragedies led to changes in public health practice that required more evidence of tuberculosis than merely an abnormal X-ray for mandatory admission to a sanatorium.

Forty percent of those infected by *Cocci* experience respiratory symptoms, but many are passed off as flu, and fewer than 10 percent develop complications.[10] Sometimes, however, Coccy can resemble a more sinister diagnosis.

I first met Larry on a hot September afternoon. He sat across the desk in my consultation room, and when I asked what brought him to the office, he blurted, "My doctor is worried I have lung cancer."

Broad-shouldered, tanned, with brown curly hair and a big mustache, he wore a short-sleeved plaid shirt that exposed muscular forearms, jeans with copper rivets on the pocket corners, and polished boots. He sat forward as he talked, filling the space between his chair and the desk front. Larry had been in good health until about four weeks before, when he began to cough and feel tired and feverish. He and his doctor at first thought it was flu, so he took a week off work, toughed it out with Advil, and cut back on cigarettes to a couple a day. But his chest started to hurt, and he found it difficult to take a deep breath. Then he spit up a fleck of bloody phlegm. A chest X-ray showed a spot in his left lung, and he was referred for pulmonary consultation.

Larry was thirty-eight years old, grew up in Arkansas, spent four years in the navy, and settled in San Diego after he was discharged. He was married, with two teenaged daughters, and employed as an operating engineer by a construction company in El Cajon, in the eastern part of San Diego County.

His temperature was 99.6, slightly high, but the physical exam was otherwise completely normal. His chest X-ray showed an irregular-shaped patch in the left midlung field, like a clump of white feathers in the dark gray background of pulmonary tissue. In addition, the hilar lymph nodes, those at the root of the lung, were enlarged. It could be malignant, but it could be inflammatory. The picture was indeterminate.

"Tell me more about your work," I asked. He informed me that he had been a member of the union for ten years and had worked for his current employer the last six. His specific job was to operate a front loader and backhoe.

"Where are you working now?" I asked.

"We're building an apartment complex on Dehesa Road," he answered, "across from Singing Hills."

"Pretty dusty, I imagine."

"You better believe it. Dusty. And hot. Thought I was gonna have a heatstroke last week, if I didn't cough myself to death first."

"I can see why your doctor is concerned," I said, "but this might be a fungus infection or even TB," which was both truthful and an effort to bring hope to a difficult situation. "I'd like to put on skin tests, do some blood work, and get a CT scan."

He arched his eyebrows. "But what about lung cancer?" he asked.

"Let's do the tests," I answered. "And in the meantime, quit smoking."

Anxiety over cancer is universal. The disease conjures images of pain, wasting, and death. Especially lung cancer in a smoker. "Why me? I should have quit smoking. Will I need surgery?" Unfortunately I faced these questions every week for my entire time in practice. And I never devised a good way to reassure a patient until I was myself sure there was no malignancy. So I hoped Larry would be one of the lucky ones. His story fit an infection, and he didn't look sick. I fell back on "Let's reserve judgment until we get all the information," the age-old platitude employed for centuries by uncertain physicians.

Larry's tests came back with equivocal results, and so I recommended bronchoscopy, inserting a miniature telescope into the lung in order to show a tumor, if one was present, and collect specimens directly from the abnormal area. The bronchoscopy showed nothing to suggest cancer, but mucus brushed out of the feathery-looking X-ray shadow was full of tiny spheres suggesting fungal spores. Larry had a fungal pneumonia, and my best guess was that *Cocci* was the culprit.

Cocci lives only in the southwestern United States, northern Mexico, and western South America, eking an existence out of the dry soil and warm climate. During the late summer, the tiny creatures send out thin-walled branches called hyphae that under a microscope look like miniature budding flowers. At their ends are clumps of spores that waft into the air when the surface soil is disturbed, spreading in an invisible cloud across the sand.

California and Arizona have been in the throes of a Coccy epidemic for the last twenty years. The number of reported cases in the United States rose from 2,265 in 1998 to 22,400 in 2011, nearly a tenfold increase. Arizona accounted for 16,600, or almost 75 percent of these, with the highest incidence in Maricopa County, which includes Phoenix and its surrounding municipalities. Most of the almost 6,000 California cases came from the San Joaquin Valley, around Fresno and Bakersfield, while Los Angeles and San Diego Counties, the two most populous in the state, contributed only 300 and 150 cases, respectively, in 2011. Because many infections go undiagnosed, passed off as the flu, the actual number of cases was likely higher.[11] Indeed, some researchers estimate *Cocci* infects more than 150,000 people per year nationwide. Mortality rate is low, averaging about two hundred cases per year, mostly from progressive pulmonary infection and respiratory failure, though deaths may result from spread throughout the body, a process called dissemination.[12] Construction workers, agricultural laborers, and archaeology students are most at risk, digging in soil being the common denominator of infection.

The California Department of Health publishes recommendations for preventing infection, like wetting the soil in areas that will be excavated and providing closed, air-conditioned cabs for trucks and earth-moving vehicles employed in construction in endemic areas. Laying paving as soon as possible after grading is completed and positioning workers upwind from dusty areas whenever possible are other preventative measures to reduce disease.[13] Despite these precautions, many cases occur without any history of overt exposure to dust.[14]

Cultures of Larry's lung washings confirmed he did have Coccy, not lung cancer. I met with him in the office as soon as the results came in. "You have an infection called coccidioidomycosis. Everyone calls it Coccy for short. It's due to a fungus, the same one that causes San Joaquin Valley fever."

He cocked his head. "How did I get it?"

"You inhaled microscopic seeds, called spores, from the air when you were grading the ground for the apartment construction," I answered. "Which reminds me, this is a work-related illness. Be sure to mention that when you fill out the insurance forms for your time off work."

"What about treatment?" he asked.

"I don't think you need treatment right now. Let's watch. I think this will heal on its own. Just stay away from tobacco."

He arched his eyebrow. "Will it come back?"

"No. You're immune."

"Can I give this to my daughters or anyone else?"

"No, you got it by inhaling spores in the air. It's infectious but not contagious."

He smiled and said, "I feel lucky, like I just got a new lease on life." I agreed. It's nice to be able to give good news. Over the next three months, Larry's lung healed, and the only footprint from his bout of Coccy was a small calcified scar in his left lung. I saw him every three months for a year after that and then turned his care back to his family doctor, so I no longer have follow-up.

Larry was indeed lucky. However, others, especially African Americans and Filipinos, are susceptible to spread beyond the lungs. For these individuals, Coccy alters their lives forever.

Hattie was a middle-aged African American woman who contracted pulmonary Coccy in 1965, which was followed by swollen lymph nodes in her back that burst through the skin and drained purulent, pus-like fluid. A year later, similar draining abscesses developed on her buttocks. *Cocci* organisms grew out of both the back and the buttocks. Dye injected into the back showed a tract that burrowed from the lung back to the spine, down along the spinal muscles, behind the pelvis, and exited in the buttock abscesses. Subjecting her to continuous pain, recurrent fevers, difficulty maintaining weight, and chronic fatigue, the unforgiving disease turned this nice lady's life upside down.

Hattie received antifungal antibiotics intravenously until her kidneys would no longer tolerate them and then irrigation of the abscesses with antibiotic solution in an attempt to treat the infection locally. I remember flushing a suspension of drugs into the sinus in her back and watching it dribble out of the hole in her buttocks, where it would collect in a gauze pad while the nurse held her hand and Hattie gritted her teeth in pain.

Occasionally, she would admit to being discouraged, but most of the time she soldiered on, raised children and grandchildren, and participated in community life. Her patience and acceptance were a lesson to me. Finally, in 1990, azoles, newly discovered antifungal drugs, finally calmed down the abscesses and helped nature to close them.

Because of her genetic background, Hattie struggled with periodic flareups of fever and increased drainage that went on for decades. Coccy came to define her life, with frequent need for toxic antibiotics and painful surgical drainage. She had difficulty maintaining her strength in the face of infection. She did live, however, into her seventies, when she finally succumbed, not to Coccy, but to dementia.

Harold Chope went on to a productive career in public health. He became the director of public health in San Mateo County, California, and was a valued steward of public trust. Chope died in 1976. In 2006, the one-hundredth anniversary of its founding, the San Mateo County Medical Association honored Chope as its physician of the century.

Charles Smith moved from Stanford to Berkeley in 1951, when he became dean of the School of Public Health at the University of California. Smith's research laboratory remained the gold standard for confusing diagnostic cases where Coccy was a possibility. It was the practice in our office to send samples of serum to Smith in any case where confusion existed or the stakes were high. Two weeks extra to get results back saved many patients from having their chests opened under a suspicion of cancer or erroneously being subjected to antituberculosis drugs.

Smith died in 1967, before I joined the practice, but Demosthenes Pappagianis, one of his proteges who was by then chair of the Department of Microbiology at the UC Davis Medical School, took over supervision of the Coccy research laboratory. I remember receiving many calls, asking how patients were doing, to compare clinical course with changing antibody levels. We relied on that lab as the highest court of appeals in Coccy.

Molds and fungi mostly cause superficial infections of body surfaces. Diaper rash, jock itch, and vaginal yeast infections affect most of us at one time or another. However, more than a dozen molds and fungi can invade the lungs and cause pneumonia, bloodstream infections, shock, and death. They are called deep mycoses. *Mycosis* means "fungus invasion," and *deep* referrs to their ability to penetrate into tissue.

North America has the dubious honor of being home to three of the most important fungal diseases that attack healthy individuals: coccidioidomycosis, histoplasmosis, and blastomycosis, called Coccy, Histo, and Blasto for short. Each has its own peculiar ecological requirements that testify to the wondrous diversity of nature, and they all regularly challenge the medical profession to recognize and treat them.

Cocci is the most prevalent of the deep fungal infections that attack healthy people and the most significant, but *Histo* and *Blasto*, which act the same way, each cause thousands of infections every year in the United States. All live in soil and produce human disease by accidental inhalation of spores. In the lungs, fungal spores become like yeast cells, budding into microscopic clumps, and the resulting inflammation is what we call disease.

Fungi have specific requirements for heat and moisture that confine them to particular geographic regions. For example, *Cocci* can live only in a hot dry climate, while *Histo* and *Blasto* grow well in moist areas and live throughout the midwestern United States. *Histo* is endemic in the valleys of the Ohio and

Mississippi Rivers and extends southwest as far as the Rio Grande. *Blasto*, but not *Histo*, inhabits soil in the eastern part of the country. Its endemic region runs as far north as Canada and extends southeast to South Carolina but not into Georgia and Florida.

These infections can be serious and, like Coccy, are often confused with tuberculosis or lung cancer, which makes them important beyond their frequency. After being inhaled, all three cause an acute pneumonia, from which most people recover without incident. As healing occurs, scars form in the lungs. These often become calcified, leaving nodules that resemble lung cancer. In addition, the fungi can cause lung tissue to liquefy and form a cavity, a thin-walled balloon deep in the lung. Cavities may persist even after the lung has healed and are predisposed to secondary infections with bacteria for the rest of the person's life. Rarely, infection progresses, and repiratory failure and death can eventuate. Even more rarely, infection spreads to other parts of the body, with disastrous results.

Diagnosis depends on recovering organisms from sputum or from biopsied tissue. The presence of a positive skin test signifies only prior infection, not disease activity. In endemic areas, the majority of the population become skin-test-positive by adulthood. For example, in some communities along the watershed of the Ohio River, as many as 90 percent of adults have a skin test reaction to *Histo*.[15] In addition, fungal skin tests can cross-react. Thus an individual who grew up in Missouri, lived in California, and then moved to New York can come down with Blasto in New York yet have positive *Cocci* and *Histo* skin tests from earlier life. To complicate matters more, rising levels of antibodies to these fungi indicate worsening infection, while falling levels reflect healing. These complexities make diagnosis more difficult, though they do create a role for pulmonary and infectious disease specialists.

Outbreaks of Histo result when humans come in contact with decaying organic matter. These have occurred around chicken coops, blackbird roosts, and caves where bats live. Archeology students excavating gravesites and spelunkers exploring caves have been well-publicized victims of infection, though urban outbreaks can result when construction projects disturb contaminated soil. The largest outbreak of Histo ever reported occurred in Indianapolis in August 1978 and September 1979.[16] Four hundred thirty-five cases resulted, with fifteen deaths, epidemiologically traced to clearing ground and excavating for a new swimming pool. Skin tests of residents in the area suggested more than 100,000 people were exposed during those years.

Blastomycosis is an even more difficult opponent to track. No reliable skin test exists to estimate its prevalence, so scientists have to rely on soil cultures and reported cases. Blasto affects mostly adults and has an attraction for people engaged in hobbies like hunting and fishing.[17] Occasionally Blasto occurs as a primary skin infection because of a cut or dog bite, but it is primarily a respiratory disease. Mike Craig, a colleague of mine at Michigan, reported a case where the wife of a man with Blasto of the prostate developed a uterine infection with the fungus, presumably transmitted sexually, a reminder that nature never lacks for ways to surprise us.[18] However, person-to-person transmission of these fungal infections is rare, and spread beyond the lungs into other tissues is uncommon.

Deep fungal infections spread like a forest fire in individuals whose defenses are weakened. Indeed, secondary fungal pneumonia is so common it is almost expected in HIV patients. Those with cancer and on chemotherapy, diabetics, renal failure patients, transplant recipients, and patients taking long-term steroids also suffer fungal infections and so require surveillance.

Individuals whose defenses are impaired are vulnerable to infection with common molds, as well. These are more frequent than *Cocci*, *Histo*, and *Blasto*. *Aspergillus*, which lives in soil; *Candida*, which lives in the human intestine; and *Pneumocystis*, which probably lives in the respiratory tract, all invade the lungs of those with suppressed immunity and can lead to fatal pneumonia, sepsis, and death.[19] These fungi are too weak to infect healthy individuals but are serious threats to those whose resistance is already compromised.

Infections are also part of the price paid for medical advances. For example, monoclonal antibodies for treatment of arthritis, psoriasis, and inflammatory bowel diseases lower resistance to fungal infections, tuberculosis, and cancer. There is no free lunch in medicine.

Because fungi prey on compromised patients, treatment is difficult. No effective vaccines exist for these marauders. Resistance to fungi does not depend on antibodies but on lymphocytes. These small cells reside in lymph nodes, the spleen, and circulating blood. They are an important defense system that complements their better-known cousins, serum antibodies.

However, since the 1980s, the azoles, including the current big gun, voriconazole, have assumed prime importance in treating fungal infections in compromised patients. Indeed, they are mainstays in oncology and intensive care units. However, judicious use of antibiotics and steroids are also important. Furthermore, isolation and hand washing, simple and time-honored, as well as gowns, gloves, and masks, are also of value to prevent caregivers and visitors from infecting vulnerable patients unable to protect themselves.

Fungal infections of the lungs, the deep mycoses, are medical curiosities to most people. It is remarkable that, of the thousands of fungal species in the environment, only a handful cause human disease. *Cocci* is a serious public health problem in Arizona and the California Central Valley, threatening agricultural and construction workers. The other deep mycoses, *Histo* and

Blasto, cause mostly sporadic infections. Outbreaks occur occasionally, like in Indianapolis in 1978, but are so rare they become news items.

In contrast, *Aspergillus*, *Candida*, and other molds are constant specters in hospitals, where cancer, HIV, and immune-deficient patients receive care. None of these give any indication of abating in the foreseeable future. Researchers are working on vaccines but have no immediate prospects of success.

Eliminating overuse of antibiotics in patients with poor resistance would reduce the prevalence of secondary fungal infection. Every prescription for antibiotics carries the danger of permitting molds and fungi to overgrow and invade the lungs and bloodstream. These are not drugs to be taken lightly.

Many of these fungi and molds have existed hundreds of millions of years and play a major role in nature's ecological balance. They can't be eradicated. We have to learn how to exist with them. Minimizing occupational and recreational contact will reduce respiratory risk from deep fungal infections. But, as with all the organisms we battle, we must have a healthy respect for their staying power and resilience.

The exotic biology of the deep mycoses and the various airborne molds makes them interesting, as well as medically challenging, and each of them are unique in their own ways. However, other unusual species of organisms exist in nature, often hidden in the most extreme locations, sometimes under our noses. These are only too happy to infect the human respiratory system, where they find a warm, moist environment in which to reside.

6

SOME LIKE IT HOT

"What has been will be again, and what has been done will be done again; there is nothing new under the sun."

—Ecclesiastes 1:9[1]

In the fall of 1976, Joseph McDade and his team of infectious disease researchers at the CDC in Atlanta were under the gun. One hundred eighty-two members of the Pennsylvania chapter of the American Legion had come down with a mysterious respiratory illness. One hundred forty-seven of them had to be hospitalized, and twenty-nine died. The public was frightened, and Congress wanted some answers.

In July, America celebrated the two-hundredth anniversary of the signing of the Declaration of Independence. Philadelphia was the site of the original Continental Congress and the place where the Declaration was signed. The Pennsylvania branch of the American Legion, the largest organization of military veterans in the country, decided to hold its annual convention in Philadelphia on July 21, 1976.

Eastern Pennsylvania was warm that week, with scattered clouds and occasional drizzle, but four thousand legionnaires attended the meeting, wearing service caps, their chests festooned with badges and medals; enjoying three days of inspirational speeches, camaraderie, and merry-making; and lubricated by hospitality suites well-stocked with beer and liquor. The convention ended July 24 amid back-slapping and teasing, as the legionnaires scattered to their homes around the state. They couldn't have known that, within two weeks, they would be at the center of a baffling medical mystery.

In late July, doctors all over Pennsylvania began to report seeing legionnaires with unexplained fever and abdominal discomfort, followed by cough, difficulty breathing, and pneumonia. When the first illnesses occurred, the Pennsylvania Health Department thought they might be influenza. But an epidemic of that disease in July would be very unusual, and none of the patients showed antibodies in their blood to indicate a recent influenza infection. Further complicating the mystery was that penicillin and other potent antibiotics didn't help. The only agents that seemed beneficial were a couple of old-timers, tetracycline and erythromycin, considered third-line drugs for pneumonia.

By August 4, a few cases that clinically looked the same popped up in nonlegionnaires, which further muddied the diagnostic waters. Pathologists found signs of bacteria in pulmonary secretions but couldn't culture any particular organisms. The CDC sent a team to Pennsylvania to assist the state public health officers. The investigators questioned treating physicians and family members all over the commonwealth. They looked for contact with animals or birds; they inquired for ingestion of a particular food and, because it was midsummer, unusual exposure to insects, such as ticks or mosquitoes. All turned out to be blind alleys. But, as they pieced together the demographics of the epidemic, the scientists noticed the sick had one thing in common: All had stayed at or visited the main host hotel in midtown Philadelphia.

A stately old building constructed in 1904, the Bellevue-Stratford at one time was the preeminent hotel in the city, nicknamed the "Grande Dame of Broad Street." By 1976, it no longer could claim an exclusive on luxurious accommodations, but it was still a well-known Philly landmark. Remodeled and air-conditioned, the hotel's seven hundred rooms, accommodations for meetings, and capacious ballroom made it an attractive site for conventions. From July 14 to 17, a society of magicians booked the hotel, followed by a candle-makers' convention until July 21, when the American Legion took over the premises. On August 1, a Eucharistic Congress succeeded the Legion. The Bellevue-Stratford Hotel was a busy place that anniversary summer.

The illness affected mainly the lungs and respiratory tract, which suggested breathing was the route of transmission. Had some visitor, perhaps a legionnaire but maybe a magician or candle-maker, been infected when they checked into the hotel and spread it to others? Epidemiologists couldn't find clustering of infections among legionnaires who shared rooms, which argued against person-to-person transmission. They queried the four hundred hotel employees. Only one, an air-conditioner repair man, had gotten sick during the time in question. However, fourteen cases of this unusual pneumonia affected nonlegionnaires, and very peculiarly, some of these had been no closer than to walk along the sidewalk in front of the hotel. These cases were called Broad Street pneumonia to distinguish them from Legionnaires' disease, the nickname given to the main group.

During August and September 1976, Legionnaires' disease ranked at the top of the list of public concerns. *Time* magazine made it the subject of a cover story and praised the efforts of the CDC chasing the elusive disease. By late September, the number of new cases dropped off. The public felt relief, but the scientists remained perplexed, and everyone felt vulnerable. Legionnaires' disease might recur. And with a 15 percent mortality rate, that could be a catastrophe. As autumn arrived and the leaves fell, so did the spirits of the researchers at the CDC.

Meanwhile, other states besides Pennsylvania began to report sporadic cases of pneumonia with no recognizable cause. Maybe they were Legionnaires' disease. If so, this was not only a Pennsylvania problem; it was much more widespread. Health authorities were concerned it might be a new form of influenza, a harbinger of an incipient pandemic akin to the Spanish flu of 1918 that killed millions. Congress authorized funds to prepare 50 million doses of influenza vaccine for immediate use.

Some raised the specter that the outbreak was the work of terrorists, maybe a Communist plot to attack America by disabling its military veterans. Though the clinical presentation indicated the disease was most likely an infection, investigators analyzed tissue samples from autopsies, seeking traces of poisons known to injure the lungs. They found nothing.

The public became impatient. Congress began to investigate, and the CDC came under fire. What were the taxpayers getting for the many millions of dollars being lavished on these high-powered scientists and these gleaming laboratories on the beautiful campus in Atlanta?

McDade was a CDC research microbiologist. He specialized in rickettsia, a subgroup of bacteria that live only inside the cells of animals they parasitize and are thus difficult to culture in the laboratory. McDade was trying to find out if a rickettsia could be responsible for Legionnaires' disease. In 1976, scientists didn't have DNA and genome sequencing, the techniques used today.[2] McDade injected guinea pigs with minced tissue from four patients that had died of Legionnaires' disease. When some guinea pigs died, he was able to see a few colonies of bacteria in their lungs but couldn't culture any specific agent. He ground up the spleens of the guinea pigs because microbes often sequester in that organ and injected the material into chicken eggs, but nothing grew. Were the bacteria he had seen in the lungs of the dead guinea pigs significant? Week after week, while public pressure increased, the unanswered question gnawed at McDade.

Myth depicts scientific breakthroughs as the result of dramatic insights occurring to brilliant investigators, as if a "eureka" moment is common in research. But progress most often results from dedication, thoroughness, and perseverance. After five months of work, McDade finally earned his "eureka." On the evening of December 28, he attended a holiday party but was unable to enjoy the conviviality. He excused himself and returned to his lab, explaining he wanted to clear up some loose ends before the year drew to a close. In isolating rickettsial organisms, McDade inserted small amounts of antibiotic into the egg-based culture medium to suppress contaminating bacteria.[3] He wondered if the antibiotic might have inhibited growth of some exotic bacteria present in the guinea pig spleen mixture. So he prepared a new batch of eggs but did not add antibiotic.

When he later withdrew liquid from the eggs and injected it into guinea pigs, they developed symptoms like those of Legionnaires' disease. This had to be it. He was sure the bacteria he had seen in the guinea pigs were the culprits. Over the next few days, he tried different culture techniques and eventually found a mix in which colonies of organisms grew. They were rod-shaped bacteria called bacilli. Fastidious in where they lived and what they ate, the bacilli were difficult to find and to culture but no longer a mystery. They were the cause of Legionnaires' disease. CDC scientists named McDade's bacillus *Legionella pneumophila*.

Meanwhile, epidemiological detectives at the CDC reviewed data from other unexplained respiratory epidemics and found two that seemed similar to Legionnaires' disease. One swept through St. Elizabeth's Hospital in Washington, DC, in July 1965, affecting eighty-one people and killing twelve. Another had occurred at a government office building in Pontiac, Michigan, in July 1968. One hundred and forty-four people became sick, but no deaths occurred.

Both of these outbreaks, like Legionnaires' disease, took place in midsummer. The CDC possessed samples of frozen serum from victims of the earlier DC and Michigan outbreaks, and in these specimens, they found antibodies to *Legionella pneumophila*. McDade was not surprised. He suspected *Legionella* was probably not a completely new species but likely already existed someplace in nature, unrecognized because of its exacting requirements for growth.

But that gave no reassurance. New cases might be decreasing as winter set in and 1977 arrived, but what would happen next summer? Legionnaires' had to be considered an ongoing threat to public health. Furthermore, McDade's discovery only solved part of the puzzle. Another important question remained: How did the victims become infected?

In early 1977, McDade contacted Carl Fliermans, a microbial ecologist with the Dupont Corporation, for help. Since the 1960s, Fliermans had been finding microbes in unusual places, such as hot springs and even in geysers at Yellowstone National Park, where water temperatures rise to nearly boiling levels. When Fliermans found *Legionella* resembled these unusual organisms (called thermophilic, or heat-loving), he focused his search on hot water.

Fliermans studied microbial growth in streams heated by human activities, such as those near electric power plants and nuclear reactors. He tested samples taken near the Savannah River Site in South Carolina, where the US Department of Energy makes radioactive hydrogen and plutonium. In the summer of 1977, Fliermans recovered *Legionella* from these streams, growing in the hot water as a biofilm, or scum. Furthermore, he injected guinea pigs with material from the cultures and caused a disease like Legionnaires', just as McDade had done at the CDC six months earlier.

Fliermans felt he was on the track and next asked himself if these organisms might reside in the Bellevue-Stratford Hotel. Aware that the Legionnaires', Washington, and Pontiac attacks had all taken place in July, when the summer heat was reaching its peak, he turned his attention to the hotel air-conditioning system. The Bellevue-Stratford employed towers that chilled water and pumped it to various cooling units throughout the hotel. From water in these cooling towers, Fliermans cultured *Legionella*. He and McDade had finally solved the puzzle. When they entered air-conditioned areas of the hotel and enjoyed the refreshing cool atmosphere, victims inhaled tiny droplets of bacteria-laden moist air from the air-conditioning ducts.

Many other outbreaks of respiratory infection caused by members of the *Legionella* family of bacteria have occurred since 1976. From 1977 to 1982, more than two hundred cases of *Legionella* pneumonia occurred at the Wadsworth VA Medical Center in Los Angeles. These were traced to contaminated water. In 1979, a mysterious pneumonia affected renal transplant patients at the University of Pittsburgh. Investigation showed the cause to be *L. micdadei*, a *Legionella* species named for Joseph McDade. The patients were receiving drugs that suppressed their immunity. These alerted the medical world that individuals who are frail or whose immune systems are suppressed are particularly susceptible to attack by *Legionella*.

Recent outbreaks took place in California and Nevada. In February 2011, two hundred people frolicking at the Playboy Mansion in Los Angeles developed a flu-like illness, and of these, four progressed to pneumonia, which was found to be caused by *Legionella*. A hot tub on the premises appeared to be the source. In 2011 and again in 2012, two guests at the Luxor Hotel in Las Vegas developed pneumonia due to *Legionella*. The 2011 patient died, and Nevada health authorities blamed the hotel air-conditioning system for both infections.

Of the thousands of reported cases, virtually all have been connected with contaminated water: cooling towers, showerheads, hot tubs, fountains, and old-fashioned swamp coolers have been sources of infection. The CDC estimates between 8,000 and 18,000 episodes of pneumonia due to *Legionella* occur annually in the United States, with a mortality rate of 15 percent, indicating a significant continuing public health threat. In the summer of 2015, eighty-one elderly patients in New York City contracted *Legionella* infection, and seven died. Organisms were cultured from water supplies in five different buildings near where the outbreak occurred.[4]

Water bugs are rarely able to attack healthy people unless some extraordinary circumstance exists, like the contaminated chilling towers during the 1976 American Legion convention. But *Legionella* infect people already sick, thus making hospitals the most worrisome sites for outbreaks. When I was medical director of respiratory care, the threat was serious enough that we followed a strict protocol to keep humidifiers and mist-generating devices safe. Respiratory therapists were required to wash their hands and wear gloves, gowns, and masks when administering treatments to compromised patients. We cultured water sources, sampled effluent from jet nebulizers, and made sure no scale or sediment accumulated in mechanical devices connected to patients. Because patients on ventilators, dialysis, and transplant recipients are among the most at risk, we could never be too careful. Fortunately, antibiotics work against *Legionella* organisms, and human-to-human transmission doesn't occur. But prevention works better than treatment, and good practices remain the best defense.

Today those responsible for safety in office buildings, hotels, and hospitals follow similar procedures required by governmental authorities. These include heating water to a temperature that reduces *Legionella* growth (the organisms die when temperatures exceed 115°F), adding chlorine to water supplies, and regular culturing of all water sources.

Legionella aren't the only waterborne microbial threats to breathing. Organisms with obscure polysyllabic names, like *Acinetobacter* and *Burkholderia*, attack patients on ventilators and those with cystic fibrosis. Also, microbes that live in the intestinal tract, though not strictly speaking waterborne, live in moist places, can migrate into the respiratory tract, make their way to the lungs, and cause pneumonia and septicemia. These include such groups as *Serratia*, *Pseudomonas*, and the infamous *Escherichia*, known by its nickname, *E. coli*.

Water bugs cause other respiratory problems besides infection. "Hot tub lung" began with complaints by previously healthy individuals of cough, fever, difficulty breathing, and weight loss. The affected individuals showed reduced pulmonary function and chest X-rays that indicated patchy inflammatory areas in the lungs, like an unusual pneumonia. Pulmonary secretions grew organisms called mycobacteria, biologically related to those that cause tuberculosis except, unlike their better-known cousins, they grow in warm water and in the soil and are not contagious.

The same type of sleuthing that uncovered Legionnaires' disease found the affected people enjoyed soaking in spas, pools, and hot tubs. This prompted the epidemiologists to culture the hot tub water, which also grew mycobacteria. The first patients received antituberculosis treatment without much effect, and public health authorities soon learned that merely removing patients from infected water was enough to make most of them improve. That implied the lung disease was an allergic reaction rather than an infection. Medical science now feels an immune reaction underlies the illness in the majority of cases of hot tub lung.

In most instances, the hot tubs were not well-maintained. Water was stagnant; sediment accumulated, and chlorine (which loses its potency above 84°F) was ineffective.[5] Hot tub lung can be an occupational as well as recreational hazard. Swedish investigators described the illness in five hotel employees who cleaned spas as part of their job.[6] A Mayo Clinic pulmonary specialist commented, "Doctors often don't think to ask their patients if they have been using a hot tub. . . . Patients also need to tell their doctors if they regularly use a hot tub if they have respiratory problems."[7] So far, no one has died from hot tub lung, but *Legionella*, *Acinetobacter*, and the other water bugs can be deadly.

The ability of these usually innocuous organisms to morph into killers relates to their invading places in the body where evolution has not provided defenses. *Legionella* can't successfully penetrate intact skin or gastrointestinal lining. But the respiratory tract, with its delicate moist surface, is vulnerable. Also, these infections represent the price of technological progress. Absent air-conditioning, organ transplantations, cancer chemotherapy, and ventilators, *Legionella* would probably be confined to tropical streams, hot springs, and geysers, where it has resided for thousands of years. No vaccines against these organisms exist, and though many strains are susceptible to antibiotics, the tried and true techniques of hand-washing, isolation, and protective clothing are the best protections against water bugs.

McDade, Fliermans, and the CDC investigators were unable to save the Bellevue-Stratford. After the July 1976 outbreak, the public became fearful that the hotel was contaminated, and bookings declined. Eventually the hotel went bankrupt. It was later refurbished and its air-conditioning system replaced, so that today it is again in business as the Hyatt Bellevue-Stratford, and as far as anyone knows, no more lung infections have occurred. But in the eyes of some, it remains tainted. Indeed, on October 29, 2008, NBC News listed it among twelve notorious hotels where Halloween celebrants could experience a creepy thrill.[8] A sad demise for the Grande Dame of Broad Street.

Legionnella and other waterborne infections show how vulnerable humans remain to the vagaries of nature. In the 1970s, with dozens of antibiotics on the market and immunization practices widespread, pundits predicted that infectious diseases would soon be a thing of the past. Legionnaires' disease dispelled that fallacy and serves today to remind us never to be smug enough to think we are in control of our environment. Vigilance is not only the price of freedom; it's also an unavoidable cost of technological progress.

7

THE VIRUS WITH NO NAME

"Alone we can do so little; together we can do so much."

—Helen Keller[1]

On February 28, 2003, Dr. Carlo Urbani met the patient who would lead to his death.[2] An infectious disease specialist with the World Health Organization assigned to Hanoi, Vietnam, his job was to investigate potential threats to public health. Authorities at the local French Vietnamese Hospital called about a patient with a strange pneumonia they thought might be bird flu. Would he come by and take a look at the situation?

Urbani visited the hospital, where he examined Johnny Chen, a Chinese American businessman who had flown to Hanoi from Hong Kong a few days earlier.[3] Shortly after arriving in Hanoi, Chen developed a cough, fever, and trouble breathing, symptoms severe enough that he was hospitalized. Urbani was concerned. Rumors had been circulating about an outbreak of a mysterious type of pneumonia in southern China, and he was worried this was more than just flu.

Two days later, on March 2, Chen became more short of breath, and several members of the hospital staff also developed coughs, with fever and difficulty breathing. Urbani at this point alerted the Vietnamese public health authorities that they had a potential emergency on their hands. He instructed the hospital to isolate all patients with respiratory symptoms and spent the next several days at the hospital, documenting findings, arranging for samples of blood and sputum to be tested, and reinforcing infection control procedures.

By March 7, twenty-two members of the hospital staff were sick with respiratory symptoms. Urbani asked WHO to send help. Over the next few days, a team of epidemiologists from WHO and the US CDC arrived in Hanoi to study the outbreak in hopes of learning how to contain it.

The scene was one of anxiety and confusion. Reports trickled in from Hong Kong about a mysterious respiratory syndrome that killed a doctor from Guangdong in southern China, who was visiting Hong Kong for a family wedding. A young woman in Singapore who had just returned from a vacation in Hong Kong was admitted to the hospital with pneumonia, and soon after, several hospital employees developed respiratory symptoms. Were these cases connected with the Hanoi case? What did they portend? The investigators had to make the public aware of the seriousness of the situation to take precautions but without causing panic. Specters of the Spanish flu of 1918 filled their minds.

Urbani was exhausted. He had spent more than a week laboring without rest. His wife, Giuliana, was concerned for his welfare. She asked him if he wasn't in danger from working so closely with patients with such a serious disease? He had responsibilities to her and their three children. He answered, "If I cannot even work in such situations, what am I doing here? Answering e-mails, going to cocktails, and pushing paper?"

Urbani was scheduled to attend a meeting on March 11 in Bangkok, Thailand, and his colleagues urged him to take a break and go to the conference. So, he kissed his wife good-bye and caught a plane to Bangkok. While in flight, he began to feel sick. A colleague picked him up at the airport, and Urbani told him not to get close; he might have the same illness as Johnny Chen.[4] Urbani called for an ambulance and took himself straight to the hospital.

An emergency response team flew in from the United States to care for him. Not only was Urbani a colleague, but he was also a possible link to understanding the illness. Scott Dowell, a team member from Johns Hopkins University School of Public Health in Baltimore, said, "Our indoctrination into this disease came in taking care of Carlo in a makeshift isolation room. He went from a really mild illness to a little respiratory distress to severe distress. Despite everything we tried, it was just an inexorable progression toward death."[5] On March 29, Dr. Carlo Urbani died of respiratory failure, a victim of severe acute respiratory syndrome (SARS), the disease he had first recognized.

Urbani lived his life to help humanity. In 1993, he joined a WHO mission to Mauritania to track the spread of hookworms and schistosomiasis, a gastrointestinal parasite prevalent in that region of Africa. In 1995, he worked in Cambodia as a member of Medecins Sans Frontieres, or Doctors without Borders, and was president of the Italian chapter of that organization. In 1999, he was one of its representatives who accepted the Nobel Peace Prize. In 2000, he was posted to Hanoi.

His ethic kept him in the French Vietnamese Hospital during the first SARS outbreak and caused him to contract the disease. When he knew he was dying, before he lost consciousness, he requested that his lung tissue be saved for science. Neal Halsey, a professor of international health at Johns Hopkins, said, "Everything Urbani did—the way he used his clinical expertise, the way he sounded the alarm, his willingness to ask for help—proved so important."[6]

Urbani's death saddened his WHO friends, but it inspired them to work even harder. From secretions and tissues of victims, CDC investigators found signs of a virus previously unknown to medical science. It was a coronavirus, a class that commonly causes colds and mild respiratory symptoms. Somehow, the SARS virus mutated into an aggressive and lethal form capable of spreading from human to human.

The epidemic accelerated. In Hong Kong, people were getting sick at the rate of fifty per day. SARS was discovered in an elderly Canadian woman who had flown to Toronto from Hong Kong in late February. Three hundred sixty-one people contracted the infection, and thirty-three died. A similar outbreak occurred in Singapore, traceable to three women who had traveled to Hong Kong in February.[7] Pieces of the puzzle started to come together. The doctor from Guangdong; Johnny Chen, the Chinese American businessman in Hanoi; the elderly lady from Toronto; and the women from Hong Kong had all stayed on the ninth floor of the Metropole Hotel in Hong Kong. The doctor from Guangdong appeared to be the source case. WHO dispatched another international team to Guangdong and on April 2 issued a travel warning recommending that all nonessential travel to Hong Kong and Guangdong be canceled.[8]

The Chinese government was initially uncooperative and restricted the virus detectives' travel. Even when the infection spread to Beijing, doctors and health authorities were pressured to say as little as possible to both the public and the outside world. By May, however, another hero emerged, this one from China itself. Jiang Yangyong, a seventy-one-year-old physician, a member of the Communist Party, and a senior medical officer in the People's Liberation Army, felt that loyalty to his 1.3 billion countrymen mandated his coming forward.[9] He e-mailed information about the epidemic to two TV stations in Hong Kong, who transmitted it all over the world. Whether it was because of his age or his Communist Party credentials or the pressure of international opinion, the government did not prosecute Jiang but loosened up and began to assist the scientists in their study of the deadly virus.

SARS spread mostly by inhalation of droplets of mucus or saliva coughed into the air, but it looked like merely touching an infected individual could transmit infection, which aggravated anxiety worldwide. It quickly showed up in Taiwan, the United States, and Australia. Television news showed travelers in Hong Kong airport wearing paper face masks to protect themselves. People were afraid to travel. The CDC issued a travel alert about visiting Toronto. President Bush signed an order authorizing public health authorities to invoke isolation and quarantine laws. Between March and May 2003, SARS showed up in 34 countries; affected 8,000 people, many of whom were hospital workers; and caused 774 deaths.[10] That is nearly a 10 percent mortality rate, higher than influenza and most respiratory viruses.

While SARS was making its global journey, investigators continued to search for a source in nature. Host animals may be infected without themselves getting sick, and humans can become accidental hosts. Coronaviruses live in bats. Armed with antibody tests and genetic markers, scientists found signs of SARS infection in horseshoe bats, common in southern China, and in civets, small catlike mammals sold in markets in that locale.

By July, public health authorities brought the SARS outbreak under control. They used the most modern techniques of immunology and genetics, coupled with standard practices of isolating suspected cases and screening travelers from areas with infection. By the time it subsided, SARS caused more than a million people to be quarantined and cost billions of dollars to manage.[11] No one knows if SARS will resurface, but like influenza, it remains a potential threat. And eleven years later, we still don't have a workable vaccine or an effective antiviral drug against it.

The SARS story may not be over yet. In May 2014, French medical authorities ordered the Pasteur Institute laboratory in Paris to suspend activities after it lost two thousand test tubes containing the SARS virus.[12] Imagine the damage those vials could do if they got into the hands of terrorists.

SARS had hardly left the news when another previously unrecognized lethal respiratory virus emerged in a different part of Asia. The Arabian one-humped camel, or dromedary, is one of the most interesting and useful beasts in the world. Domesticated for four thousand years, the "ship of the desert" transports heavy loads and gives its milk as drink, its meat as food, and even its dung as fuel for cooking fires. Adapted over eons to life in the hot, dry sands of Asia and north Africa, it can carry a four-hundred-pound load a hundred miles a day in the sweltering desert heat and can pace at twenty-five miles per hour or sprint at forty miles per hour.

In June 2012, a sixty-year-old man from Bishah, a small town in Saudi Arabia near Jeddah, became sick with a cough, fever, and difficulty breathing. He was admitted to his local hospital and, when he worsened, was transferred to a referral center in Jeddah. There, his chest X-ray showed patchy shadows, indicating bilateral pneumonia. He received antibiotics and antiviral drugs, but several days later, his lungs filled with fluid and his oxygen level plummeted, so he had to be moved to the intensive care unit. Medical staff inserted a tube into his trachea and attached a mechanical ventilator to breathe for him, but their efforts failed, and eleven days after being admitted, the man died of respiratory failure.[13]

Dr. Ali Mohamed Zaki, the consulting infectious disease specialist who cared for the man, was concerned. He had seen many patients die of overwhelming respiratory infections, but this case troubled him. What caused it? Tests for the usual bacteria and viruses, including swine flu and HIV, were unrevealing. Could it be a hantavirus? Tests for that turned out negative, as well. Zaki was determined to track down the responsible agent. He sent a letter describing the case to *Pro MED*, a newsletter published by the International Society for Infectious Diseases, to alert doctors elsewhere about the illness. He sent samples of the man's sputum to Rotterdam, home of the Erasmus University Medical Center, one of the top virology labs in that part of the world.[14]

This led to the first breakthrough. Scientists at Erasmus isolated a new virus, one never before seen, from the man's secretions. It was a coronavirus, a member of the same biological group from which SARS had arisen in 2003. It wasn't identical to the SARS organism but similar enough that the Rotterdamers contacted the Saudi Ministry of Health and requested permission for a team to fly to Bishah to study the infection. They also persuaded Jonathan Epstein, a New York–based veterinary epidemiologist, to join them.

Epstein was an expert on the biology of bats. Bats were a known reservoir for SARS, and the new virus was in the same family, so he recommended they search the neighborhood where the man, now called the "index case," had lived. They saw sheep, cows, and goats but no traces of bats. Someone also noticed four camels, apparently pets, in a paddock adjacent to the home of the dead patient. But the sleuths were focused on bats and weren't sure the camels had any significance.

Through the summer, the great Arabian bat search continued without progress. Then in September 2012 came the next breakthrough. A Qatari man who had been in Saudi Arabia was admitted to a hospital in London with a strange respiratory illness reminiscent of the Jeddah patient. Tests of his blood and sputum showed evidence of infection with the same virus. With memories of SARS haunting their minds, the team in Bishah ramped up its search for a source from which the new virus might be spreading to humans. Finally, in an abandoned building in a nearby village, they found a cluster of five hundred roosting bats. They immediately swabbed the throats of the bats, a tricky undertaking, and sent the specimens to New York for analysis. Some of the bats harbored genetic material like that of the virus that killed the Jeddah patient.

Over the next few months, Zaki's efforts to publicize the infection paid off. Doctors in Saudi Arabia, Qatar, and Jordan spotted additional cases of the syndrome, recognizing the characteristic signs: fever; shortness of breath; and bleeding; followed by kidney and respiratory failure; and, in nearly half of the patients, death. Through the winter and spring of 2013, more patients with the same unusual constellation of symptoms appeared in Britain, France, and Germany. All had visited the Middle East or had contact with someone who had been in that region.

Meanwhile, Zaki's enthusiasm cost him his job. In November 2012, he and the Dutch virologists had published an article on the virus in the *New England Journal of Medicine*, one of the most widely circulated journals in the biomedical world. Soon after, Zaki was fired by the Saudi Ministry of Health for publicizing the case.[15] He returned to his native Egypt, where he is now a professor at the medical school of Ain Sharm University in Cairo and continues studying the disease that he was the first person to recognize.

By May 2013, forty-four cases had been diagnosed, and the World Health Organization christened the disease Middle East respiratory syndrome, abbreviated to MERS-CoV, to denote it came from a coronavirus.

But gaps in understanding remained. None of the victims of MERS-CoV had contact with bats. Was it passing from human to human? The high mortality rate made the investigators shudder just to consider the question. Or could there be another species of animal that harbored the virus without becoming sick itself and was transmitting it to humans? Sheep, cows, and goats showed no signs of infection. That was a blind alley. So attention eventually turned to camels.

This led to another breakthrough. Researchers found MERS-CoV genetic material in nasal swabs from Arabian camels and antibodies in their blood.[16] Veterinarians next tested samples from camels in other regions of Saudi Arabia and found most of them had antibodies to MERS-CoV.[17] They wondered how long the virus had been present in camels, so they obtained frozen samples of camel serum and thawed it for testing. To everyone's surprise, they found signs of MERS-CoV infection going back as far as 1992. The virus had been circulating in camels for over twenty years.

How did MERS-CoV originally infect camels? No one knows for sure. Perhaps bats transmitted it by biting camels. Maybe camels inhaled particles of dried bat urine or feces. Camels have respiratory illnesses, like most animals, but no lethal epidemic of respiratory failure has been recognized in camels.[18] So, this remains an unsolved question.

Jonathan Epstein and his team continue to investigate the genetics and ecology of MERS-CoV: how it mutates, how it spreads, and where it resides.[19] Is it seasonal, like influenza? Are there other animal reservoirs? Like in so many areas of science, answering one question creates multiple new questions.

How did the virus make its way to humans? In Saudi Arabia, people eat camel meat, drink camel milk, groom camels, ride them, and sleep near them, so opportunities for the virus to infect humans abound in that region. In addition, many human cases have occurred without camel contact but always after contact with an infected person. Thus, humans can infect other humans by coughing, sneezing, or maybe simply touching. This is worrisome because it means family members; caregivers, like nurses and physicians; and even neighbors are in danger.

As of May 2014, more than five hundred cases have been identified worldwide, including two in the United States. Many have occurred in health care workers. At this point, no vaccine and no treatment exist. Prevention depends on standard infection control techniques: isolation, hand-washing, masks, and avoiding unnecessary contact with exposed individuals.

As frightening as SARS and MERS may be, they are recent versions of another equally lethal respiratory virus, this one indigenous to North America. For a while, it was so mysterious it didn't even have a name.

The borders of Colorado, New Mexico, Utah, and Arizona intersect at a single place called the Four Corners. The area is rugged, mountainous, and graced with spectacularly beautiful skies that demonstrate the ever-changing power of wind and water. When thunderheads roll in from the west over the San Juan and Sangre de Cristo Mountains and lightning bolts streak the atmosphere white, it is easy to see why the native people thought First Man and First Woman were formed from these clouds. Nearby Monument Valley, with its jagged sandstone buttes, testifies to nature's versatile artistry. Mesa Verde National Park and Canyon de Chelly tell the silent story of the Anasazi, the ancient people who dotted the cliffs with cave houses a thousand years ago. The mile-deep, six-million-year-old Grand Canyon of the Colorado River to the west reminds visitors of how old the land is. Most of the region belongs to Native American nations: Navajos, Hopis, Utes, and Zunis.

The spring of 1993 came to Navajo country wet and warm. Chaparral greened and pinyon trees bore nuts, welcomed by all in that arid land. Animal life flourished, especially deer mice, ubiquitous residents in the area. Then a perplexing event occurred. A young Navajo man developed a strange illness. His muscles ached, he felt feverish, and then he began to have difficulty breathing. His family rushed him to the reservation hospital, but he deteriorated rapidly and died within a day.

Autopsy revealed his lungs were full of bloody fluid, the result of overwhelming infection. Doctors in the Indian Health Service were mystified. They thought it might be influenza or even plague. Someone told the doctors that the young man's fiancée had similar symptoms and had died five days earlier, which accentuated the mystery.[20] Over the next few weeks, more cases occurred, and by mid-June, twenty-four patients contracted a similar illness. Most were young, healthy Navajos, though nine were white, and one was Hispanic. Half of them died.

The New Mexico Department of Health and the CDC joined the investigation.[21] In blood samples and autopsied lung tissue, they found antibodies to a group of viruses called hantaviruses. Hantaviruses are rare and known to cause fever and kidney failure in parts of Asia and Europe. But for the virus to cause respiratory failure in a remote area of the United States was surprising and ominous.

The scientists knew hantaviruses infect deer mice and spread to humans by inhalation of microscopic droplets of mouse urine or fecal matter. They trapped deer mice in hogans on the Navajo reservation and found antibodies to hantavirus in many of them. The investigators then postulated that the wet weather and spring warming had increased the food supply and permitted deer mice to increase in number, which put some in closer-than-usual contact with humans.

Later that summer, more cases occurred in Nevada and California. The clinical histories were similar: fever, muscle aches, and a cough, followed five days later by difficulty breathing and respiratory failure. The germ was called *virus sin nombre* in Spanish (the "virus with no name"), or VSN for short. It remains rare; only 160 cases have occurred since 1993; however, the mortality rate is 50 percent. No antiviral treatment has shown any significant effect, and management depends on early diagnosis and aggressive use of respiratory support. Scientists have worked to develop a vaccine but to date have been disappointed with results.

Nearly all cases have been traced to contact with deer mice, and human-to-human transmission is virtually nonexistent. The most recent outbreak in the United States occurred in 2012, when ten campers in Yosemite National Park in California contracted the disease from deer mice that had infested cabins in Curry Village, a popular place for visitors to stay in the park.

SARS, MERS, and VSN frighten us because they rise up unexpectedly, spread fast, kill indiscriminately, and are not treatable at this time. But added together, these infections have struck only a few thousand patients and killed only a few hundred since their original recognition. Influenza, in contrast, leads to the death of thousands every year and, when pandemics occur, many more than that.

Eventually science will develop vaccines to control these marauders, but until then, controlling them depends on combining sophisticated technology and age-tested, low-tech public health practices. This means administering antiviral drugs and assisting ventilation when needed but, in addition, prompt case reporting, isolating infected individuals, and educating the public.

These lethal respiratory infections frighten us because they are alive and, in an era of global travel, no more than a plane ride away. But forces in nature that threaten to suffocate us include dusts, fumes, and toxins, as well. These are not alive and thus not able to propagate and reproduce themselves, but they are ubiquitous in the environment and deserve as much attention and concern as infections. And they are preventable.

II
KILLER AIR

8

SUFFOCATING WORK

"Concern for the man himself and his fate must always form the chief interest of all technical endeavors; concern for the great unsolved problems of the organization of labor and the distribution of goods in order that the creations of our mind shall be a blessing and not a curse to mankind."

—Albert Einstein[1]

An insurance company asked me to examine Rick, a young man who was applying for disability. Rick was thirty years old and had been employed as a painter in an automobile body shop for eight years. He had no history of respiratory problems and had never smoked. Two years before, he began to have spells of wheezing. These episodes tended to occur late in the day, subsided in the evening, and improved on weekends. He consulted his doctor and was treated with inhalers, which helped him to feel better.

However, when he worsened, Rick began to suspect something at work was responsible. His doctor agreed and said that he had to change jobs. His employer had no other position to which he could change, and so Rick filed a workers' compensation claim.

When I examined Rick, he was free of symptoms, so I asked him to explain what he did at work. He described how he sanded the metal surface, cleaned it with solvent, applied a primer, and finally sprayed the finishing coat. "Every manufacturer has its own formula," he said. "I follow the instructions. You have to be careful to thin the paint just right. Otherwise it looks dull."

I told him I needed to review the safety data sheets for the paints and hardeners that he commonly used in his work. (The National Institute of Occupational Safety and Health mandates that employers maintain logs on all substances in the workplace.) In the meantime, I recommended he be considered temporarily disabled until I sorted out the possible exposures and informed him I was concerned he had asthma.

Respiratory disorders are the most common occupational illnesses, and asthma is the most common occupational respiratory disease. Exposures to chemicals, dust, and fumes are estimated to cause between 15 and 20 percent of cases of new adult asthma. One in six cases of asthma originates or is worsened by occupational exposures.[2] Diagnosis is often difficult because asthma is common, and symptoms may not develop until several days after the person leaves work.

Over three hundred different substances are recognized to cause occupational asthma.[3] As many as eleven million workers are exposed to these agents.[4] Many occupations besides spray-painters involve working with substances that bring on asthma. Bakers, woodworkers (including those at sawmills), farmers, and pharmaceutical workers, to name just a few, are all vulnerable. The costs of time lost from work, disability payments, and medical care are enormous, estimated at $1.6 billion annually in the United States.[5]

To complicate the matter further, the lungs can sometimes tolerate a serious injury for several hours and then become overwhelmed, eventuating in severe respiratory distress. The respiratory tract has a limited number of ways it manifests injury, but that doesn't lessen or simplify the challenge of detecting offending agents.

Rick's problem was eventually traced to the hardener used to cure paint. It contained toluene diisocyanate, or TDI, a recognized cause of occupational asthma. Isocyanates are one of the most widely used agents in industry worldwide. The NIOSH estimates that 280,000 workers are exposed to this group of compounds, and in some industries, 15 to 20 percent of workers are sensitive.[6] Besides their role in spray-painting, isocyanates are used in making polyurethane, which is applied to many products as a protectant and as foam for packaging and insulation. Isocyanates are used to coat fiberglass, cement, wood, steel, and aluminum in cars, trucks, and ships. Thus, they are nearly ubiquitous in manufacturing.

Isocyanates irritate the cells that line the respiratory tract, but even more important, they act as allergens and, like ragweed pollen or house dust, cause the bronchi to constrict, swell, and weep mucus, thus blocking airflow. Furthermore, both an immediate and a delayed allergic reaction can occur, so the exposed worker may have an immediate asthmatic reaction and then several hours or even days later have another. This combination of types of reactions leads to confusing patterns of symptoms, with improvement, followed by worsening, followed by apparent tolerance, followed by aggravation. But if these reactions continue unchecked, permanent damage to the bronchi can occur, with airway obstruction becoming irreversible.

Another insurance company asked me to examine a hotel housekeeper who filed a claim because of coughing and wheezing. She dated her problem to an episode two months previously in which, while working in a small closet, she accidentally mixed bleach and ammonia in a bucket, which caused smoke to rise in the air and immediately made her choke and cough. She had no history of asthma or allergies and was not a smoker. Her chest was clear on exam, but when she took a deep breath, she began to cough, which can be a sign of hypersensitive airways.

I felt she had an entity akin to asthma called reactive airway dysfunction syndrome, or RADS, and that it was occupationally caused. The active ingredient in bleach is sodium hypochlorite, and combined with ammonia, chlorine is released, which irritates the respiratory tract lining.

RADS differs from ordinary asthma in that it relates to a single exposure to an irritant. The reaction is like asthma, with constriction of the airways, inflammation of the cells lining the bronchi, cough, mucus, and wheezing. Treatment is with bronchodilators and steroids, like asthma, but the irritated bronchi can remain overly sensitive for months or years after the exposure.

I saw several more RADS cases afterward in hotel housekeepers. In San Diego, tourism is a big business. Hotel maids are mostly immigrants and mostly women, who are hard workers but often have difficulty understanding English. They developed persistent wheezing and coughing, were helped by asthma treatment, but not made well. They presented difficult problems to manage because they couldn't perform a heavy job and couldn't work around any irritating substance. In addition, those without legal status in the United States were reluctant to push the system, which aggravated their predicament.

RADS is not confined to hotel workers. Firefighters, farmers, construction workers—anyone who breathes fumes, dusts, or aerosols—all are vulnerable. Some epidemiologists feel it is more prevalent than statistics indicate and is a significant cause of disability in many industries. Mustard gas, the infamous poison used in World War I, killed and maimed its victims by producing severe RADS. (More on poison gases later.)

In 1932, British physician J. M. Campbell published a report of a group of farmers who became short of breath after pitching hay.[7] Why it happened was a mystery. Symptoms didn't occur until several days after exposure. In addition, Campbell heard crackling sounds over the lungs of those affected, as though pneumonia was present, rather than the wheezes that signify asthma or RADS. In addition, chest X-rays revealed unusual changes resembling cobwebs in the lungs. These also suggested a type of pneumonia. It became known as farmers' lung.

Researchers identified an immune reaction to mold spores as the cause of the problem and broadened the name to hypersensitivity pneumonitis, or HP. They showed certain species of fungi, which germinated mostly at high temperatures, induced an allergic response that caused the lung air sacs to become inflamed rather than the airways, as in asthma. In addition, the reaction took several hours or days to occur, accounting for the delay in onset of symptoms. Furthermore, investigators found antibodies in the serum of these patients chemically different from those seen with ordinary asthma. Avoiding moldy hay worked to reverse the problem in its acute stages, but if unrecognized, the inflammation caused lung scarring and irreversible impairment in breathing.

Soon, descriptions of similar reactions followed in sugar cane cutters, cotton processors, and sawmill workers, as well as in exotic occupations, like malt workers, mushroom processors, and cork strippers. When I was in Wisconsin, our laboratory performed pulmonary function tests for our allergist colleagues, who were studying hypersensitivity pneumonitis in pigeon breeders, caused by proteins in the birds' feathers and their droppings.

Occupational health experts recommend that employers screen the workplace for agents known to cause occupational asthma and HP and eliminate them or substitute other substances if possible.[8] They also advocate protective respiratory equipment as an additional precaution. Considering how occupational asthma, RADS, and hypersensitivity pneumonitis are prevalent and serious, employers, unions, physicians, and public health agencies all have a stake in controlling these threats to breathing.

Before the advent of the modern chemical industry and the rise of occupational asthma, the most frequent occupational respiratory illnesses were pneumoconioses, lung scarring due to mineral dusts. Silica, asbestos, and coal dusts were the most prominent. These remain as workplace threats to breathing, as well as other metals, from aluminum to zinc, that also cause lung inflammation and scarring. Furthermore, these diseases are preventable.[9]

The New River, so named because it wasn't explored until late in the eighteenth century, is one of the geologically oldest in North America, predating the tectonic collisions that formed the Appalachian Mountains. It flows north from its source in North Carolina, through western Virginia, and across the hills of West Virginia to enter the Ohio River. The New River Gorge, which cuts a path through the Appalachian Plateau in West Virginia, is one of the most scenic areas in the eastern United States. As it descends, the river offers white-water rapids that challenge rafters and kayakers. Hawks Nest State Park, through which the gorge runs, attracts hikers and photographers with picturesque overlooks above steep walls topped by pine and maple trees.

Near Hawks Nest, the New River flows around Gauley Mountain, then drops precipitously. In the late 1920s, this made it a prime candidate for a hydroelectric power project.[10] The goal was to boost the state's economy, and the Union Carbide and Carbon Corporation secured a contract to blast tunnels through Gauley Mountain, construct dams to divert the river flow, and build power stations to generate electricity. The centerpiece of the project was the three-mile-long Hawks Nest Tunnel. However, four-thousand-foot-high Gauley Mountain, an ancient mass of compressed sandstone, was rich in silica.[11]

Silica is the name for silicon dioxide, or quartz. It comprises 10 percent of the earth's crust and is the main constituent of sand. Silica crystals are tiny, between two and five microns in diameter. One micron is one-thousandth of a millimeter. For comparison, red blood cells, among the smallest in the body, are eight to ten microns in size. Thus, if inhaled, silica particles are minute enough to penetrate deep into the lungs.

Construction at Hawks Nest began in 1930. Union Carbide ignored the known dangers of tunneling through silica and pushed the project forward.[12] The company recruited 1,500 nonunion laborers from the rural South to work on the tunnel. Seventy-five percent were African Americans. Workers toiled six days a week, ten hours each day. They alternated three-hour shifts inside the tunnels, drilling holes in rock, planting dynamite in holes, blasting rock loose, and hauling out debris, followed by three hours outside clearing the dust from their eyes, noses, and mouths.

Carting out debris was the worst. The workers inhaled high concentrations of silica-laden dust. Managers and supervisors used respirators and masks, but the laborers had no protective apparatus, no dust-suppressing agents, and no mine ventilators. Few workers lasted more than a year on the job. They either left on their own accord or were turned loose because they couldn't keep up. The workers were itinerant, and medical information on why they quit was scanty or nonexistent.

By 1932, tunnel workers began to file lawsuits alleging they had acquired acute silicosis from the Hawks Nest Tunnel. Their chest X-rays showed nodules of scarring that resembled tuberculosis. Indeed, silicosis and tuberculosis often coexist, so many tunnel workers likely had both. And many died of respiratory failure.

No one knows exactly how many workers succumbed to silicosis on Gauley Mountain. A historical marker at the site indicates 109 deaths. A congressional hearing placed the total at 476. In 1986, Martin Cherniack published an account of the tragedy entitled *The Hawks Nest Incident*, in which he estimated at least seven hundred workers died of silicosis during tunnel construction.[13] Union Carbide paid a local undertaker fifty dollars per body to collect the remains of dead workers and bury them. The graves that have been found contain no headstones to remember the fallen.[14]

For a dust particle to cause disease, it has to be small enough to reach the tiniest passages that abut the air sacs in the lungs, plus be durable enough to resist being broken down. Such dust particles are foreign material, and nature tries to get rid of them or wall them off. The lungs swell and weep fluid. Scavenger cells migrate to the area and engulf particles if they can and then transport the offending particles to lymph nodes to be eliminated. If these defenses don't work, then the body tries to sequester the particles, putting layers of scar tissue around them. As these areas of scar coalesce, the lung loses its natural elasticity and becomes stiff, like a crusty, dried-out sponge.

Thus, breathing becomes progressively more difficult. Oxygen can't diffuse through the scarred areas into the pulmonary capillaries. Eventually respiratory failure results. This process usually occurs slowly, over years and decades, but if massive amounts of dust are inhaled, then scarring can develop rapidly over a period of weeks or months. In either case, the end point is destroyed lung tissue and death by suffocation. Whether the inhaled culprit is silica, asbestos, or coal dust, the lung's reaction is the same: inflammation, walling off, and scarring.

The summer before I started medical school, I worked in upstate New York as a laborer in the construction of the St. Lawrence Seaway. I lived in the town of Massena and roomed with a pipe coverer. Pipe coverers were the envy of the carpenters, masons, and other tradesmen. Their work was not heavy, and their pay scales were high. However, the most widely used pipe-covering material was asbestos, and pipe coverers were surrounded by it. When my roommate emptied his work clothes into the laundry bag, we both likely sniffed a few million fibers.

The group of minerals we call asbestos (Greek for "unextinguishable" because it was used in lamp wicks) are silicates, compounds of silicon, oxygen, and hydrogen. Humans have used asbestos since ancient times because of its durability, resistance to heat, and fibrous nature that allows it to be spun into fabric.[15] Mined in Canada, Russia, Brazil, China, and South Africa, asbestos commercial use began in the nineteenth century and grew exponentially during the two world wars. Production peaked in 1976, when more than five million tons of the mineral were mined, and then began to fall in the 1980s, when the public became aware of its dangers.

Asbestos forms crystals that are long thin rods, like microscopic needles. Their diameter is only three microns (one-third the diameter of a red blood cell), and thus they are able to penetrate to the depths of the lungs when inhaled. They are particularly vexatious because the body tries to encase them with fibroblasts, scar-forming cells, to wall them off. But the effort never succeeds; the needles are too thin. So, the process continues inexorably over decades, as layer upon layer of scar cells form a leathery cocoon around the tiny fibers. The resulting disease is called asbestosis.

Asbestosis causes one major symptom: difficulty breathing that slowly squeezes life out of its victims. Insulation workers, miners, ship fitters, construction workers, and cement makers comprise the groups most at risk, but asbestos has been mined, milled, transported, and used in so many industries that millions of workers around the world have inhaled the deadly fibers. Those who work in the vicinity of asbestos, like carpenters, welders, and electricians, are also vulnerable. In addition, spouses of asbestos workers have an increased incidence of lung scarring and pleural cancer attributed to washing contaminated work clothes. Even residents of neighborhoods near asbestos mines or plants are more likely to die from mesothelioma, a cancerous tumor of the pleura, than the general population.

Because asbestos has been used in insulating homes, offices, and schools, as well as in water pipes, ceramics, and automobile brake linings, concerns about the danger to the public have received much attention. Data on prevalence are irregular, and conclusions are difficult to draw. Epidemiologists know the more exposure, the more disease, and low-level exposures, like in schools or office buildings, appear not to entail risk.

Asbestosis mortality has declined in the United States since government-mandated controls went into effect, but new cases continue to show up due to exposures before 1980. Asbestosis has no treatment. The offending agent remains in the lungs until death. In the developed world, substitutes for asbestos, like fiberglass and rock wool, have emerged. They have potential problems as well but much less than asbestos.

From time to time, I remember that summer in Massena, New York, and wonder about my pipe-coverer roommate. Did he get asbestosis? Did he get lung cancer? I must have at least a few tiny fibers burrowing into the lining of my lungs. However, nearly sixty years have passed without signs of trouble, so I am optimistic for myself.

Mose Peltier, my grandfather, was a coal miner. He grew up in Spring Valley, Illinois, and had to drop out of school at the age of thirteen to help support his family. He and his brothers worked underground in the local mine. Old family photo albums show him in work clothes, smiling, and wearing a hard hat with a headlight on it. In time, he took correspondence school courses in mining engineering and worked his way out of underground digging into operations, but he remained in the coal business his whole life. He married my grandmother, who came from New Straitsville, a mining town in southern Ohio, famous for the underground fire started by dissident miners in 1884 that still burns, 130 years later.

I visited the Ohio relatives several times in the 1940s when I was growing up and remember the burning mines. My aunt took me to the outskirts of town, where I gazed at fire and smoke coming from the ground. I was terrified when she told me never to go near the area because the ground could collapse, sucking me into a deep hole from which I could never escape. My mother confirmed that occasionally someone's cow would wander into a dangerous area to graze and disappear forever into the smoky flames beneath the ground's surface.

My grandfather never developed lung disease from his years spent working underground. I attributed this, when I grew old enough to know about respiratory disorders in coal miners, to the fact he did not smoke cigarettes.

All urban dwellers inhale microscopic specks of carbon in soot and dust, which are deposited in their lungs. These tiny nubbins cause no ill effects and are too small even to show up on chest X-rays. Coal miners, in contrast, breathe enough carbon dust to form larger clumps called coal macules. Over time, these coalesce, and the miners' lungs fill with nodules like a sponge containing gravel. This is coal workers' pneumoconiosis, known commonly as black lung.

The bronchi become irritated, and the affected person coughs up mucus. He (most miners are men) becomes short of breath with exercise. Colds settle in the chest, sometimes leading to pneumonia. If dust exposure continues, the carbon nodules enlarge further, and scar tissue envelops the lungs. This brings about what is called progressive massive fibrosis, the most severe version of black lung, which affects about 3 percent of miners. The lungs become more and more leathery until the victim can't breathe even at rest and dies of respiratory failure.

The first reports of lung disease in coal miners appeared during the early nineteenth century. René Laennec, the French physician who invented the stethoscope, wrote a treatise on miners' respiratory problems in which he described how their lungs contained pigment he called *la matiere noire pulmonaire,* or "black material of the lungs."[16] However, for the next 140 years, medical authorities debated whether coal dust caused lung injury. Many felt respiratory impairment in miners was due to silica dust or tobacco smoking. This was what I learned in medical school in the 1950s. But as miners' breathing problems became more obvious, investigators began to question if coal dust was benign, and by the 1960s, researchers recognized coal dust causes a particular type of lung injury, though silicosis and tobacco-related damage often coexist.

Coal consumption in the United States has been declining as oil and natural gas compete to fuel power plants. Nevertheless, more than 1 billion tons a year are mined annually, compared to 600 million tons in 1920, when coal burning was at its peak. In 1920, when my grandfather was active, coal mining employed 784,000 Americans, while now the number is approximately 85,000. Giant drills, cutting machines, and scoops now permit miners to bore through seams of coal that are miles long and generate more particles to be inhaled. So, fewer miners dig more coal but have greater dust exposure. In 2014, the Coal Workers Health Surveillance Program reported that progressive massive fibrosis is on the rise again in Appalachia.[17] Thus, though the United States has made strides, coal dust–induced lung damage remains a serious respiratory threat.

China is the world's largest coal producer, mining more than 3.5 billion tons a year.[18] The *Wall Street Journal* reported in 2014 that the incidence of black lung in China is rising fast.[19] Between 2005 and 2013, the number of cases rose from 100,000 to 750,000. In 2013, China recorded 23,152 new cases of pneumoconiosis in miners, which is likely an understatement because most miners in China do not have labor contracts that would include them in official health surveys.[20] The founder of a pro-worker organization called Love Save Pneumoconiosis reportedly told the *WSJ* that the true number of black lung cases could be as high as six million throughout the country.[21]

Many job-related respiratory deaths come, not from specific diseases like asbestosis or silicosis, but from acceleration of preexisting COPD and asthma or lung cancer. Hazards to breathing lurk in many different jobs. Rick, the patient with paint-hardener asthma, the hotel maids with ammonia-bleach RADS, and miners with black lung illustrate the breadth of occupations that entail respiratory threats.

A century ago, when my grandfather and great-uncles were miners, most people lived in small towns or on farms. They faced respiratory threats from infections and irritants in whatever jobs they could obtain, and dying at a young age was common. My grandchildren live in an urbanized society, where hundreds of new products in electronics, pharmaceuticals, manufacturing, and agriculture enter the marketplace every year. As they embark on their work careers, they will face both old and new risks to breathing. Most occupational threats can be prevented if we pay attention to Albert Einstein's words from 1931: "Concern for the man himself and his fate must form the chief interest of all technical endeavors."[22]

9

CODE RED

"In all natural disasters through time, man needs to attach meaning to tragedy, no matter how random and inexplicable the event is."

—Nathaniel Philbrick[1]

In 2001, my daughter Mary Ellen and her husband lived in Tribeca in New York City, three blocks from the World Trade Center. Their apartment faced east, with an unobstructed view of the Twin Towers. They were away in early September, and the apartment was cleaned while they were gone. On Tuesday morning, September 11, my daughter left the window in their bedroom open about three inches and walked to the World Trade Center, where she thought her polling place was located, to vote in the Democratic primary for mayor. She couldn't find the polling place, so she decided to vote later. At 8:15, she caught a subway north to the UN headquarters, where she worked. She was underground when the first plane hit at 8:41.

After the attack, the neighborhood where they lived was off-limits, and so my daughter and her husband spent the first few nights afterward couch-surfing with friends and then moved into a hotel, where their neighbors for the next few weeks were firefighters and rescue workers who needed to shower and rest between shifts. In mid-October, when they were finally able to inspect their apartment, they found that, from the one slightly open bedroom window, dust and debris from the imploding Twin Towers had covered everything, all the way into the kitchen and living room. Their home was unlivable. They had to hire a fire restoration company to clean up the mess.

In early November, they moved back into the apartment. Fires were still smoldering at Ground Zero, and they worried about potential damage to their lungs. My daughter remembers Environmental Protection Agency head Christine Todd Whitman assuring everyone that the air was safe. My daughter then asked what I thought. I said probably she and her husband were far enough away that they would not be affected.

Most of the people in their building opted to move. But the two of them felt the patriotic thing to do was to stay. For the next year, they watched giant chunks of concrete and massive beams of twisted metal being hauled out and loaded onto barges in the Hudson River. Fortunately, my daughter and her husband did not have any cough or wheezing to indicate respiratory injury after 9/11. She was concerned about the people who worked removing rubble and said, "How could they not suffer lung damage, considering the amount of stuff that was incinerated in the collapse of the Towers?"

When the Twin Towers collapsed, they created a massive dust cloud of pulverized cement, metal, and plastic. Aerosolized jet fuel added to the toxic brew, causing fires with core temperatures of 2,000°F. The extreme height of the towers made concrete, asbestos, and steel compress as they smashed to the ground. Electronic equipment, including computers, cables, and wires, exploded, spewing metal particles everywhere. For days afterward, smoke, fires, and a dense fog of dust enveloped Ground Zero.

Not only did 2,751 innocent American civilians and 343 firefighters die in the New York, Pennsylvania, and Virginia crashes, but 15,000 first responders, including firefighters, police officers, and emergency medical technicians, also inhaled toxic substances in the rubble of the Twin Towers. The Fire Department of New York City (FDNY) arrived on the scene immediately and set up a triage center.[2] Firefighters described the atmosphere as dark with smoke and dust. Almost everyone was coughing. Few had adequate respiratory protection, and several days elapsed before effective respirators became available. Ninety percent of exposed workers initially complained of cough. Those who arrived earliest and had the most prolonged exposure developed the most symptoms. Medical officers were among the first responders and dispensed steroid inhalers to combat inflammation triggered by the extreme lung irritation.

Public health authorities in New York knew that, going forward, lung injuries would be a major problem during the rescue and cleanup; consequently, they instituted medical monitoring of exposed firefighters and paramedics. Doctors and nurses worked seven days a week to evaluate those most heavily exposed. Medical workers examined more than 10,000 FDNY personnel during the cleanup. Six months later, wheezing and difficulty breathing affected nearly one-third of responding firefighters and paramedics.[3] Pulmonary tests showed drops in breathing capacity five times what would be expected under normal exposures to urban dusts.

Dr. Benjamin Luft, director of the World Trade Center Health Program at Stony Brook Medicine on Long Island, treated many of these injured first responders. "They were told the environment was safe, that there was no real risk in terms of toxins, that the air was clear," Dr. Luft said in a 2014 interview with National Public Radio.[4] "They were not given the appropriate protective equipment, and then what was found, subsequently, was that the opposite occurred. The environment was full of carcinogens and toxins."

FDNY has periodically published results of their continuing observations of 12,000 rescue workers.[5] Reports released in 2010 indicated 10 percent had persistent asthma or bronchitis. The most recent follow-up, published in June 2016, demonstrates persistent decline in firefighter lung function thirteen years after the 9/11 attack, with smokers worse than nonsmokers.[6]

In addition, upward of 50,000 civilians joined in the recovery efforts, either immediately or over the next several weeks after the attack, and they breathed many of the same dust and asbestos and chemical end products as early responders. What about the nearby residents and those who worked or went to school in lower Manhattan, like my daughter and her husband? Unfortunately, most of what we know about this group is anecdotal.

Sister Cynthia Maloney, an Episcopalian nun and chaplain, attended many of the responders at Ground Zero. She worked amid the dust and rubble for five months, consoling survivors and assisting the coroner's office, which necessitated that she handle parts of burned bodies. As time passed, Sister Cynthia started wheezing and became short of breath. She was diagnosed with reactive airway dysfunction syndrome (RADS), asthma, and COPD. Unable to continue working, Sister Cynthia returned to her home in South Carolina and slowly deteriorated. She believed her problem was related to the months of toxic exposures she sustained after 9/11, and so as she faced impending death, she asked her attorney to be sure her body was autopsied in hopes of helping others. Sister Maloney died in 2006 at the age of fifty-four.

In 2011, Congress passed the James L. Zadroga 9/11 Health and Compensation Act,[7] which created a compensation fund for those injured while helping after the September 11 disaster. The bill was named after a New York police detective who worked hundreds of hours at Ground Zero amid the rubble and dust. A nonsmoker with no history of asthma, James L. Zadroga died in 2006 at the age of thirty-four of what the Ocean County, NY, medical examiner called respiratory failure attributed to toxic exposures. But a second autopsy by New York City's chief medical examiner disagreed, saying Zadroga's death was more likely due to misuse of a prescription medication. A firestorm of anger followed, triggering debate on whether the many claims for compensation filed after 9/11 were valid. Thousands of claims were eventually filed and more than a billion dollars awarded.[8] Even today, the anger still rages on in the blogosphere.

The attack of 9/11 was a horrific disaster, an act of terrorism, of war. The collapse of the Twin Towers, which was unique, illustrates how buildings contain substances that can damage the respiratory tract in such disasters as earthquakes, hurricanes, and wars. When fire is involved, combustion products aggravate lung injuries. Survivors and rescue workers may suffer years later from respiratory problems traceable to these toxic exposures. The aftermath of 9/11 dramatizes the importance of respiratory protection, including filters and self-contained breathing units for rescue workers of all types, including chaplains and nurses, as well as firefighters.

The most lethal industrial disaster in history occurred in India. In the 1970s, Union Carbide Corporation opened a plant in Bhopal, a city of one million people located in central India, to manufacture carbaryl, an insecticide common in much of the world. When crop failures in the 1980s led to farmers having less money to invest in insect control and plant revenue decreased, the company cut back on safety procedures to keep costs low. The local authorities were aware of this, and the Indian government was a part owner of Union Carbide India.

Methyl isocyanate (MIC) was used to make carbaryl.[9] At 11:00 PM on December 2, 1984, when most of Bhopal was asleep, an operator noticed a leak of MIC gas and increased pressure in a storage tank. The safety valve had been turned off three weeks earlier, and the refrigeration coolant for the MIC storage tank had been drained to be used elsewhere in the plant. MIC gas mixed with water, which increased heat and pressure in the system.

Two hours later, thirty tons of MIC exploded, spewing a giant cloud of gas skyward. Immediately, those in the vicinity began to choke. One survivor said, "Then I started coughing, with each breath seeming as if I was breathing in fire. My eyes were burning."[10] At least four thousand people died soon after, asphyxiated by the poison gas formed by hot MIC. Five hundred thousand people were exposed, and as many as fifteen thousand deaths eventually occurred.

MIC was so caustic it caused the cells of the lungs of those who inhaled the gas to weep fluid, leading to pulmonary edema, so that the victims drowned in their own lung fluid. In addition, chemical breakdown of hot MIC led to formation of hydrogen cyanide, a notorious nervous system poison. Another survivor said, "It felt like somebody had filled our bodies up with red chillies [*sic*], our eyes had tears coming out, noses were watering, we had froth in our mouths. The coughing was so bad that people were writhing in pain."[11] Bodies were thrown in graves or incinerated without precise counting. Most of the victims were citizens unlucky enough to live near the plant.

In 1989, Union Carbide agreed to pay out $470 million in partial settlement, but almost thirty years after the accident, thousands of Bhopalis still can't work and live with tons of remaining toxic waste in the water and ground around the contaminated area.

Bhopal was an extreme example of RADS. This asthma-like reaction results from exposure to irritating vapors or fumes.[12] Most instances occur in the workplace and affect small numbers of individuals, though in Bhopal, thousands of residents of the area around the plant absorbed the damage. Not only do breathing problems develop nearly immediately after injury, but also the key part of the syndrome is that the airways remain overly sensitive for months or even years afterward, causing coughing, wheezing, and difficulty breathing.

The collapse of the hundred-story-high Twin Towers and the Bhopal disaster combined massive explosions and searing fire with corrosive dust and toxic inhalants. They illustrate the power of disasters, natural and man-made, to suffocate us. In addition, fire and smoke inhalation kill thousands every year. The US Fire Administration reports that in 2013, the most recent year for which figures are available, 3,240 people died from fires.[13] Most of these suffocated to death.

Brendan McDonough was nineteen years old when he found his calling as a firefighter and became a member of the Granite Mountain Hotshots, a special team based in Prescott, Arizona. Hotshots crews are elite firefighting units, analogous among firefighters to the Navy Seals among sailors. Two years later, on Sunday, June 30, 2013, the Hotshots' firefighting skills were put to the test. A fire broke out near Yarnell, a small town in the mountains sixty miles northwest of Phoenix. Thunderstorms generated lightning that ignited brush, followed by twisting winds that caused flames to shift and dodge like elusive ghosts. Six hundred firefighters were deployed to manage the blaze, the Granite Mountain Hotshots among them.

McDonough was assigned as lookout. His job was to report to the other firefighters where to attack the flames and, if necessary, when and how to escape. Late that afternoon, from his post high on a rugged slope near Yarnell, McDonough felt the wind change directions and saw the fire front turn toward where his buddies were working. With his colleagues in danger, McDonough radioed them an alert.[14] Within a few minutes another wave of flames swept over McDonough's own perch. Following protocols for this kind of crisis, he radioed again, informing the team that his observation point was on fire. He told them he was retreating from his lookout spot and urged them to implement their escape plan as quickly as possible.

McDonough withdrew and hitched a ride from another team to a safe area. There he heard the Hotshots' superintendent on the radio telling a fire manager that nineteen men, now trapped by flames, were "deploying," setting up fire shelters to protect themselves. However, their fire shelters weren't enough to protect the men from the intensity of the fire. The Hotshots never made it out.

When a state police paramedic later helicoptered into the area, he found their bodies. Eighteen of the dead were from the Granite Mountain team, and the nineteenth was from another team helping them. Most were in their twenties, many husbands and fathers. It was the worst loss of firefighters in the United States since the 9/11 attack. After performing autopsies, the Maricopa Medical Examiner's Office officially stated that the Hotshots died from burns, oxygen deprivation, and carbon monoxide inhalation.[15]

Fire victims die from heat, asphyxiation, and carbon monoxide. In a fire, air is hot, dry, and low on oxygen. When the lungs are burned, their cells weep fluid. What little oxygen is present cannot move from the atmosphere into the blood, and because the brain depends on the lungs for oxygen, victims quickly pass out and suffocate.

What do individuals being overcome by flames experience? Survivor accounts vary. For some, loss of consciousness from lack of oxygen comes quickly, and they cannot recall details of their ordeal. Others describe the agony of waiting, able to extract enough oxygen to breathe but facing the prospect of slowly dying. Some remember mainly darkness, with smoke and dust making it impossible to see, and increasing feelings of impending doom. Others emphasize being smothered and unable to breathe, which may relate to inhaling heated air or air lacking oxygen. Many recall choking, gagging, and coughing up soot.[16]

One survivor of the 2003 West Warwick, Rhode Island, nightclub fire, which killed one hundred people, awoke pinned beneath a pile of bodies that had collapsed on top of him as he tried to escape. He realized, if he stayed on his back, he would surely suffocate. He instinctively rolled on his side and curled up, with his knees close to his chest. This likely kept his abdominal organs from pressing against his diaphragm, thus allowing him to breathe.[17] This survivor's experience explains why firefighters entering a burned-out area often tell of finding dead bodies in the fetal position.

To be lethal, a fire does not have to be a conflagration. On a winter evening in the early 1980s, I consulted on a family of newly emigrated Vietnamese who developed dizziness, confusion, and difficulty breathing. Because it was chilly outside, they had closed the doors and windows of their apartment while they prepared supper over a charcoal wok. Not aware of the danger of carbon monoxide, they fried their food, apparently putting up with the smoke. Some-one eventually passed out, and they called 911 in a panic. All were taken by ambulance to our hospital emergency room, where the staff quickly diagnosed carbon monoxide poisoning and administered oxygen to everyone. The father, who was unconscious, had the highest levels of blood carbon monoxide. He was taken to the hyperbaric chamber, where I saw him. In a desperate effort to wash out the lethal gas, we administered oxygen under pressure three times that of the atmosphere, equivalent to descending sixty-six feet below sea level. The mother and children recovered, but despite these heroic efforts, the fa-ther died.

When substances containing carbon burn, they emit energy in the form of heat and light, plus water and carbon dioxide as end products. If combustion is incomplete, not all the carbon combines with oxygen, and carbon monox-ide forms. The gas is odorless, tasteless, invisible, and deadly. When inhaled, carbon monoxide chemically binds to hemoglobin in the blood, displacing oxygen. Because the bond between carbon monoxide and hemoglobin is 250 times stronger than the bond between oxygen and hemoglobin, it's difficult to eliminate carbon monoxide from the body. Preventing cells from receiving the oxygen they need to remain alive, carbon monoxide kills by a form of cellular asphyxiation.

Each year, this silent assassin slays 400 people across the United States and sends 15,000 to emergency rooms for care.[18] Accidents or attempted suicide cause most cases of carbon monoxide poisoning, but residential fires and wild-fires also kill their victims by carbon monoxide asphyxiation.[19]

Many victims of the 9/11 attacks died from being crushed or falling from high elevations. But many others died from suffocation caused by breath-ing dusts and toxic chemicals. The common factor in the deaths of the 9/11 victims, the Bhopal residents, the Granite Mountain Hotshots, and the Viet-namese family was that they inhaled substances that prevented oxygen from doing its job of keeping them alive. The 9/11 attack and the Bhopal disaster crushed, burned, and suffocated thousands immediately and also crippled the breathing of many more thousands who did not die but still suffer today. These catastrophes expose the vulnerability of breathing in disasters.

Fire is a powerful natural force that has enabled humans to create civiliza-tion. But the accompanying heat and smoke have also suffocated humans since our ancestors lived on the savanna thousands of years ago. In minutes, fumes can engulf a burning residence, or shifts in the wind can choke off the air in a forest. Furthermore, complex construction materials used nowadays make fires an even greater threat to breathing than in times past, when buildings were made of wood and stone.

The ancients recognized fire and air as two of the fundamental elements in nature. Breathing, the movement of air, was to them a sign of life. When they cremated their dead, the rising smoke symbolized the return of life to its source. Fire and air, breathing and smoke, became intertwined as metaphors for life and death.

10

CLEOPATRA REINCARNATE

"Man has an inborn craving for medicine. Heroic dosing for several generations has given his tissues a thirst for drugs. The desire to take medicine is one feature which distinguishes man, the animal, from his fellow creatures."

—William Osler[1]

In the mid-1990s, Jasmine became my patient when one of the other physicians in the office retired. I saw her mainly because of recurrent episodes of coughing and wheezing that were aggravated by tobacco addiction. But to her, respiratory problems were a minor part of her myriad medical difficulties. She suffered from anxiety, sleeplessness, and allover aching that she was sure was some form of arthritis.

Jasmine was in her midfifties, divorced, unemployed, the mother of three adult children. She was tall and slim and presented an exotic appearance, with long hair hung over a heavily made-up face and colored eye shadow with black lines that outlined the edges of her lids. She wore flowing gowns with bizarre patterns and baggy sleeves that nearly reached her waist. Dangling earrings, brass necklaces, bracelets, and rings on multiple fingers accented her flamboyant costuming.

Gayle, my medical assistant, often the receiver of interesting information not told to me—or overlooked—pointed out that Jasmine's clothes still had the tags on. I thought that was just a sign of her quirky personality, but Gayle felt it was more likely because she returned them after a few wearings. Gayle also informed me with a straight face that Jasmine confided to her that she was the reincarnation of Cleopatra.

Jasmine's and my relationship was difficult. I was focused on her coughing and wheezing. I felt sorry for her because she seemed unhappy and unable to figure a way to change, but I wished she would stop smoking or change doctors. A typical office visit usually began with my asking how she felt. She would respond, "I still have this cough."

"How're you doing in the battle against tobacco?"

"Still a few."

"I'm afraid the medicines aren't strong enough to block the irritation of smoking."

"My back hurts. Can you give me something for it?"

And so the interplay went on, neither party satisfying the other. Every office session ended with Jasmine asking for painkillers or sedatives and me resisting. Eventually I told her I would treat her chronic bronchitis, but she had to find another physician for the many other symptoms that afflicted her. Sometimes she would disappear for several months and then show up with a list of complaints that never changed.

At the end, I didn't see Jasmine for a long time. Then I received a summons suing me for prescribing drugs that wrongfully killed her.

Two million people in the United States take prescription narcotics for nonmedical purposes at least once a year.[2] Sixteen thousand die from overdose. What kills them? They stop breathing. Narcotics act like opium, the dried residue of fluid contained in poppy seeds. They reduce transmission of pain impulses, so they are great analgesics. However, they suppress cells that control wakefulness and so cause sleepiness, stupor, and coma. When narcotics block the nerve centers that control breathing, they can also kill.

Overdose with respiratory suppression is a constant threat. Prescription drugs cause more deaths than street drugs like heroin and cocaine.[3] The most abused of these is long-acting oxycodone, whose trade name is OxyContin, called Oxy by its users. Since its release in 1996, it has spread like a wave throughout the country. Many of those who overdose are doctor-hoppers and take multiple prescriptions. Rural dwellers and those of low income are at the highest risk for prescription drug abuse and therefore self-inflicted suffocation.

For a while I was a consultant to the health care division of a large international company. In March 2001, I was part of a team that visited a hospital in a small coal-mining town in southeastern Kentucky, near the Virginia border. Driving from the regional airport in a rented car, I wound my way through beautiful mountain passes, green with pines and budding hardwoods. I stopped in Big Stone Gap, the home of John Fox Jr., who in the early twentieth century wrote stories like *The Trail of the Lonesome Pine* that told the outside world about the pioneers of Appalachia and how the discovery of coal affected their way of life.[4]

When I crossed into Kentucky and arrived at my destination, I came upon hills that had been scalped, their summits a dusty yellow tan. The town was gray-brown, with strip malls, and small bungalows that needed painting. The hospital, recently constructed with state and federal funds, was bright and well-equipped. It looked to me like the nicest building in the area.

After the consultation finished three days later, the team, two nurses, a pharmacist, a medical records librarian, and myself, shared a drink at the airport while we waited for flights to our home cities around the country. One of the nurses, whose job had been to analyze hospital drug use, told us, "I swear this whole town is on OxyContin. Half the records I reviewed showed the patient was receiving Oxy." The pharmacist agreed, and we all frowned in dismay.

"Why are you surprised?" she asked, looking around the table. "The people are poor; half of them are out of work. Their countryside has been strip-mined bare. No wonder they're depressed. It's easier for doctors to give out painkillers than to spend time on counseling."

A couple of weeks after my trip to Kentucky, I was surprised to read a report in *Newsweek* magazine that suggested the town we had visited was at the center of OxyContin abuse in the United States.[5] More Kentuckians die of drug overdose than traffic accidents.[6] What the nurse saw in March 2001 was the breaking wave of drug abuse in rural Appalachia that has inundated the country.

OxyContin is synthesized from thebaine, a chemical in poppy seeds. It is of great benefit to patients with cancer and postsurgical pain. It causes a highly pleasurable feeling of well-being along with pain relief. Unfortunately, it's highly addicting and difficult to withdraw from. And in large doses, it suppresses breathing.

Military veterans are at particular risk. A 2016 PBS report indicated more than 500,000 ex-military take opioids, and of those, one in eight have opioid-related problems.[7] A 2011 Texas study reviewed records of 53,000 veterans applying for disability; 266 later died, and nearly a third of these were due to drug overdose (i.e., stopping breathing).[8] Indeed, the study reported, among males under thirty-five, the rate of death from overdose was 2.6 times higher than that of the overall population. Veterans are also likely to be receiving antidepressants and tranquilizers for posttraumatic stress disorders and are vulnerable to alcohol abuse, which aggravates the respiratory depressive effect of narcotic pain pills.

Meanwhile, according to CDC data, drug overdoses from illegal drugs, like heroin and cocaine, are on the rise as well. Heroin is diacetylmorphine, a chemical relative of morphine but with a greater tendency for addiction. It also works fastest if injected intravenously. This makes its users constantly need to increase the dose to achieve the same feeling of pleasure they previously enjoyed. Unfortunately, this is a recipe for stupor, coma, respiratory suppression, and death.

Both prescription painkillers and street drugs cause other respiratory injuries besides suppression of breathing. Blunting protective reflexes allows microorganisms to be inhaled into the lungs and bring about pneumonia. Addicts often dilute intravenous heroin by mixing in starch, sugar, powdered milk, and even chalk. Particles of these substances enter the blood and flow into the lungs, where they plug the tiny capillaries and lead to microscopic scars called granulomas. These increase pressure in the pulmonary circulation and eventuate in heart failure. Heroin is versatile: It can destroy breathing in several ways.

Codeine, another chemical cousin of morphine, is also present in opium poppies. In the body, it is metabolized to morphine, so it is an excellent pain reliever and good for suppressing coughing but has the same risks and side effects as morphine. It is also popular on the street as a substitute for morphine and heroin and, like them, kills by respiratory suppression.

Illegal drugs account for nearly 22,000 of the 36,000 deaths each year in the United States from overdose. Most are due respiratory and cardiac arrest.[9] But for every fatal celebrity overdose trumpeted in the media, hundreds of anonymous addicts succumb every year, their brains doped so they stop breathing.

When Jasmine stopped breathing, her children took her to the emergency room, where she died. The coroner's medical examiner determined she had elevated levels of codeine and sedatives in her blood and that she died of respiratory suppression from a drug overdose. According to the coroner's report, nothing I prescribed caused her death. My lawyer found out that Jasmine had been seeing multiple doctors and had filled prescriptions for painkillers and tranquilizers at several pharmacies around the city. When that became known, Jasmine's children's attorney resigned, and the judge dismissed the suit.

Jasmine abused drugs and stopped breathing. The rural Kentuckians used painkillers to assuage depression and stopped breathing. Traumatized veterans used narcotics to blunt their suffering and stopped breathing. The tragedies march on. Disaffected adolescents numb the pain of everyday life by sniffing glue and paint thinner, which mimic anesthetic gases and stop breathing or induce cardiac rhythm abnormalities. For many of these sufferers, suffocation or cardiac arrest are just a whiff away.

In 1992, presidential candidate Bill Clinton was asked if he ever smoked marijuana. He answered, "I experimented with marijuana a time or two, and I didn't like it, and didn't inhale, and never tried it again."[10] The "I didn't inhale" remark became a joke that persisted years afterward. Twenty years later, the former president clarified his statement and said, "I didn't say I was holier than thou. I said I tried. I never denied that I used marijuana." Times have changed, and when he was a candidate for the presidency, Barack Obama openly admitted experimenting with pot as a teenager and suffered no political damage. In 2012, nearly a quarter of high school seniors surveyed admitted they had tried marijuana in the month before.[11] And according to the surgeon general, 7 percent use it on a regular basis.[12] Indeed, more teenagers smoke marijuana than tobacco.

Marijuana can be a medicine. Its active ingredient, tetrahydrocannabinol (THC), has mild bronchodilator properties. But marijuana is not an ordinary medication.[13] Evidence favoring its use rests on anecdotes and testimonials rather than on prospective studies. Its optimum dosage is uncertain. The concentration of active drug varies widely, so that determining potency is difficult. While ordinary prescription medicines, like those for antibiotics, contain single active compounds, marijuana contains more than one hundred chemicals. If pot were a usual drug, it could never pass muster. For these reasons, the Drug Enforcement Administration continues to place it in schedule I, meaning no legitimate use known.

Marijuana cigarettes contain fillers whose source is often weeds. It's not called grass without reason. Studies have shown that tobacco smokers who also inhale marijuana suffer reduced lung function.[14] Proponents of the drug claim any impairment to breathing is small. I know I've seen patients referred for bronchitis where the only recognizable potential offender was marijuana, so I consider pot a respiratory irritant.

Marijuana is not only inhaled in cigarettes. It may be baked into cookies, brownies, or other sweet treats. The amount of active drug in a cookie or candy bar is unknown. This makes children especially vulnerable from accidental ingestion. In 2014, the *Annals of Emergency Medicine* reported an increase of marijuana overdosing among children residing in states that have legalized medical marijuana.[15] Association doesn't prove causation, but it surely makes one wonder.

A comprehensive review of the effect of marijuana smoking on the lung published in 2013 emphasized that pot smoke contains carcinogens, but epidemiologic studies have not shown a significant increase in lung cancers among light or moderate users.[16] Because many marijuana smokers also smoke tobacco, sorting out responsibility is difficult. A 2015 study suggested adenocarcinoma, the type of lung cancer seen in nonsmokers, occurred more often in individuals who smoked both tobacco and pot than in those who only smoked tobacco.[17] The verdict is not in yet. Pot appears less dangerous than tobacco, and there is no sign that weed harmed the lungs of Bill Clinton or

Barack Obama. But those who reassure themselves that marijuana smoking is safe are playing Russian roulette with their lungs as well as their brains.

Toxic inhalation occurs through industrial and household exposures as well as medical or recreational contact, sometimes with tragic outcomes for innocent bystanders. Nadia and Lalia came to San Diego to study. Residents of Saudi Arabia, the friends lived near Nadia's cousin Ahmed while they attended university and learned English. They rented rooms in a modest house not far from the University of San Diego campus and learned to take a bus to class. Ahmed drove them when they needed to go elsewhere to shop and buy groceries.

They had been in San Diego only two months when they received a letter from their landlord saying the house was infested with termites and was to be fumigated. Unacquainted with this procedure, the two continued in their daily routines. One afternoon when they returned from class, they found the house covered with a tent of brightly colored rubber sheets. A sign staked beside the walkway from the street contained "Danger" in large bold letters and urged readers to stay out.

Not knowing what that meant, they looked for a way to enter. They somehow slipped inside the tent and into the house. Almost immediately, they felt their eyes burn and their stomachs churn. Knowing something was wrong, they tried unsuccessfully to reach Ahmed. Then Nadia passed out. Panicked, Lalia dragged her friend outside and went to the house next door, where she pounded on the door. Luckily, she found someone home. The neighbor called 911.

Suffocation due to breathing fumigant gas is fortunately rare. But this tragic story illustrates that substances encountered in everyday living can injure the lungs if inhaled. Certain industries, like construction and oil and gas, carry the most risks. Most of us in pulmonary medicine have cared for workers exposed to sewer gas, hydrogen sulfide, which is highly toxic. In addition, workers whose job is to measure oil and gas levels in storage tanks after the fracking process have died unexpectedly, likely from inhaling evaporated hydrocarbons.[18] The list of injurious substances is long, though the types of injuries are few: acute asphyxiation, lung irritation, aggravation of asthma, fluid in the lungs, pneumonia with scarring, and cancer.

In the emergency department, the doctor listened to Nadia and Lalia's story and quickly knew what had happened. They had inhaled Vikane, a commercial pesticide widely used in termite fumigation. Tom Farrell, my associate, was called. He checked with the local poison control center and learned that Vikane contains sulfuryl fluoride, a colorless, odorless gas that causes nausea, headache, and central nervous system depression. In high concentrations, it can also inflame the respiratory tract, causing pulmonary edema, fluid buildup in the lungs. The manufacturers often add a small amount of chloropicrin, a type of tear gas, to discourage unwary individuals from remaining in the toxic air. Tom also learned sulfuryl fluoride–induced pulmonary edema may not become manifest until hours after exposure. He thus admitted both women to the hospital for observation.

The two women were put in separate rooms and started on oxygen and intravenous fluids. That evening both of them began to cough and feel short of breath. A nurse called Tom, who transferred them to the intensive care unit. In the unit, Lalia was uncomfortable but in no distress, and her vital signs were normal. Nadia, who had the most intense exposure, quickly worsened. Her pulse rose. Respirations became more rapid and labored. Her color went from pink to ashen. Then Nadia suddenly stopped breathing. Staff called a code blue and began resuscitation. They inserted a tube into her trachea, and pink, frothy fluid bubbled up, a sign of pulmonary edema.

Nadia continued on oxygen, and a mechanical ventilator pumped air under pressure into her wet lungs. Despite these efforts, over the next couple of hours, she went downhill. Her lungs became so boggy that, even with high pressures, it was impossible to oxygenate her blood. Her heart rhythm became rapid and irregular. Cardiac arrest followed. Intravenous antiarrhythmic drugs and electrical countershock were not able to restore cardiac action, and she was pronounced dead shortly after midnight.

Meanwhile, Lalia was a few beds away, receiving supportive care and slowly improving. Over the next twenty-four hours, she slowly stabilized and survived without any sign of impairment. Tom had the painful job of telling her that her friend had died. Lalia returned to Saudi Arabia soon after and was lost to follow-up.

Poisonous gases like sulfuryl fluoride damage the air sacs, where gas transfer occurs. The borders between cells become porous. Plasma leaks from pulmonary capillaries into the space surrounding the air sacs and prevents oxygen from being absorbed. The fluid also makes the lungs wet and boggy, like a soaked sponge, and this forces the person to work more to inhale and exhale. Between difficulty in oxygenation and increased work to move air, victims drown in their own body fluids. This is what happened to Nadia. Lalia probably had mild pulmonary edema, but with extra oxygen and time, she was able to recover.

Nadia resembled the victims of the Bhopal disaster described earlier, many of whom died, and Lalia's injury was more like that of the hotel housekeeper who inhaled a bleach-ammonia mixture. These stories also illustrate how the lungs can often resist the corrosive action of poison gas or vapor for several hours, but in time the defenses give way, and the victim drowns. Oxygen and ventilators help, but the best treatment is prevention.

Nadia and Lalia's story reminds us of the vulnerability of the respiratory system. Occasionally cases occur that are so unpredictable and strange they define categorization. I once cared for a patient who not only demonstrated how medical sleuthing works but also confirmed how right William Osler was when he talked about the human desire to take medicines, whether by mouth or otherwise.

Maude was eighty-seven. She was referred because of two months of coughing, wheezing, and difficulty breathing. She had never smoked, had been a homemaker all her life, and had not been exposed to any known lung toxin. In addition to her respiratory symptoms, she had severe degenerative arthritis, with continuous aching in her knees, hips, elbows, and back. She treated these with many proprietary remedies, including liniments and a heating pad. Maude was widowed and lived most of the year in San Diego with her two daughters. She came from a small town in Indiana and spent summers there visiting relatives and old friends.

Maude was heavy and walked with difficulty, using a cane for assistance. She had to rest after traversing the short distance from the consultation office to the examining room.

"I apologize for being so slow," she said. "Between my sore knees and hard breathing, it takes me a while to get anywhere."

"It's okay. Take your time," I answered, while I watched her. Her respiratory rate was at least half-again higher than normal. When I put a stethoscope on her chest, I could hear crackling sounds, as if someone was crunching cellophane as she inhaled, a characteristic of scarred or inflamed lungs. Her fingers were knobby, with pea-sized bumps at the knuckles. Described by British physician William Heberden in the eighteenth century and seen especially in women, these nodes are a tip-off to the presence of osteoarthritis.

Maude's lab work was unremarkable, but her chest X-ray showed collections of wavy white lines at the bases of the lungs, indicators of lung scarring. Her pulmonary function tests were 60 percent of normal for her age, and her blood oxygen was reduced as well.

I wondered what was going on. Perhaps Maude had an unusual type of pneumonia that left scars in the lung. Maybe this was a diffuse malignancy. Could she have unknowingly choked on something that inflamed her lungs? I was at a loss for a diagnosis, so I recommended a bronchoscopy, with biopsies of the scarred areas and collection of secretions for cultures. As I explained this, Maude's daughter, herself in her sixties, interrupted, "You know, Dr. Glynn, Mom uses WD-40 on her sore muscles, and I worry about that."

My eyebrows rose, and my eyes widened. I turned to Maude. "Tell me about that."

She smiled a little wan grin and didn't answer. She looked at her daughter, who continued talking. "It's common back in Indiana. Lots of older folks massage WD-40 on their sore joints. I worry because my mother gets carried away."

"But my neck and fingers are so sore," Maude interjected.

The younger woman spoke to me. "When I go into her room I can hardly see because there's a cloud of WD-40 spray everywhere. That can't be good for Mom's lungs."

I nodded assent. "Thanks for telling me. When I do the bronchoscopy, I'll examine the lung fluid for oil." Probably a red herring, I thought to myself.

The procedure went fine, and I was able to get plenty of specimens. The biopsies and cultures showed nothing conclusive, but the fluid from the bases of the lungs showed histiocytes, cells that mop up foreign matter. And they contained globules of oil.

Maude had a form of lung inflammation called lipoid pneumonia. Seen predominantly in the elderly, it's an uncommon but significant medical problem, resulting from oil seeping into the airways and making its way via gravity to the lower regions of the lungs. It's been described in users of oily nose drops and waxy lip gloss. A variant occurs in carnival fire-breathers, who breathe in volatile hydrocarbons and ignite them as they exhale. Oil irritates the lungs and causes inflammation that can lead to irreversible scarring. Maude's lungs were inflamed and scarred from inhaling droplets of lubricating oil in WD-40.

I recommended she stop WD-40 and prescribed steroids and oxygen for her breathing. Maude's breathing improved over the next couple of months but never became normal, and the cough remained. She lived another two years before dying of an unrelated problem.

Was William Osler right? Is the desire to take medicines hardwired in humans? Can we help the Jasmines, the Kentuckians, and the ex-military among us? One hundred people continue to die each day in the United States because painkillers and street drugs make them stop breathing. The problem won't end soon: Chronic pain, depression, and anxiety are real illnesses and will increase in prevalence as the population ages. Reversing this epidemic will require changing public policies. Drug abuse treatment is now segregated from ordinary care and considered a problem for public health agencies to solve rather than for private doctors to attack.[19] In his 2015 book *Dreamland*, reporter Sam Quinones recounted this discouraging story but also reported how people in communities from Oregon to Appalachia are fighting back against opiate abuse by improving economic conditions and throwing off the culture of drug dependence.[20]

In contrast, the stories of Nadia, Lalia, and Maude are medical curiosities. These idiosyncratic tales exist as counterpoints to the drug poisoning cases. They remind us how threats to breathing lurk amid the mundane activities of day-to-day living and how innocent actions can be fatal.

Toxic breathing also illustrates the marvelous complexity of the respiratory system. Narcotics kill by suppressing the brain's signals to breathe. IV heroin additives kill by plugging lung capillaries, preventing oxygenation. Vikane kills by causing the lungs to leak fluid and drown victims. Oil irritates the lungs and produces scars that impair oxygen transfer. Collectively, these threats form a lesson in abnormal pulmonary physiology. And they make us aware of the fragility of one of our basic functions of living.

⑪

SMOKING BEAGLES

"The roles I play in movies are far from easy on my voice—I can't risk throat irritation. So I smoke Camels—they're *mild*."

—John Wayne[1]

In the late 1960s, I had the good fortune to participate in the annual Tri-State Therapy Conference, a meeting of respiratory physicians in Minnesota, Michigan, and Wisconsin. Originated to discuss the best treatment for tuberculosis, the conference evolved to focus on other major lung diseases, as well. Held the weekend after Labor Day at a resort in northern Wisconsin near the little town of Pembine, it came to be called the Pembine Conference. Seventy lucky pulmonologists got to debate and learn in an informal, bucolic setting. As a youngster in the specialty, I could pick the brains of professors from the universities in the three states as well as from major groups like the Mayo Clinic.

The schedule left afternoons open for informal discussions. Sunny skies invited hiking in the forests, pine and spruce sprinkled with maples and oaks, whose leaves were turning yellow as the lengthening evenings cooled the air. White clouds moving south from Canada accentuated the late summer colors. Those who liked golf got to enjoy a course on the resort property, and I made sure I brought my clubs when I packed for the trip. It was not often I got to spend leisure time with senior professors in such a beautiful surrounding.

Among visiting lecturers, one of the stars was Oscar Auerbach. A pathologist interested in lung diseases, he was a senior investigator at the East Orange VA Hospital in New Jersey. Auerbach's presentations consisted mostly of slides of lungs of smokers who died of lung cancer or COPD. A meticulous examiner, Auerbach sectioned the bronchi, the place where most lung cancers start, and the air sacs, where emphysema destroys the lungs, looking for abnormalities. He made photographs of the microscopic changes he found and showed them to us.

The room was dark and the audience attentive. In a didactic tone, with a New York style of delivery, he pointed out changes occurring in the bronchial walls, cells becoming large, dark, and irregularly shaped, indications of cancerous degeneration. He showed air sacs whose architecture was torn apart, resulting in giant air spaces where a fine mesh of lacy cells belonged.

Auerbach's most compelling presentations were slides of his famous smoking beagles. In one series of experiments, he performed tracheostomies on dogs and taught them to smoke.[2] He gradually increased consumption until the dogs were up to twelve cigarettes daily, a large amount considering a beagle weighs about one-sixth as much as an adult human male. Auerbach sacrificed the dogs at various intervals up to fourteen months and showed that, the longer a dog smoked, the more atypical nuclei were found in the lining of the bronchi, cellular changes that lead ultimately to cancer. Even with dry, academic descriptive language, like "There is variation in the size, shape, and staining character of the nuclei," Auerbach's presentation was graphic and convincing.[3]

He performed a similar series of experiments to look at how tobacco smoke produced emphysema. Some dogs smoked as many as four thousand cigarettes during the year-long study, and when Auerbach autopsied the dogs, their lungs showed "connective tissue surrounding dilated air sacs," hallmarks of early emphysema.[4]

Epidemiologists had been claiming since the early twentieth century that there was a connection between smoking and both lung cancer and emphysema. In 1949, Ernst Wynder and Evarts Graham put smoking and lung cancer in the spotlight when they compared the smoking habits of 684 lung cancer patients and a group of 780 patients without cancer. They found the cancer patients were much more likely to be smokers.[5] This seems so simple and obvious to us today we wonder why the fuss, but in 1950, it was front-page news.

Soon afterward, British researchers Austin Bradford Hill and Richard Doll performed a similar study, and oceans apart, they obtained the same results. Hill and Doll queried 41,000 British doctors about their tobacco use. The researchers followed the physician subjects to see who would die and how. During the two years of the study, 789 doctors died, 36 from lung cancer. All the lung cancer victims were smokers. Hill and Doll published their work in

1956, which happened to be near the apogee of smoking prevalence. That year, 45 percent of adults in the United States used tobacco.

Meanwhile, scientists studying COPD collected similar data that indicted smoking as a causative factor in bronchitis and emphysema. In 1959, C. M. Fletcher at the London Postgraduate School of Medicine claimed chronic bronchitis, common in the United Kingdom, and emphysema, common in the United States, were both COPD with different manifestations, and both were heavily influenced by tobacco smoking. Fletcher wrote, "The disease (chronic bronchitis) is, in fact, seldom seen in men who have never smoked."[6]

I was in college around that time and remember the controversy these reports stirred up. Yet like most young people, I paid little attention. And every Sunday evening, the Winston man came through the fraternity house where I lived, dispensing free samples that supported their slogan, "Winston tastes good, like a cigarette should."

But association does not prove causation, and so science awaited studies that would show exactly how cancer and emphysema developed in the lungs of smokers. Auerbach provided actual pictures of lung tissue undergoing malignant degeneration and progressing from bronchitis to emphysema. His work confirmed the epidemiological investigations and refuted tobacco industry claims that smoking was innocuous.

Auerbach remained an active teacher and investigator for the rest of his life. A week before he died at the age of ninety-two, he was still lecturing and training residents at the University of Medicine and Dentistry of New Jersey.[7] Today medical science recognizes Auerbach as a pioneer in understanding the natural history of lung cancer and emphysema. However, in 1967, he was a prophet showing how these diseases start, and his smoking beagles can be thought of as martyrs for medical science.

Tobacco smoke irritates the cells that line the airways of the lungs. At first, the cells react by swelling, producing mucus, and trying to sweep the toxic particles out. As the process goes on, molecules of tar accumulate. Tar is the oily, sticky residue of burning tobacco leaves. It contains chemicals that slowly seep into the nuclei of the cells and disrupt DNA synthesis. This goes on for decades, until the DNA becomes so deranged that it disrupts the intracellular mechanisms for growth and reproduction. Eventually a clone of cells develops that grows wildly, like weeds in a garden, sapping nutrients and blocking attempts by the body to destroy them. This is cancer.

Slowly these monster cells invade adjacent capillaries and lymph vessels. They break off and travel to other organs, such as bone, liver, and brain. This process, called metastasis, crowds out normal cells, siphons energy, and eventually kills the person.

Similarly, as nicotine and tars from tobacco smoke inflame bronchial cells, recurring infections and scarring cause irreversible bronchitis and destroy pulmonary air sacs. These become clinically manifest as COPD, chronic obstructive pulmonary disease. Lung cancer and COPD have the same root source, tobacco, and frequently coexist in the same patients, a lethal form of double jeopardy. I can't even count the number of patients I've seen who could not undergo lung cancer surgery because they had such severe COPD they could not withstand the operation. Medicine could offer these patients only radiation or chemotherapy in hopes of slowing cancer growth.

Humans have used tobacco for centuries. Reports from the time of Columbus indicate Native Americans practiced inhaling its smoke. Smoking was part of religious as well as social ceremonies because the Indians believed their gods manifested themselves in the rising fumes.[8] Columbus and his companions made notes in their journals of how the natives rolled dried tobacco inside palm leaves and "drank" the smoke. In the sixteenth century, explorers returning from the New World introduced tobacco and smoking into Europe, where it caught on fast and never lost its popularity.

By the seventeenth century, critics indicted tobacco as a noxious weed that worked by "evaporating man's unctuous and radical moistures" and compared inhaling tobacco smoke to breathing soot.[9] Indeed, references to cigarettes as "coffin nails" date at least to the 1800s.[10]

In the mid-nineteenth century, cigarettes, little cigars made of shredded tobacco wrapped in paper, became popular in Europe among the upper classes, who could afford the cost.[11] Skilled cigarette rollers catered to their patrician desires, while ordinary people had to buy a little bag of tobacco, make a funnel of paper, pour in the shredded leaves, cinch closed the neck of the bag with their teeth, roll the mixture into a cylinder, lick the paper to make it stick, and finally light a match to the end to inhale the pungent smoke. Then in 1880, Virginian James A. Bonsack invented a machine that rolled cigarettes a hundred times faster than hand-rolling could. This revolutionized the tobacco industry.

With cigarette manufacturers promoting their products, cigarettes caught on among the masses. Subsidiary industries sprouted to make safety matches, lighters, cellophane packages, and ashtrays. Everyone could afford to buy cigarettes by the box, carry them in a pocket, and grab a quick smoke at lunch or catch a puff while working. The aesthetics of smoking also changed because cigarette butts were less messy than cigar stubs. In addition, cigarettes became popular among the military, reinforcing the notion that manly men smoked cigarettes.

James Duke, whose Duke of Durham brand would evolve into the American Tobacco Company, saw the potential of machine-rolled cigarettes and installed Bonsack machines in his factories. In 1884, Duke was able to produce 744 million cigarettes, more than the entire US output the previous year.[12] Unfortunately for those manly men who smoked, manufactured cigarettes increased the amount of tobacco they inhaled, as well as the carcinogens contained therein.[13]

Aggressive marketing propelled sales skyward during the first two decades of the twentieth century.[14] This was the era in which my father and uncles took up the habit. Average annual consumption of cigarettes increased from 54 per capita in 1900 to 4,345 in 1963, almost a one-hundred-fold jump.[15]

Women were tobacco targets as well. As far back as the 1920s, extolling cigarettes as "torches of freedom," Big Tobacco exploited women's aspirations for independence and equality with men.[16] Cigarette advertisements emphasized smoking as a sign of style, sophistication, and fashion. Lucky Strike promoted "Reach for a Lucky instead of a sweet" to connect cigarettes with the allure of slimness. (Smoking suppresses appetite and reduces weight, but lung cancer and COPD are surely not worth the benefit.)

With dozens of brands available for smokers to choose from, tobacco companies needed forceful strategies to sell cigarettes and so used incessant promotion to increase smoking. In the 1940s and '50s, they connected smoking with health and medicine. Ads in the major weekly magazines, like *Life* and *Look*, showed a clean-cut man in a white coat wearing a doctor's head mirror, attesting to the refreshing power of Camel cigarettes. A few pages away, competitor Lucky Strike featured pictures of a fatherly looking physician testifying to the merits of its product.

Another Camel ad emphasized the "T-zone," an imaginary space that went across the face and down the throat, as if created by nature to be cleansed and refreshed by the beneficial mists of smoldering tobacco. Still another ad claimed, "More doctors smoke Camels than any other cigarette."[17] Reportedly, 113,597 physicians participated in the survey quoted in the ad, so the medical profession had its share of nicotine addicts.

While cigarette makers exploited the medical profession to promote their products, they also relied heavily on athletes and movie stars. One ad showed Bob Hope, Bing Crosby, Perry Como, and Arthur Godfrey, popular entertainers of that time, wearing elf hats like Santa's helpers, smiling and urging readers to "Make 'Em Happy. Treat 'Em Right," by giving them a carton of Chesterfields as a Christmas gift. Even Ronald Reagan, the future president, pitched their merits for holiday cheer, claiming, "I'm sending Chesterfields to all my friends."[18]

Other ads showed female movie stars like Rita Hayworth and Betty Grable smoking, which added to the glamor. The tobacco industry even sold brands specifically aimed at women, like Virginia Slims and Eve. These implied health-conscious women could both smoke and be responsible to their families by using low-tar "light" cigarettes. After these campaigns, tobacco consumption among teenaged girls and young women doubled.

Tobacco companies sponsored radio and television programs, as well. We listened to *Your Hit Parade*, a weekly replaying of the most popular tunes, coming to us through the good wishes of Lucky Strike. Chesterfield played a song that began, "A, B, C. Always Buy Chesterfield." When television arrived, the commercials became visual. Old Gold, whose motto was "Not a cough in a carload," sponsored *The Amateur Hour*. Its ads featured a woman inside a box with the Old Gold label on it, only her legs showing, who tap-danced to snappy slogans that announced, "A treat instead of a treatment . . . made by tobacco men, not medicine men." Sometimes a small girl in a matchbox accompanied her. I always wondered how they synchronized their steps without being able to see each other.

As warnings about smoking dangers accumulated, cigarette makers changed composition of their products. They featured cigarettes with filters and "light" products purportedly lower in tar. These claims were mostly bogus. Researchers measured saliva levels of cotinine, a nicotine metabolite, to estimate the actual inhaled dose and showed that "light" cigarettes did not decrease nicotine intake, industry propaganda notwithstanding.

The tobacco titans also fought back against Auerbach, Wynder, Graham, and the other scientists indicting smoking by challenging the validity of their research. By creating their own institutes to study the question of tobacco dangers, they implied the issue was in doubt.[19] For a while, the strategy worked, but then Congress passed laws that required labeling cigarettes with the health risks involved. These ultimately resulted in the famous surgeon general's warning, "Smoking Causes Lung Cancer, Heart Disease, Emphysema, and May Complicate Pregnancy," stamped on cigarette packages.[20] These laws also led to banning advertising tobacco products on radio and television, and the CDC began issuing annual reports on the public health consequences of smoking.

Tobacco smoking kills slowly. Most of its ravages don't occur until more than twenty years after victims start to smoke, which means long-term studies are necessary to identify trends. In 1964, the US Public Health Service stated that tobacco smoking was a definite cause of lung and laryngeal cancer in men and a probable cause of lung cancer in women.[21] By the end of the 1960s, more than seven thousand reports had accumulated in the medical literature indicting tobacco smoke as a cause of lung and throat cancer, as well as leading to chronic obstructive lung disease.[22]

I entered practice in 1969 and experienced the front-line effects of the smoking epidemic. Lung cancer and COPD became frequent in my small corner of the medical world, and women began to show the ravages, as well. Dorothy was a sixty-year-old woman I saw in 1990 because she was coughing up blood. She had been a smoker since she was in her twenties. She had no history of any serious diseases but when questioned admitted she had been troubled by a "cigarette cough" for several years and had become short of breath in the previous year. Her chest X-ray showed a lung mass the size of a baseball, that on biopsy was squamous-cell cancer.

Dorothy's pulmonary function was too poor even to consider the thought of surgery; she had COPD, as well. And so, she began radiation, which unfortunately was of little help. Divorced and with no children, she was alone, which aggravated the sadness of her predicament. Over the next few months, I became Dorothy's primary doctor, and one of the themes in our discussions was her wistful regret about having smoked. I played that down—feeling more guilt was the last thing she needed—and connected her with hospice as soon as I could, which helped ease her last weeks.

Looking back, it wasn't surprising Dorothy had lung cancer. She had been born in 1930, started smoking in the 1950s, and by 1990 was due to get in trouble. I saw her two weeks before she died, and she was at peace, resigned to the future, and appreciative, which I credited to the excellent support she received from San Diego Hospice more than to anything special I did for her.

By the later decades of the twentieth century, cigarette use declined among adults in the United States as antismoking campaigns ramped up. Nevertheless, lung cancer and COPD mortality rates continued to climb, reflecting the time lag between smoking and onset of lung diseases. In 2001, the National Cancer Institute concluded that changes in cigarette manufacturing over the previous fifty years had not benefited public health, despite Big Tobacco's claims that cigarettes were safer than ever.[23]

Smoking affects those around smokers, as well. Beginning in the 1980s, reports alerted the medical profession about the increased risk for lung cancer among wives of smokers, who themselves had never smoked. Data suggested being married to a smoker or working around smokers increased one's chances of acquiring lung cancer by 20 percent. This meant thousands of people were dying each year in the United States from secondhand smoke.[24]

Forty-five million Americans still smoke. More than eight million live with chronic lung or heart disease resulting from tobacco smoke. In addition, even if a longtime smoker stops, twenty years later, the risk for lung cancer is still double that of someone who never smoked.[25] Thus, lung cancer and COPD will not soon go away. The CDC estimates that more than 400,000 people die prematurely every year from tobacco-related diseases in the United States, nearly half of these from lung cancer and the rest from COPD, cardiovascular diseases, and other inflammatory lung diseases, like pneumonia and pulmonary fibrosis.[26]

Tobacco companies continue to court potential smokers in developing countries throughout the world.[27] And they are succeeding. For example, in the United States, 20 percent of adult men smoke, while in China, smoking rates among adult men exceed 50 percent. These smokers pay a price: Their average lifespan is reduced by thirteen years.[28]

Hon Lik comes from northeastern China. A pharmacist by profession, in the 1990s, he became concerned because his father had died of lung cancer, and he, himself, was smoking a pack of cigarettes a day. So, he determined to do something. His goal was to make a cigarette that didn't create smoke. It took him a while, but in 2003, he invented a way to vaporize a nicotine solution so that it could be inhaled.[29] This was the original e-cigarette. Hon was the first, but competitors quickly marketed similar devices, and soon vaporizing pens, waterpipes, and electronic cigars became available all over the world. E-cigarettes have become a $2-billion-a-year industry in the United States alone; they appeal to those who want to stop smoking cigarettes and have caught the attention of teenagers curious to try nicotine.

Proponents assert that e-cigarettes work as well as nicotine gum or patches to aid in stopping smoking. They also stress that, by eliminating the tar contained in cigarette smoke, e-cigarette users have less risk of getting cancer or COPD. E-cigarette opponents insist they are far from safe. They concede e-cigarettes may decrease nicotine craving but worry about adolescents becoming addicted to nicotine via e-cigarette use. In addition, they note that e-cigarette vapor isn't just nicotine and water. It contains propylene glycol, which is irritating to the lungs, and other chemicals to impart flavors and colors to nicotine that are potential respiratory toxins.

In 2009, Congress passed legislation that gave the Food and Drug Administration (FDA) power to regulate tobacco products, but due to industry lobbying, the law excluded e-cigarettes.[30] Thus began a struggle between regulators and manufacturers. The FDA continued to attempt to increase its authority over e-cigarettes and water-pipe tobacco devices and in May 2016 succeeded in prohibiting sale of e-cigarettes to minors.[31] In addition, forty-one states passed their own laws prohibiting sale of e-cigarettes to individuals younger than eighteen. But if adolescents want to try something, prohibiting it merely increases their curiosity.[32]

Conventional cigarette smoking among teenagers has been decreasing in the United States, but e-cigarettes are on the upsurge.[33] E-cigarette manufacturers have played up the differences between vaporized nicotine and tobacco smoke and have suggested e-cigarettes are safer and that it's cool to vape. They have created flavors like cherry crush, bubble gum, and chocolate treat to appeal to youngsters. It's working. Reports from the CDC indicate that as many as a quarter of high school students have tried e-cigarettes.

In addition, reports of children being poisoned by unintentionally ingesting nicotine liquid are rising. Because of the sweet fruity flavors added, the nicotine loses its bitter taste, and thus small children are at risk. The CDC reported that poison control centers noted a two-hundred-fold increase in e-cigarette-related calls between 2010 and 2014.

E-cigarettes are too new to have information on long-term toxicities. Even the medical profession is divided: Some doctors feel e-cigarettes are safer than smoked cigarettes and that they help in smoking cessation, while others worry about addiction and late toxic effects. No one knows the definitive answers. It will be years before medical science knows for sure whether vaping plays a role in lung cancer and COPD, but the odds are it will.

The battle goes on. Cigarette consumption has declined in the United States over the last decade. Twenty-one percent of adult Americans smoked in 2005, and this figure dropped to 17 percent in 2014, the most recent year for which figures are available. But 20 percent of young adults smoke, so youth are trying tobacco.[34] The CDC and voluntary health organizations, like the American Lung Association and the American Cancer Society, have publicized the dangers of tobacco, lobbied Congress, promoted smoking cessation, and produced public service advertisements that discourage adolescents from using tobacco. The tobacco industry has responded by increasing marketing efforts abroad in countries like China.

Today, Hon Lik works for a subsidiary of the Imperial Tobacco Company of the United Kingdom, which bought his e-cigarette patents. Hon sees no irony in this and says he is content, with no regrets.[35] Living comfortably and traveling as a spokesman for Imperial, Hon is pleased that his e-cigarette idea has caught on so well and that he has made a difference in the world.

Nicotine continues to be a prominent feature in global culture, regardless of the troubles it may cause. Over the years, many patients have asked me about the contribution of dusts, toxins, and air pollution to their medical conditions. I answered that the most injurious form of air pollution they needed to worry about was cigarette smoking. If everyone on planet Earth stopped smoking, longevity would increase for millions of us. It wouldn't happen immediately, but the effect would be profound. It would turn diseases like lung cancer and COPD into medical rarities. And society would breathe a sigh of relief.

⑫

DAD, AND THE WEREWOLF

"We shall draw from the heart of suffering itself the means of inspiration and survival."

—Winston Churchill[1]

"You gain strength, courage, and confidence by every experience in which you really stop to look fear in the face."

—Eleanor Roosevelt[2]

More people in the United States die from lung cancer than any other type of malignancy.[3] It causes 160,000 deaths a year, more than breast, colon, and prostate cancers combined.[4]

I watched my father die from lung cancer. Dad was easygoing and witty, a master fixer who could repair just about anything in the house. The son of a carpenter, he was unafraid to tackle any project. From him I learned this lesson: You can take almost anything apart and put it back together if you are careful. I still have many of his tools, some dating from the 1920s.

Dad was also a heavy smoker for as long as I could remember. He kept at least one carton of Lucky Strikes in his top dresser drawer at all times and smoked almost two packs daily. To be sure he had a ready source of tobacco available, he kept a tin of pipe tobacco in that same drawer, though he smoked his pipe much less than cigarettes. I still have pictures of him smiling, with a cigarette between his second and third fingers. After supper, he would light up while he made a joke or told a story, his coffee cup and ashtray in front of him on the dining room table. He used to cough a lot; they called it catarrh, and my mother blamed it on his working in the steel mills during the Depression.

Shortly before Christmas 1952, a month before he was to turn forty-eight, Dad's cough worsened. He developed a lump in his neck. After he went to the doctor, Mom said it was a lymph node, which meant nothing to me at the age of sixteen. A series of X-rays and tests followed, and a surgeon removed the lymph node. Mom said he had a lung tumor and that he was to have X-ray therapy.

I saw an article in the *Saturday Evening Post* suggesting that smoking was linked to lung cancer and showed it to Mom. She nodded but said little. Meanwhile Dad worsened. He was quiet and less outgoing; quips became a rarity. He began to lose weight and moved more slowly. It seemed like he was aging every week. I was the only one of the kids old enough to drive a car, and so I was enlisted to take Dad to the hospital for the radiation treatments. I remember him huddled in the passenger seat, buried beneath a scarf and thick overcoat, a frail figure in the January cold of that bleak Chicago winter.

Radiation didn't work. The skin over his chest turned red, like a severe sunburn, but the cough was deeper and harder. He couldn't go to work and remained at home, resting in a chair. His feet began to swell, and his freckled Irish skin paled. Soon he was staying in bed most of the day. Medicine bottles, spoons, and water glasses collected on his bedside table. In the middle of the night from my bedroom, I could hear him coughing.

He abandoned the X-ray treatments in February, two months after the lymph node biopsy. I never learned whether they were finished or whether it was too difficult for him to get to the hospital or whether they were simply judged a failure. That marked the beginning of the end. Visiting nurses came to help, and Dr. Kelly, who lived three blocks from us, made house calls. I fantasized that would help in some magical way, but it didn't. Dad's feet swelled more until he could hardly move. His breathing became labored. Even shifting his weight in a chair looked like it was painful.

He slept most of the time, and when he was awake, he couldn't muster enough breath to talk. With his face contorted into a frown and his movements so slow they resembled a creaky machine, I could see his suffering and wished I could do something. I kept telling myself that maybe he would turn the corner and recover. Mom told me to come home right after school every day, which made me worry more.

Finally, he lost consciousness, and each breath became a struggle. On March 27, four months after Dad first became sick, the Friday a week before Easter, I was called to the principal's office at my high school and told to leave class and go home immediately. When I arrived, Mom said Dad had died soon after lunch. I was not to see his body. The morticians were coming. I waited for a miracle, thinking maybe they made a mistake, but there was no mistake and no miracle.

I felt a deep, icy emptiness that sank to the bottom of my stomach. It was as if the chill of late March had squelched the promise of increasing sunlight and reverted to the dark frigidity of winter. Self-centered adolescent that I was, I focused on what life without Dad meant for me: no one to take me to play golf, no father to advise me about college. Then I realized that it must be worse for my brother and sisters, who were younger than I and still needed help with homework and to learn to drive a car. What would Mom do? Was there enough money for us to stay in our house? Would she have to go to work? Only later did I come to realize how deeply she would miss him for the rest of her life. Only later did I appreciate how he had been her love.

Many years later, my sister shared a copy of Dad's death certificate with me. It said he died of bronchogenic carcinoma, referring to the fact that many lung cancers start in the bronchi, the small tubes through which air moves in and out of the lungs. By then, I had treated hundreds of lung cancer patients myself, understood the natural history of the disease, and didn't need official confirmation to reconstruct his last four months.

Lung cancer is not a single entity. Oncologists distinguish two broad categories: small-cell cancers and non-small-cell cancers. Small-cell cancers make up only 10 percent of lung cancers but are the most aggressive, sometimes killing the patient in a few weeks. Non-small-cell cancers are the most frequent, further divided into adenocarcinomas when they contain gland-like cells, squamous-cell carcinomas if they look like skin cells, and large-cell carcinomas if the cells are big but don't look like glands or skin cells.

Small-cell cancers arise from primitive tissues whose normal function is to connect impulses from the nervous system (brain) and the endocrine (hormonal) system. These primeval cells are scattered throughout the bronchi and play a role in lung growth and in how the lung responds to oxygen. Under the microscope, small cells are spindle-shaped, resembling miniature bottles or flasks. For a long time, they were called "oat cell" cancers because someone thought they looked like cereal grains.

Small-cell and non-small-cell cancers cause similar symptoms, except in small-cell tumors they occur faster. Small-cell cancer patients often develop symptoms of metastasis early, and bone pains or mental changes may be the first signals that bring the person to the doctor.

Small-cell cancers frequently secrete strange hormone-like compounds that cause bizarre findings. Ozzie was a forty-four-year-old man who sought help for a one-week-long headache, with dizziness so severe that he was staggering about like a drunk. He had been feeling weak for a month or two, and his weight dropped fifty pounds in that short time. Ozzie was a longtime heavy smoker but had no other pulmonary history. On examination, he was confused and uncooperative, with flabby skin folds that denoted extensive weight loss. Ozzie's most remarkable finding was that he looked like a werewolf. He said he had noticed fuzzy hair growing for the past couple of years, and his brother corroborated this.

His chest X-ray showed a mass in the left lung, indeterminate as to whether it was a tumor or pneumonia. The next day Ozzie spiked a fever of 102° and was started on penicillin. Despite this, he quickly became lethargic, then comatose, and died within two days. Autopsy showed a small-cell cancer in the left upper lung. However, the most striking finding was Ozzie's skin. His body was covered with fine hairs, some as long as four inches. The palms, soles of the feet, and genital organs were spared, but otherwise he was furry, like an animal.

Ozzie's case was so unusual that George Hensley, the pathologist, and I published it in the journal *Cancer*.[5] George found five similar cases in the literature of excessive hair growth with cancer. Ozzie died before sophisticated immunoassays for various protein fragments in serum became available, and genomic analysis was decades in the future. Nevertheless, Ozzie's bizarre hair growth made a strong case that small-cell lung cancers elaborate some hormone-like substance that suppresses growth of adult hair and stimulates baby hair.

Among non-small-cell cancers, adenocarcinomas are the most frequent subtype, accounting for 35 percent of lung cancers. These occur in the outer portions of the lungs, often arise in lung tissue scarred by previous infections, and may develop in people who have never smoked or whose exposure to tobacco is restricted to living with a smoker, so-called passive smoking or secondhand smoking.

Squamous-cell carcinomas, in contrast, tend to occur in bronchi nearer the trunk of the bronchial tree, likely because the most carcinogen-laden air passes over them during breathing. These make up 25 percent of lung cancers. This is probably what my father had.

The vast majority of squamous-cell cancers occur in smokers or former smokers. Carcinogens in tobacco smoke slowly change the cells lining the bronchi, first turning them from a regular shape, like miniature bricks, into large, darkly colored particles that cling together like fried eggs in a skillet. Soon these cells grow into adjacent capillaries and lymph ducts and then eventually spread to other organs beyond the lungs.

Genes play a major role in most types of lung cancers. Altered genes that drive malignant changes, called oncogenes, cause tumorous change, while other gene alterations turn off natural cancer-suppressing functions, enabling tumors to grow. As a malignancy enlarges in the lung, it often causes the patient to become short of breath, and when the tumor obstructs a major bronchus, pneumonia develops as well. When spread to bones occurs, pain becomes severe, and if the cancer sends satellites to the brain, headaches, confusion, seizures, and loss of consciousness result.

My father's story was typical for someone with non-small-cell lung cancer, likely squamous type. He had a nagging cough for several months, chest pains, loss of appetite, drop in weight, and profound tiredness. He complained about that more than shortness of breath, but he surely had difficulty breathing as his disease progressed.

The mortality rate from all these lung cancer varieties is high because the disease is ordinarily not discovered until it is in an advanced stage. Even small lung spots have already metastasized by the time they are recognized as cancerous. About one-third of small-cell lung cancers are in a "limited" stage at the time of discovery and carry a five-year survival rate no better than one out of three. For non-small-cell cancers, the outlook is more optimistic, but regardless of cell type, if the tumor has spread outside the lung, which is the situation most of the time, prognosis for five-year survival is less than 10 percent.

Surgery is the preferred method of treatment, and if the tumor load is light, meaning absence of symptoms, size less than one inch, no lymph node involvement, and no spread beyond the lung, removing the affected lobe offers a 40 to 50 percent five-year survival.

Radiation and chemotherapy offer some benefit to patients whose overall status is good. This means minimal weight loss, ability to exercise, and enough strength for activities of everyday living. In small-cell cancer, radiation and chemo actually produce better results than surgery, except in the occasional case where the tumor is detected accidentally and has not caused any symptoms.

Recently, monoclonal antibodies against proteins called PD, or programmed death, have shown promise in non-small-cell lung cancers. These antibodies block the ability of cancer cells to hijack the body's own immune-protective mechanisms, thus retarding tumor growth and spread. It is too early to know for sure, but these immunologic approaches may have more to offer in lung cancer than standard chemotherapy.

While more than 80 percent of lung cancers are associated with tobacco smoking, other environmental agents play a role, as well. Asbestos exposure is the most prominent occupational risk for lung cancer. Asbestos causes scarring of the lungs, as discussed earlier, but also incites lung cancer in smokers. Experts debate whether asbestos directly makes bronchial cells become malignant or whether asbestos-caused scarring facilitates cancerous degeneration.[6] A person who has smoked and worked around asbestos carries nearly a thirty-fold increased risk of lung cancer compared to someone who has never smoked and never been exposed to asbestos.[7] Earlier I mentioned my pipe-coverer roommate in Massena, New York, and his risk of asbestosis; he was a smoker and so in danger of lung cancer, as well.

Mesothelioma is a rare malignancy of the pleura that occurs nearly exclusively in people exposed to asbestos and can occur without tobacco playing a role. Because the pleura covers the lung but is not anatomically part of the lung, mesothelioma is not technically a lung cancer but is usually discussed with cancers arising in the bronchi and air sacs. Also, it is acquired via inhalation and affects breathing.

Medical science only knows part of how asbestos produces mesothelioma. Asbestos fibers are both small enough to be inhaled deep into the lung and durable enough that defense mechanisms cannot break them into less injurious parts. As the tiny fibers burrow into the pleura, the body attempts to wall them off, and low-grade inflammation goes on for decades. In time, genetic changes occur that lead to unchecked growth and spread; in other words, cancer of the pleura.

Other mineral dusts are less associated with lung cancer, likely because their fibers are larger and less penetrating. Silica, the most prevalent, is not generally considered a carcinogen, though some evidence indicates iron and steel foundry workers, sand blasters, and metal molders who have intense contact with crystalline silica have increased rates of lung cancer.[8] Chromate workers also have an increased risk of cancer, and the American Cancer Society suggests arsenic, beryllium, and cadmium may be work-connected carcinogens, but the evidence is less persuasive.[9] Summing all the available data, authorities consider occupational exposures to be responsible for less than 10 percent of lung cancers.[10]

Radiation can also cause lung cancer.[11] A seventy-two-year-old Navajo man lived by himself in a small cabin on the reservation in northeastern Arizona. The area is stark but beautiful. He would have been able to wander through land occupied by his ancestors for hundreds of years, watch the majestic clouds roil over the mountains, and enjoy the ever-changing colors on the red rocks as the sun crossed the sky. He would have been able to feel the wind tousle his hair and smell the ozone when lightning crackled above the stormy summits. He would have been close to nature.

Without modern conveniences, like running water or electricity, he was isolated but was active enough to herd a few sheep in the nearby hills. Then in 1990, he got sick. He began to vomit and over six months lost thirty pounds, which his children attributed to his poor eating when he was away from home herding sheep. He started to cough and to have difficulty breathing, which led to his being admitted to the local Indian Health Service hospital. The doctors found pneumonia in his right lung, a pocket of infected fluid between the lung and chest wall, and a hole between his esophagus and his windpipe. He was immediately transferred to the University Hospital in Albuquerque, New Mexico, where bronchoscopy showed a cancer in his right lung had blocked the bronchus, permitting pus and infection to build up and to erode through the wall of his esophagus.

Because he spoke no English, his son supplied the past history. He had high blood pressure and arthritis, as well as a past exposure to tuberculosis, but had never smoked and had no lung disease in his background. However, for seventeen years, he had been a uranium miner. He shoveled ore into wheelbarrows and hauled it out of the mine. During this underground work, he had no personal protective gear and often inhaled the dust and smoke that welled up after dynamite blasted the ore-bearing rocks loose.

The elderly man went downhill fast. Infection spread throughout his system, and he died less than three weeks after first being admitted to the Indian Health Service hospital. An autopsy confirmed a squamous-cell lung cancer with extension into the chest and erosion into the esophagus. Uranium exposure got the blame.

As uranium undergoes radioactive decay, it turns into radium, which decays further to become radon, a gas that emits electrically charged particles called ions. These particles damage DNA in genes. This leads to mutations that set in motion a cancerous growth cycle in cells. Because radon is a gas, humans inhale it, and so the lung is the primary organ damaged. The Environmental Protection Agency (EPA) considers inhaled radiation to be the second-most frequent cause of lung cancer after tobacco smoking, responsible for more than 20,000 deaths a year in the United States.[12]

Uranium, radium, and radon have been present in the earth's crust for millions of years, and their concentration in soil and atmospheric air is low. However, the EPA estimates that about 6 percent of homes have levels of radon high enough to be potential causes of injury and recommends all homeowners check radon levels periodically. Smoking increases the cellular injuries caused by radon. Indeed, the risk of radon-induced lung cancer is ten times higher in smokers than in nonsmokers. So, the best way to reduce the risk of lung cancer from radon is to be sure one's home is well-ventilated and that no one inside smokes.

Uranium was first isolated in the late eighteenth century in central Europe. It was initially used in pottery and glass making, but in the 1890s, Antoine Becquerel and Marie and Pierre Curie, working in Paris, discovered its radioactive properties. Marie Curie isolated radium, which is formed when uranium decays. (Marie Curie later died of bone marrow poisoning from her exposure to radium, and her daughter Irene, who worked with her, contracted leukemia.)

Around the same time, archeologists exploring in the southwestern United States recognized uranium ore in mineral formations on the Colorado Plateau, a geological area encompassing parts of Colorado, New Mexico, Utah, and Arizona. The Navajo and Hopi Reservations are located in the western portion of the Colorado Plateau in the Four Corners region.

During World War I, when the military began to use radium to make luminescent dials for nighttime warfare, demand for uranium rose sharply. Soon Congress decided to open tribal lands to uranium mining. This led to a dramatic rise in mining on the Navajo Reservation during the 1930s.

After Hitler invaded Czechoslovakia in 1938, Germany controlled the largest deposits of uranium known in the world at that time. In addition, scientists fleeing the Nazis informed the US government that the Germans were working on an atomic bomb. In 1942, President Franklin D. Roosevelt authorized the Manhattan Project, and the United States went into high gear to extract uranium from the Colorado Plateau. From 1940 until the 1960s, 2,500 uranium mines were dug on and near the Navajo Reservation. These mines employed as many as 3,000 Navajos, among them the man who became the lung cancer patient forty years later.

After World War II, studies of atomic bomb survivors in Japan showed they had increased incidence of several types of cancer, including in the lung. Radiation appeared responsible. By the 1950s, government officials became concerned enough about the risk of cancer among uranium miners that they commissioned the US Public Health Service to study the question.[13] These studies confirmed the association between uranium mining and lung cancer.[14]

Uranium today is used for nuclear power. Mining in the United States has gradually decreased over the past thirty years, and only about 5 percent of the uranium consumed by nuclear plants in this country is mined in this country.[15] In the United States, 1,200 individuals are currently employed in mining uranium.[16] Most of the world's uranium comes from Australia, Kazakhstan, Russia, and Canada, with some from southern Africa. In these countries, the risks of uranium lung injury persist.

Nearly 160,000 Americans this year will die from lung cancer.[17] Tobacco smoking will be responsible for more than 80 percent of these, with radiation and occupational exposures, especially asbestos, causing the rest. That is a huge number, more than homicides, suicides, and motor vehicle deaths combined.[18] Also, lung cancer spreads early; even those whose cancer is localized and less than one inch in size have only a 50 percent five-year survival.[19] However, reports of screening heavy smokers by means of CT scans are encouraging and offer hope of improving the outlook by picking up cancers earlier.

Lung cancer is also costly. The US health care system spends $88 billion each year diagnosing and treating lung cancer, plus the country loses $150 billion in economic productivity from the depredations of the disease.[20] These figures indicate the massive public health problem lung cancer presents but say nothing about the suffering and grief the disease causes to patients and their families. I can testify to that from my Dad and from my own experience in practice.

Earl was my former piano teacher and friend who became my patient. Earl consulted me because he was coughing up blood.[21] He had served as a GI in World War II and settled in San Diego afterward, playing the piano in various bands and teaching music. He smoked his entire adult life. Through a tobacco-stained moustache, he reminded me of how obtuse I was when I began lessons. "I still remember when you came to me," he said. "You thought the music came from the piano. I couldn't believe someone smart enough to get through medical school would think music came from a box of wires and hammers."

"Like it was magic," I answered with a smile.

Earl had a newspaper clipping taped to the wall of his studio. It quoted Arthur Rubenstein, who said if he didn't have a couple of slips in a performance, he hadn't given his best effort. That was an important lesson for me: Trying to be perfect leads to being mechanical. Over time, as Earl showed me how to feel music, not analyze it, he helped me become a better doctor, husband, and father.

Earl's chest film indicated a large lung mass, and biopsy confirmed advanced squamous-cell cancer. Earl said he did not want radiation and wanted to remain at home. I partially repaid my debt to him by arranging for hospice care and making house calls as he was dying. Thirty years later, I still have sheet music with notations scribbled by Earl with his felt pen. The pages are dog-eared and stained from turning, but they are treasures to me. They remind me of not only losing a friend and teacher but also a time when I was learning about myself and medicine and the world.

Earl is but one of the hundreds of lung cancer patients I treated during the cigarette smoking epidemic. Every morning for thirty years, I went to the hospital, greeted the nurses and ward clerks, made rounds, taught interns and residents, and saw consultations. At least once a week, lung cancer was involved. For me, it was part of the job, but for the patients, it was dread, their lives on hold while work-up proceeded. Sometimes the diagnosis would turn out to be nonmalignant, and I could feel the relief that flooded the room when I brought the good news. But more often, studies confirmed the dreaded disease, and patients' lives and the lives of their families were upended forever.

Even if surgery was possible, which it usually wasn't, the specter would preoccupy and distract them, that sick feeling that things will never again be right in the world. No longer would a chest cold be a simple, self-limited problem. Maybe it portended cancer returning or growing. Life became uncertain, never to be taken for granted. For some, the disease led to seclusion and depression; for others, it promoted reconciliation with estranged relatives, closeness with family and friends, and gratitude for the gift of life.

I coped by concentrating on what I could do to inform, reassure, and encourage. As the end approached, my focus changed to saying good-bye and helping loved ones let go. That seemed better than squeezing a few extra days of life from another round of chemotherapy or watching my patient die in the intensive care unit on a mechanical ventilator.

It is an irony of clinical medicine that my memories of one of the worst diseases to afflict humans fasten on these experiences of friendship and concern. Maybe a lesson of lung cancer can be not just suffering but also hope. The number of smokers is decreasing, and with continued effort, public policies to reduce exposure to respiratory carcinogens will succeed. Learning the genetics and immunology of cancer formation will lead to effective treatments, with therapy tailored to individual needs. It won't happen quickly and will require perseverance, but it's attainable. So, let that hope be a memorial to lung cancer patients like Ozzie, Earl, and my father.

⑬

THE LETHAL BROWN CLOUD

"Water and air, the two essential fluids on which all life depends, have become global garbage cans."

—Jacques-Yves Cousteau[1]

Western Pennsylvania is hilly and densely forested. Hemlock, fir, oak, and maple trees grow well on the Allegheny mountain slopes. Heavy rainfall supports thick forests, and the ground beneath the hills is rich in bituminous coal. Major rivers, like the Monongahela and Allegheny, flow west out of the mountains and provide access to the Ohio-Mississippi River system. In the mid-nineteenth century, this helped Pittsburgh become a major manufacturing center, and the availability of coal to heat blast furnaces led to a concentration of steel mills in the area.

Donora, Pennsylvania, sits on a horseshoe bend in the Monongahela River, twenty miles south of Pittsburgh and surrounded by hills. On October 26, 1948, Donora went from obscurity to infamy when the worst mass of polluted air in US history descended on the little town.[2]

Since 1915, American Steel and Wire Company operated a steel mill and zinc smelter in Donora. From the onset, dust and chemicals tainted the air, but the factory offered jobs to nearly half the residents, so they tolerated the smoke and congestion for more than three decades until that fateful October. Then calamity struck. Warm air high in the atmosphere above the hills trapped cool air below in an invisible canopy that meteorologists call a thermal inversion. Corrosive acids and oxides from the blast furnaces in the steel mill and zinc works combined with river fog to form a dense yellow-brown blanket of immobile air over Donora. As the factories continued to pour smoke and chemicals into the air, townspeople began to complain of coughs and difficulty breathing.[3]

Eileen Loftus, the company nurse at the steel mill, later recalled when the first affected worker staggered into her office: "He was gasping. I had him lie down and gave him oxygen. Then another man came in, and another."[4] By early evening, wheezing, panicky workers filled every bed and examining table on the premises. The eight physicians in the town rushed around to people's homes, examining patients with respiratory problems.[5] The fire chief and his staff responded to calls for oxygen, soon depleted their supply, and had to resort to borrowing tanks from nearby municipalities. The chief said, "I didn't take any myself. What I did every time I came back to the station was have a little shot of whiskey."[6]

The anxious Donorans were choking in a haze of smoke. One resident reported he had to drive his car on the left side of the road and use the curb to see the edge. The town Halloween parade became a ghostly line of shadows moving through the gloom.[7] The high school football team had to run the ball because the players couldn't see to attempt a pass.

Polluted air usually kills slowly by accelerating underlying lungs diseases, like emphysema, or heart diseases, such as coronary artery sclerosis. It is only with highly concentrated levels of pollutants that acute symptoms occur in people with normal lungs. Then, inhaling air contaminated by dust, corrosive acids, and chemical products of combustion burns the cells that form the delicate lining of the lungs. The cells react by swelling and secreting fluid. White blood cells migrate to the area and begin devouring foreign matter. A form of acute pneumonia follows, not an infectious process like with influenza but a chemical inflammation. The bronchi constrict in an attempt to protect the air sacs from injury. Oxygen can't move from the atmosphere into the bloodstream. The lungs quickly become wet and boggy, making it more difficult to inhale and exhale.

Those exposed experience cough, wheezing, and hard breathing. They feel dizzy and light-headed as their brains react to the lack of oxygen. In the most severe instances, exposed individuals drown in their own body fluids.

The first death in Donora occurred on October 29. By the next day, the three funeral homes in town had more corpses than they could handle, and the town set up a temporary morgue to cope with the casualties.[8] Before rain finally cleared the air on October 31, 20 people had choked to death, and 6,000 of the 14,000 townspeople became sick. The *New York Times* called it one of the worst environmental disasters in American history.[9]

Federal and state investigators blamed Donora's topography and the unusual weather pattern for the catastrophe and minimized the role of fumes from the steel mill and zinc smelter. The report satisfied no one except the factory owners. It based estimates of permissible levels of noxious gases on observations of healthy young workers, while those who died were over fifty and had asthma or underlying heart problems. The local paper editorialized that one didn't need scientific reports to identify the culprit; common sense and a set of eyes were enough. It was the toxic smoke.

Lawsuits followed that accused U.S. Steel, owner of both factories, of negligence. Company representatives claimed the steel mill and zinc works had been there since 1915 and procedures had not changed since then. Eventually the company settled without accepting blame. The public was outraged. Citizen groups sprang up to fight for more strict regulations, but it took two years, until 1950, before President Harry Truman convened the first national air pollution conference and cited Donora to exemplify the need. Illustrating how slowly the legislative process works, it was not until 1963, fifteen years after the Donora disaster, that Congress passed the first Clean Air Act.

In 1956, the Donora steel mill and zinc plant closed, and the town never experienced a recurrence of that horrific week. But the population shrunk to six thousand, and ironically, some residents still blame the air-quality movement for destroying the town. Donora epitomized the constant clash between the public demand for products and services and the need to breathe clean air. Donora also illustrated the requirements for an acute attack of air pollution: location in a valley or river basin, fossil fuel combustion, and a weather aberration in which winds stop blowing.

Donora was a wake-up call about the dangers of air pollution but at a terrible price. Devra Davis, writer and former Donora resident, noting a memorial plaque to those who died, said, "The thousands who died over the following decade are nowhere counted. And there is no counting of the thousands . . . who went on to suffer in various poorly understood ways."[10]

In May 2016, the World Health Organization reported that global air pollution is worsening, especially in poor countries.[11] But contamination of the atmosphere also threatens breathing in the most affluent parts of the world, like my home state of California.

We are on our way to northern California. We'll see Yosemite and Sequoia National Parks and Lake Tahoe, among nature's masterpieces, and the wine country, reminiscent of Tuscany at its most charming. As we head north from La Jolla, we navigate the smoky maze of freeways that comprise Los Angeles, cross Tejon Pass at the western edge of the Tehachapi Mountains, and descend into the Central Valley, that flat, dry table of dirt through which flows the San Joaquin River on its way to San Francisco Bay.

Traversing the valley, we enjoy the spectacle of its diversity. Canals, some paved with concrete, shimmer with ribbons of life-giving water for the green fields of vegetables and grapevines. Orange and lemon trees, fragrant with blossoms, wave at us. Orchards of peach, cherry, and apricot trees, leaves set in motion by the westerly breezes, dance as we pass. Olive groves and mounds of almonds waiting to be processed form the background. We enjoy a picnic lunch near the banks of creeks flanked by oak and sycamore and cottonwood trees that shade us while we eat.

Suntanned workers wearing wide-brimmed hats and kerchiefs to cover their necks bob up and down, pitching broccoli, lettuce, and chard into wagons. Tractors pull hoeing machines, and irrigation wheels with rotating sprinklers punctuate the green expanse of fields. Giant loads of tomatoes in open-bed trucks speed along the highways. Farmers in pickup trucks spin trails of dust into the air as they bounce along the access roads. Roadside kiosks sell sweet corn, strawberries, and blackberries to passing tourists like us.

Along Interstate 5, eighteen-wheeled rigs tear along the road, the fabric skin of their trailers shimmying in eddies of air created by trucks and buses speeding in the opposite direction. If we take State Route 99, we know that Mount Whitney, the highest peak in the lower forty-eight states, points its summit to the sky not much more than a hundred miles east in the Sierras. That reminds us that only a hundred miles away lies Death Valley, the lowest and hottest place in North America.

We drive under cloudless skies so blue they appear to have been painted, and sometimes lightning flashes over the hills and then the subtle, sharp odor of ozone follows. Later showers that drop great water drops on the parched land pummel us. After the storms pass, rainbows follow. In the winter, we inch our way through ground fog so thick that, even with headlights on, it is impossible to see more than a few feet ahead. Birds swarm along the margins of the fields, swooping to pick up gleanings. And on rare occasions, the V-shaped patterns of Canada geese emerge in the sky. Perhaps they will winter in California near the tributaries that meander out of the Sierras and flow into the Sacramento and San Joaquin, eventually to merge in the marshes of the California Delta.

We notice many more people, cars, and trucks in the Central Valley than when we first passed through forty years ago. We also notice the air looks more like Los Angeles than Lake Tahoe. (My wife classifies the sky at Tahoe as blue, Los Angeles as yellow, and the Central Valley as brown.) We stop to rest south of Stockton. The sun is a blurred halo in the murky brown haze of a windless afternoon. It seems like tiny particles of soot hit my throat when I inhale, and I wonder if I will wheeze tonight. We sleep in an air-conditioned motel and early the next morning head north to the wine country, fleeing the smog as quickly as possible. Our experience confirms what we have read: Air pollution in the valley is severe. That makes us sad.

What exactly does the term air pollution mean? The atmosphere contains many injurious chemicals, but the National Primary Air Quality Standards consider six the major pollutants: small particles of carbon, sulfur dioxide, nitrogen dioxide, carbon monoxide, ozone, and lead.[12] These result from burning coal and petroleum. The air-quality index published in many daily newspapers results from counting the quantities of these in the atmosphere and recording their levels. Smog is a mix of atmospheric pollutants thick enough to create haze or fog.

These chemicals irritate the lungs. When present in high concentrations, they cause even those with normal breathing function to cough, wheeze, and experience tightness or burning in the chest. But air pollution mostly kills by accelerating the downward spiral of such chronic lung diseases as asthma and COPD or cardiovascular diseases, like coronary sclerosis. So, it doesn't appear on death certificates as a direct cause of death.

Fresno and Bakersfield, both in California's Central Valley, are among the two most polluted cities in the United States.[13] Westerly winds blow dust particles across the fields. Speeding trucks and cars belch exhaust into the air. From Stockton in the north to Bakersfield in the south, a haze of particles stains the air gray, obscuring the view east toward the Sierras.[14] When high-pressure air ridges off the Pacific Coast prevent the usual winter storms from cleaning the air, pollution levels spike throughout California but especially in the Central Valley. A dry winter means, the next summer, fungal spores in the air will cause more cases of valley fever.

Southern California is vulnerable, as well. In their book *Smogtown*, Chris Jacobs and William Kelly described growing up in 1960s LA. They said, "Air pollution was a devil at once ironic and insidious. Over the decades it became an almost natural state requiring unnatural vigilance. Hundreds of thousands of people died from it, mostly from slow acting diseases in a toll dwarfing local losses to war, traffic accidents, and gang bloodshed."[15] California also has its share of oil refineries. These emit less sulfur oxides but more carbon and nitrogen than eastern industries that burn coal. So, California smog is different from that in eastern cities because it contains less sulfur oxides and more ozone, the pungent irritating gas formed by sunlight acting on automobile exhaust fumes. This has medical consequences.

Asthma rates among Fresno County children are three times the national average. One of seven Los Angeles school-age children has asthma, and the problem is worst among minorities and those of low income, who have greater exposure to dust, tobacco smoke, and ozone. Infants in the Los Angeles–San Bernardino–Riverside–Orange County region exposed to high levels of air particles have twice the respiratory death rate as nonexposed babies.[16] Two of my grandchildren live in Orange County. I worry about what air pollution may do to them.

Air pollution is not a new concern. Wherever humans congregate, smoke and soot follow. As far back as the third century BCE, Theophrastus, a student of Aristotle, noted that, in Athens, the "smell of burning coal was disagreeable and troublesome."[17]

The Roman historian, Seneca in 60 CE commented on the oppressive condition of the air in the city of Rome. Smog has plagued London since the middle ages. In 1285, town leaders created a commission to remedy the severe air pollution associated with sea coal–burning kilns. (Sea coal is coal washed up on beaches. It contains large amounts of sulfur.)

Charles Dickens described the city, saying, "Not only does a strange and worse than Cimmerian darkness hide familiar landmarks from the sight, but the taste and sense of smell are offended by an unhallowed compound of flavours, and all things become greasy and clammy to the touch."[18] In 1911, Dr. Harold De Voeux reported at a scientific meeting that lethal accumulation of smog had been associated with 1,100 deaths in London two years earlier.[19]

Los Angeles has been creating smog since it was first settled. As early as 1905, the city council was passing ordinances to battle smoky air.[20] When a major "gas attack" in 1943 turned the skies dark and stung the eyes and throats of residents, the war on smog began. In 1953, a blue ribbon committee appointed by the governor recommended a campaign to cut vapor leaks from refineries and filling stations, ban open burning of trash, and encourage trucks and buses to burn propane instead of diesel fuel. As the Los Angeles basin grew in size and population, pollution worsened. In 1959, scientists estimated 120,000 gallons of gasoline evaporated daily from refinery storage tanks and fuel pump nozzles at filling stations throughout Los Angeles. In southern California, the problem was cars.

I spent the summer of 1956 in Los Angeles. I lived on campus at the University of Southern California and rode the bus to work. The afternoon sun turned the air a yellowish color but did not aggravate my asthma. In retrospect, I was lucky.

In the 1960s, California put limits on tailpipe emissions and reduced the amount of lead in gasoline. By 1975, catalytic converters were mandatory in the Golden State. The state created an Air Quality Management Board to set policies and slowly improved the air Californians breathe. Ozone levels are now less than half what they were in the 1950s. Nevertheless, despite these forward-looking policies, air quality continues to preoccupy southern Californians, and Fresno, Bakersfield, and Los Angeles Counties remain near the top of the most polluted regions in the United States.

Many urban areas in the United States have experienced severe air pollution as part of the increase in population and as a consequence of the Industrial Revolution. Just as epidemics focus public attention on important infectious diseases and workplace disasters awaken consciousness of occupational hazards, smog attacks have been needed to galvanize public action to fight air pollution.

Prior to 1980, the conventional wisdom was that low-level particulate air pollution did not have any significant adverse health effects.[21] In 1979, the *American Journal of Epidemiology* reviewed the health effects of particulate air pollution and concluded there was no evidence for negative health effects from inhaling atmospheric air, at least in the United States. Conventional wisdom was wrong.

C. Arden Pope is an environmental economist at Brigham Young University. In the 1980s, he noted an association between hospital admissions for respiratory problems and the number of fine particles emitted into the air by a steel mill in the Utah Valley.[22] Strikes caused the steel mill to close intermittently, which enabled Pope to compare the fluctuations of air particles versus hospitalizations. Pope found preschool-age children were twice as likely to be hospitalized for bronchitis and asthma when the steel mill was operating versus when it was not. When he expanded his studies to include residents of several other Utah counties, he found similar trends, as well as spikes in hospital admissions for pneumonia when air quality deteriorated.

In 1992, Pope joined a group at Harvard studying air pollution and health. The researchers had access to a huge American Cancer Society database of 1.2 million people, with information on 552,138 available for review. They found, to no one's surprise, that lung and heart diseases are most prevalent among smokers, but adjusting for that factor, they found air pollution and mortality rates are connected. Most important, air pollution is related to lung cancer, chronic lung diseases, and heart disease.[23]

In 1993, the Harvard researchers published a study that showed an increase in mortality rates in cities affected by air pollution.[24] The study followed a population of eight thousand adults and children over seven years; monitored air samples; and controlled for sex, age, smoking, and job exposures. Thus, it was a very strong indictment of air pollution as a hazard to health.

Pollution, of course, is a global problem. It is particularly bad in China. Newspaper and video clips show Beijing residents wearing face masks to protect themselves from contaminated air. Studies indicate that northern Chinese live five years less than their countrymen in the south because of widespread burning of coal in the north.[25] One analysis suggested air pollution in China contributes to as many as 1.2 million premature deaths, mostly from lung and heart diseases.[26] Recently an eight-year-old girl was hospitalized in Shanghai with lung cancer, an astoundingly young age for that disease. Her physician attributed it to air pollution.[27]

Conditions in India are even worse. Studies suggest that Indians have lower lung function than their Chinese neighbors and children of Indian immigrants born and raised in the United States have better lung function than those born and raised in India.[28] While the Chinese have begun to agitate for change and the government has responded, India has been slow to deal with its pollution problems.[29] Furthermore, the situation in India exposes an added problem: indoor pollution.

We think of air pollution as coming from factories and vehicles, but cooking fires are as much a risk. In low-income countries, people burn wood, animal dung, and dry stalks of harvested crops to prepare food. These heat sources are low in energy and high in contaminants.[30] In addition, they particularly expose women and children to toxic smoke because they are the ones who use them to keep warm, as well as to do the family cooking.

Satellite photos show a huge blanket of polluted air that covers much of Southeast Asia during the winter months.[31] Called the Atmospheric Brown Cloud, it is due to particles from forest fires, burning farm wastes, vehicle emissions, soot from factories, and home cooking stoves. The haze reduces the solar energy that reaches Earth's surface and has been accused of reducing rice yields in India. The brown cloud is not confined to Asia—this soupy ceiling shows up over other parts of the globe as well. The United Nations Environment Program has indicted it as a cause of premature deaths worldwide.

Air pollution is a moving menace. Seasonal changes in temperature, wind patterns, and rainfall influence where and to what extent small particles and gases settle in the atmosphere. Climate scientists compare it to an imaginary railway that encircles the globe.[32] Think of freight cars filled with pollutants loading and unloading at various points along the route. Everyone is vulnerable.

It is not difficult to imagine that tiny specks of carbon, sulfur, and nitrogen can injure the delicate cells that line the air sacs in the lungs. But it is amazing that these supersmall particles appear to pass through the lungs, enter the circulation, and cause damage to blood vessels and the heart, as well. In 2004, the American Heart Association stated that long-term exposure to polluted air triggers heart attacks and reduces life expectancy in cardiac patients.[33] It seems these molecules cause inflammation that leads to clots and thickening of arterial walls, with risks of sudden death. Even short-term exposure appears injurious. The observations from Utah suggest that, during weeks when air quality goes down, hospital admissions for coronary events like angina and heart attacks go up.[34] It may be that exposures of only a few days are enough to trigger coronary events.

World Health Organization figures claim seven million people died in 2012 from breathing contaminated air.[35] That exceeds the number killed in traffic accidents. Most of the deaths result from contaminated air worsening lung and heart diseases. However, the seven-million figure is frightening because it is twice previous estimates, which suggests a growing problem. Imagine what it means if one out of every eight deaths that occur worldwide is partially caused by dirty air. It means we have the makings of a crisis.

The battle against pollution requires leaders to carry the banner for clean air. Professor Veerabhadran Ramanathan is director of the Center for Atmospheric Sciences at the Scripps Institution of Oceanography, part of the University of California, San Diego, located in La Jolla. A native of Madras, India, he wrote of how his grandmother would cough when she was cooking family meals over a wood-fired stove.[36] Perhaps that is why, after emigrating to the United States, he focused his research on the atmosphere. He is one of the scientists who discovered the Atmospheric Brown Cloud.

Ramanathan sees air pollution and climate change as different faces of a common enemy. He notes that black carbon, ozone, methane, and halocarbons (chemicals like Freon in spray cans and refrigerator cooling systems) cause 40 percent of the greenhouse gases that cause both air pollution and climate change. Unlike carbon dioxide, which remains in the atmosphere for hundreds of years, these pollutants have life spans of a few weeks to a few years. This means, if we reduce their atmospheric levels, we will improve air pollution and soften the effect of climate change.[37]

China, India, and the United States contribute most of the global air pollution. Under the aegis of the United Nations Environment Program, thirty nations, including the United States, have formed a Climate and Clean Air Coalition to control short-lived pollutants. We in the developed countries have access to coal, oil, and natural gas for our energy requirements, while in low-income parts of the world, people have to rely on burning wood, animal wastes, and crop residues. In these countries, most black carbon comes from cooking stoves.

Professor Ramanathan estimates India could lower its carbon emissions by half if efficient, up-to-date cooking stoves replaced traditional stoves that burn firewood and dung. This is not an exaggeration. In twenty minutes, a solar cooker that costs less than thirty dollars can heat water close enough to boiling to cook a cup of rice.[38] I proved it on my backyard patio, and it wasn't even a sunny day. A huge potential exists to reduce air pollution in the developing world.

China and India claim western-led efforts to reduce short-lived pollutants are ways to disavow responsibility for decades of carbon dioxide pollution. This has made international cooperation difficult. In addition, foreign aid to battle pollution has focused on large-scale projects. These have not succeeded because managing atmospheric pollution is a local activity. Ramanathan stumps for diplomatic policies that connect communities all over the world so they can learn best practices in controlling pollution from one another.[39]

Ramanathan is a political activist as well as a climate scientist. He advocates measuring wealth not just by gross domestic product but also by including clean air, clean water, forests, and health as assets.[40] With this in mind, he launched

Project Surya (Sanskrit for "sun"), whose goal is to substitute clean-fueled cooking stoves in households in India. In 2013, he earned the United Nations' highest environmental honor, the Champions of the Earth Award. In his acceptance remarks, he discussed cutting emissions of short-lived pollutants and said, "The response of the climate system would be fast, and the relief to human health would be fast because people would be breathing cleaner air."[41]

California cut carbon emissions from diesel engines nearly in half in the past twenty years by requiring better fuels and engine filters. Los Angeles reduced ozone levels to one-third of what they were in the 1950s by lowering emissions from power plants, oil refineries, and vehicle exhausts.[42] This has decreased the incidence of bronchitis in children.[43] In the San Joaquin Valley, similar campaigns reduced toxic emissions by 90 percent in the past twenty years.[44] But geography and internal combustion engines are formidable obstacles, and despite these major efforts, Fresno–Bakersfield and Los Angeles–Orange–Riverside–San Bernardino remain among the most polluted regions in the United States.

Public policy in the United States has made strides in the war against air pollution, but there is a long way still to go. This will require discipline, perseverance, and ingenuity by everyone: industry, government, and individual citizens. Mortality rates for lung and heart diseases have improved in communities that adopted measures to reduce fine particles in the air after the Harvard study was reported.[45]

Science can invent medical devices like filters and oxygen extractors, but these alone will not solve global air pollution. We don't have the time our predecessors did to clean up the air we breathe. Population increases around the globe mean more people need air to breathe and heat to warm and feed themselves. That means we have to be that much more inventive in our strategies to reduce ozone, nitrogen oxides, dusts, and sulfates in the atmosphere. Furthermore, air pollution aggravates climate change. World leaders understand this. In November 2015, representatives from 190 countries convened in Paris to fight climate change. Despite the wide political differences among participants, they approved a plan to reduce carbon emissions over the next decade.

Improving air pollution will ameliorate global warming. Both depend on lowering atmospheric carbon dioxide. Carrying out these commitments will give us breathing room for the future and lessen our chances of becoming a global Donora. Climate change skeptics worry that reducing burning of coal, petroleum, and natural gas could trigger a worldwide economic collapse. But cleaning up the air we breathe will decrease asthma and COPD around the globe. Cardiovascular deaths will diminish. These should lower health care costs and increase productivity. Even the incidence of premature births may diminish. The stakes are high, and the choices are ours.

III
VULNERABLE BREATHING

⑭

PANTING FOR AIR

"The face is pale, the expression anxious, speech is impossible, and in spite of the most strenuous inspiratory efforts, very little air enters the lungs."

—William Osler[1]

"It's strange that words are so inadequate. Yet, like the asthmatic struggling for breath, so the lover must struggle for words."

—T. S. Eliot[2]

Polluted air, toxins, infections, and carcinogens are external threats to breathing. They arise from the outside environment. But many forms of chronic lung disease have an internal component as well. Asthma belongs in this category. Only 10 percent of the population has asthmatic tendencies. Thus, something must be deficient in the lungs of certain people to make them vulnerable to asthma.

Mike worked as a respiratory therapist, and I was his medical director. He had asthma. One night at eleven o'clock, Mike arrived at the emergency department, panting for air. He had been fighting an asthma attack for two days and that evening deteriorated. His fiancée immediately drove him to the hospital and summoned me.

Mike was so breathless he couldn't speak. Drops of perspiration collected in his hair and trickled down his neck. His skin was pale, his tongue dry, his pulse rapid. Neck muscles bulged as he strained to exhale. Mike was on the brink of respiratory arrest and needed help right now.

Asthma is chronic reversible inflammation of the bronchi, the tiny tubules that transport air in and out of the lungs. During an asthma attack, these airways constrict, their walls swell, and mucus accumulates, obstructing flow of air. Asthma attacks cause cough, wheezing, and difficulty breathing. However, when an attack subsides, symptoms disappear and pulmonary function may become normal. Most asthma begins in childhood, and attacks recur throughout life in the majority of sufferers. A few unlucky patients develop permanent irreversible obstruction and evolve into COPD.

Asthma is formidable. It results in more than 500,000 hospital admissions every year in the United States. Ten percent of hospitalized asthmatics require treatment in an intensive care unit, and one-fifth of these need mechanical ventilation to survive. Asthma can also be lethal. It causes 3,000 deaths each year in the United States, mostly among adults, and an estimated 250,000 worldwide, especially in developing countries.

Earlier I described my first emergency room visit as a ten-year-old battling the disease. Two of my grown children and two grandchildren also have asthma. Improved treatment has enabled them to lead normal lives with minimal restrictions. Inhaled bronchodilators and steroids have warded off disability, but when hit by an upper respiratory infection, they can overnight choke up enough to force a visit to the emergency department. Fortunately, I am the last Glynn to have required hospital admission for asthma, and that was sixty years ago. But many asthmatics fare worse.

Asthma is an ancient disease. The word comes from a Greek verb meaning "to pant or to experience difficulty breathing." Chinese manuscripts from 2500 BCE mentioned it, as did Egyptian scrolls written several hundred years later. Hippocrates was the first to define it as a medical problem, and many famous medical writers over the centuries discussed its manifestations and treatment. Thus, asthma appears to have been a common problem throughout history.

In 1860, British physician Henry Hyde Salter, himself an asthma sufferer, wrote the authoritative textbook of that era on the disease, which he defined as "Paroxysmal dyspnoea of a peculiar character, generally periodic with intervals of healthy respiration between the attacks."[3] In 1892, William Osler, in his famous textbook of medicine, described asthma as due to spasm of the bronchial muscles, with associated swelling of the airway walls. Always a sharp observer, he connected it with hay fever and observed that it ran in families.[4] Osler influenced medical thinking on both sides of the Atlantic, and during the first half of the twentieth century, medical science emphasized "bronchospasm" as the mechanism of asthma.

Most treatments consisted of drugs to dilate the bronchi, to relax the constriction felt at the root of the difficulty breathing. I remember taking many of them. In addition to receiving adrenaline injections, I also drank elixirs containing ephedrine and aminophylline. Ephedrine is an adrenaline-like stimulant that opens airways, but it makes the user shake and can kill by causing abnormal cardiac rhythms. It also happens to be used to make methamphetamine, so the FDA has banned it from ordinary clinical use. Because better medicines now exist, patients with asthma aren't the worse for its removal.

Aminophylline is a stimulant widely prescribed until recently to combat bronchial spasm. Because of its risk of seizures and fatal cardiac rhythm disorders, it's out of favor today. When I was a resident in the 1960s, we struggled with respiratory patients developing tachycardia (rapid heartbeat) from adrenaline and theophylline combined. Sometimes they died.

The focus on bronchial constriction as the most important factor in asthma led to some strange remedies. When I was twelve, I was prescribed Asthmador, cigarettes made from an herb called stramonium, also known as stinkweed. It was reported the soldiers of Alexander the Great in the fourth century BCE smoked it to "relax" the lungs, and it endured into the twentieth century as a way to deliver bronchodilator directly to the lungs for fast action. My father showed me how to put the medicated cigarette into my mouth and breathe in. But when I smoked Asthmador, I coughed so hard I brought up blood, which scared my parents and limited its use in our house.

I was also ordered to drink hot coffee to alleviate asthma attacks. It tasted bitter and made me nauseated, but it did help. Caffeine is related to theophylline and is a weak bronchodilator. Unfortunately, near-toxic doses are required to observe any beneficial effect on bronchial obstruction, so don't look for Starbucks to enter the asthma business any time soon.

The worst asthma treatment of them all was syrup of ipecac. A brown liquid that looked and smelled terrible, it made me vomit. That was the idea. Extracted from the root of a poisonous plant that grows in Central and South America, ipecac induces immediate vomiting. Pediatricians used it at one time to make children eliminate poison, and many households kept a bottle on a shelf for emergency use. Its role in asthma was to create a massive outpouring of nervous impulses that caused the patient to sweat and the bronchial muscles to relax. Though it gags me just to remember it, the awful stuff did work. After retching until I thought my stomach would turn inside out, I would break into a drenching sweat but would soon breathe easier. Later generations of children can rejoice that pediatricians no longer prescribe ipecac syrup.

While wheezing children like me were chug-a-lugging ipecac, research scientists were coming to realize bronchospasm didn't explain the whole pathology of asthma. Autopsies of patients dying from asthma showed bronchi that were swollen, edematous, and clogged with thick mucus. These are hallmarks of inflammation, not spasm. Some argued of course spasm wouldn't show at autopsy; constriction and relaxation are dynamic processes that can't be seen in dead tissues. Indeed, this was the state of the art when I entered medical school in the late 1950s.

Asthma is complicated. It runs in families, affects children more than adults, and often occurs in conjunction with hay fever and skin allergies. It often occurs after workplace exposures and overlaps with bronchitis and emphysema but is different from them. Thus, researchers have sought ways to tie together these disparate observations. One avenue of thinking has pursued a connection with allergies.

Physicians have known for a long time that hay fever results from allergies. The name *allergy*, which means in Greek "another working," was coined in the early twentieth century. It described an altered type of immunity in which antibodies cause harmful inflammation instead of protection. In the 1860s, British physician Charles Blackley suspected hay fever was due to grass pollen and showed he could produce an allergic reaction in the skin by rubbing pollen particles on a scratched area.[5] In the 1920s, German researchers discovered a substance in the serum of allergic patients that produced an inflammatory bump if injected into the skin of nonallergic subjects. Skin-testing for the presence of an allergic state became popular, and pollens from grass, trees, and weeds were identified as responsible for seasonal hay fever.

Researchers also discovered inflammatory substances in eosinophils, a subgroup of white blood cells that occur in asthma, which raised further doubts about bronchospasm as the fundamental abnormality in the disease. For example, certain types of white blood cells release histamine when stimulated by allergens. Histamine produces an inflammatory response. Soon pharmaceutical companies developed histamine-blocking drugs like diphenhydramine, marketed as Benadryl, to treat allergies. These helped hay fever but had little benefit for asthma.

Allergists sought to prevent asthma by injecting tiny amounts of offending substances, like weed and grass pollen, to induce the body to create antibodies that would block the allergic reaction. This is called immunotherapy. I recall during the 1940s receiving allergy injections twice a week in hopes they would reduce asthma attacks. No one could be sure how much they helped, and I continued to wheeze. Years later, however, clinical trials showed immunotherapy does help asthma due to pollens, dust mites, dogs, and cats.

Sometimes asthma research has circled back and gained insights from drugs that work in unrelated ailments. In 1948, Hench and Kendall isolated cortisone from adrenal gland tissue.[6] It had remarkable ability to reduce the painful inflammation of rheumatoid arthritis. (Hench and Kendall won the Nobel Prize in 1950 for their discovery.) Cortisone belongs to a group of naturally occurring compounds called steroids. Vital in many areas of body metabolism, steroids exist in plants, animals, and fungi. Cholesterol and the sex hormones testosterone and estrogen are examples of important naturally occurring steroids.

Knowing rheumatoid arthritis involved immune reactions in the joints, researchers tried cortisone in other diseases where immune-induced inflammation was suspected, and asthma was among them. They figured, if anti-inflammatory drugs helped asthma, inflammation must be part of its genesis. They were right, and soon pharmaceutical manufacturers synthesized other steroid compounds, like prednisone and prednisolone, which proved to be lifesaving anti-inflammatory agents and remain widely used to this day in many areas of medicine but especially in asthma.

Meanwhile bronchospasm continued to share the spotlight with inflammation in asthma research. In the 1960s, potent, long-acting adrenaline derivatives came on the market to treat bronchospasm. Some were even sold over the counter. Soon fatalities among asthmatics increased. Asthma researcher Stephen Holgate observed, "These asthma death epidemics drew into sharp focus the shortfalls in asthma treatment and emphasized how little was understood about why the airways of asthmatics were so liable to bronchospasm."[7]

And so the asthma debate continued. Was it bronchospasm or inflammation? Allergic or nonallergic? Environmental or intrinsic? As the science of immunology progressed, investigators came to appreciate that globulin, a major protein component of blood, carries hundreds of antibodies that affect inflammation. They called them immunoglobulins. Most protect from infection, but some cause allergic reactions. They were associated with life-threatening attacks of anaphylactic shock, like after bee stings and penicillin injections. These could kill within minutes. But often it took a day or two after exposure to molds and pollens before sneezing and wheezing developed. Occasionally, it could take as long as a week for asthma to occur among workers exposed to sawdust or moldy grain. Maybe asthma was actually several entities.

Scientists learned that based on molecular size and electrical charge, at least four different types of immunoglobulin were responsible for these various reactions. Then in 1966, Kimishige Ishizaka discovered a new immunoglobulin he called immunoglobulin E, abbreviated IgE, because it was the fifth immunoglobulin recognized. IgE was elevated in asthmatics allergic to dust and pollens but not in the majority of people. If some misdirected form of immune reaction was causing inflammation in the bronchi, that would help explain what the pathologists had been saying for decades when they looked through the microscope at the lung tissue of dead asthma patients.

Epidemiologic studies shed light on who was susceptible to asthma but added to the complexity. Researchers were aware that asthma occurs more frequently in city children than in those raised in rural areas. Asthma is also more prevalent in the industrialized West than in developing countries.[8]

Maybe modern urban society, with its emphasis on cleanliness and avoiding infection, prevents infants from acquiring natural immunity to environmental agents. Perhaps exposure to animals and dusts early in life stimulates the immune system to develop resistance. For example, children in Hutterite communities, whose religion permits modern, industrialized agricultural practices, have more asthma than their Amish relations, who eschew modern agriculture in favor of traditional farming.[9] These types of observations have become known as the hygiene hypothesis and spawned a popular movement that recommends toddlers play in dirt and have household pets in order to build immunity to infections and allergens.

Population studies also suggested inhaled irritants are major asthma triggers. Tobacco smoke is by far the most important, and children growing up in a house with smokers have more asthma than children not exposed to tobacco. (Both my parents smoked.) Microscopic fragments of detritus from the bodies of insects, like mites, present in house dust, can also trigger asthma. The list of culprits goes on and on. Almost anything may be capable of becoming an allergen.

Yet asthma remains mysterious. Children have a higher prevalence of asthma mediated by IgE than do adults. But adult-onset asthmatics may develop disease from allergies or following viral infections or from working around irritants, toxic dusts, chemicals, or tobacco. Reflux of acid from the esophagus and heavy exercise may also precipitate wheezing. Adult asthma is often year-round and may progress to irreversible airway obstruction that evolves into COPD. In addition, obese people are prone to asthma. As scientists peel away the layers of asthma epidemiology and physiology, the puzzle remains unsolved.

What about genes? Because asthma often clusters in families, it's natural to explore the role of genetic factors. Take my family: Three successive generations have asthma. According to family lore, my grandmother lost several siblings from respiratory problems. But there is no way to know if any of them had asthma.

Researchers have discovered nearly one hundred genes connected with asthma.[10] However, no single gene controls inheritance of asthma or how asthma acts.[11] Some genes influence the responses of other genes to environmental stimuli. So, if a cluster of genes in certain people were defective, those individuals might react differently from normal, and an allergic reaction might be the end result.

Furthermore, genes alone aren't enough to create asthma. Susceptible individuals must also be exposed to some environmental trigger to provoke airway obstruction in asthma. Don Stevenson, allergist at Scripps Clinic in La Jolla, said that, when he was at the University of Michigan in the 1960s, many Asian students without a family history developed ragweed hay fever or asthma soon after arriving in Ann Arbor. Their families likely had the genes but not the exposure, living in a part of the world where there was no ragweed pollen in the air.[12]

In 2004, British investigators described a gene called $ADAM_{33}$ they linked to hyperreactive bronchial constriction.[13] Individuals with $ADAM_{33}$ coughed and wheezed when they breathed cold air or were exposed to dust and allergens (i.e., they were asthmatic). "Airways in asthma patients undergo a number of changes such as thickening of the airway walls and subsequent narrowing of the airway passage," said Prof. Stephen Holgate, leader of the group. He added, "[I]t is looking increasingly as if $ADAM_{33}$ is a gene involved in multiple aspects of airway modelling and remodelling."[14]

Current understanding of asthma emphasizes the idea of remodeling. The term means that repeated bouts of inflammation, whether caused by allergens, tobacco smoke, viruses, or dust, leave the bronchial walls thickened. Their inner surfaces become irregular and develop scars, like pockmarks. Also, bronchi are more than just tunnels for air. Their walls contain tiny spiral muscles that contract and relax to flex the airways open to help inhale or constrict to protect from irritants. In asthma, these become musclebound; they are twitchy and tighten under circumstances that don't affect most people, like breathing cold or dry air or exercising.

Asthmatics face risks to breathing everywhere they go. Imagine the precariousness of confronting respiratory distress whenever the weather changes. That's the predicament of severe asthmatics. I always made sure I had a supply of inhalers at my bedside, in my office, and in my car. Even as a mature physician, I still worry about being caught without a means of prompt relief when I travel. No wonder physicians used to think asthma was a psychosomatic disease caused by anxiety. Anxiety isn't the cause of asthma; it's the result.

When I saw Mike in the ER that night struggling to breathe and about to have a respiratory arrest, I had no time to reflect on the science of how he came to be in such distress. But I did know I was dealing with both airway obstruction and inflammation that were about to kill him. I didn't consciously think of the times I myself had struggled like Mike to pull air into my lungs, wondering how I could keep going, but I did understand his situation and knew the bond we shared as asthma sufferers. I had to act.

I passed a tube into his trachea and attached him to a mechanical ventilator. Using a bronchoscope, I sucked out spaghetti-like cylinders of thick mucus that formed casts of the inside of his inflamed bronchi, and I irrigated his lungs with saline solution. He quickly improved and by the next morning was able to come off the ventilator. The day after that, Mike went home. Mike married his fiancée, and the two of them moved to the Midwest. Mike has done well. He has not needed to be hospitalized since that nearly fatal night twenty years ago and follows a strict schedule of medicines daily that permits him to live without physical restrictions. He is currently a manager in the respiratory department of a prominent academic medical center and leading a normal life, a credit to himself and his profession.

We never pinpointed why Mike developed respiratory failure. It might have been a virus or an allergen or an irritant or all of these. But if his fiancée hadn't taken the initiative to bring him to the hospital, his story wouldn't have had a happy ending. Mike probably got in trouble because he tried to tough it out too long at home. Severe asthmatic patients, even knowledgeable ones like Mike, need an action plan, so that when symptoms worsen, they know exactly what to do. That is why the National Asthma Education and Prevention Program emphasizes recognizing warning signs and urges all asthmatics to have a specific written plan, like the checklists that pilots use to ensure safety in flight.

Asthma is increasing in frequency. Is it because of air pollution or novel viruses or urbanization? Science is working to understand. With improved treatments, asthma deaths are decreasing, except among African Americans, where they are rising.[15] In addition, asthmatics are twelve times more likely than the general population to develop COPD.[16] The risk for Mike and for my grandchildren is that repeated asthma attacks will lead to irreversible airway obstruction.

We have the tools to control asthma but need to deploy them widely enough to reach all those at risk. Avoiding irritants, especially tobacco, and also reducing workplace dust and household allergens remain bedrocks to prevent asthma. Drugs to relax airway constriction, adrenaline derivatives, are helpful, and new ones come on the market every year. Steroids and medicines to alter the inflammatory response remain pillars of therapy as well. In recent years, injectable monoclonal antibodies against IgE and other inflammatory triggers have been released for severe asthmatics. Investigators are just beginning to use gene therapy to tailor treatments for some causes of asthma.

In addition, innovative procedures, like heat-searing the thickened irregular surface of the large bronchi, called bronchial thermoplasty, have shown promise in situations where nothing else works. The high temperatures somehow affect the elasticity of the tiny muscles in the airway walls to diminish their reactivity.

Asthma treatment has progressed a long way forward in just two generations from smoking stinkweed and gulping ipecac to injecting steroids and monoclonal antibodies. Maybe the future Mikes of the world, as well as youngsters like my grandchildren and the children of the inner city, will enjoy a healthy adulthood because of what we are learning. What a great legacy that will be.

⑮

LUNGS THAT DO NOT COLLAPSE

"The respirations are often harsh and wheezy, and expiration is distinctly prolonged."

—William Osler[1]

"The pulmonary tissue loses entirely the slight rose tint which is natural to it, and becomes of a pale, grey color; it is denser and heavier than in its sound state, and does not collapse on opening the chest."

—René Laennec[2]

Ray was a seventy-year-old retired golf professional referred to me because of difficulty breathing.[3] He had been coughing for many years and short of breath for five years, which prompted him to stop smoking. He had lost ten pounds and recently noted his ankles were puffy in the late afternoon. The day we first met, he wore faded yellow golf slacks, a threadbare blue sweater, and a terry-cloth bucket hat perched on a curly hairpiece he left on even in the examining room. His brown and white shoes were large for a small man with a spare frame. He sat with arms braced forward and exhaled through pursed lips. Sunken hollows above his clavicles belied his emaciated state. He showed me an orange and yellow inhaler and said, "I take a whiff on this when I'm choked up. I think I have emphysema."

X-rays and pulmonary-function tests confirmed that Ray had severe obstructive lung disease, so I prescribed medications and referred him for pulmonary rehabilitation. I saw him every two months in the office, and we gradually became friends.

Ray was widowed and childless and supplemented his retirement income by giving lessons at the practice range of a golf club not far from my office. He asked me if I played golf, and I replied that I liked it but had little time to play and wasn't very good. At the end of every visit, after we discussed his respiratory status, he would invite me to come to see him for lessons.

After a while, I took him up on the offer. Because of his impaired breathing, Ray conducted teaching from a canvas director's chair. When explaining how to make shots, he stood and, with visible effort, demonstrated some aspect of the swing. On that rare occasion when I struck it just right, he would exclaim, "That's pure."

Unfortunately, over the next year, Ray's lung function deteriorated, and he went on continuous oxygen therapy. He had to stop giving lessons and began to cancel office appointments, claiming he was too weak to drive, so I made house calls. Ray lived in a tiny studio apartment near the ocean, with surfers for neighbors. It had a Pullman kitchen, a musty bed in the corner, and a single closet covered by a curtain.

Knowing the natural course of his illness was downward and concerned about his isolation, I asked him for a playing lesson to get him out. We took a cart, and near the greens, Ray would remove his oxygen tubing to chip and putt. Despite his difficulty breathing, he seemed to enjoy himself. After we finished nine holes, he told me, "That was pure."

"Let's do it again one of these days," I said, though I knew he probably didn't have enough wind to repeat the outing and that he was running out of time.

Ray's story was typical of COPD. Bronchitis usually comes first. This means the tiny tubules that transport air in and out of the lungs become chronically inflamed. The lungs have twenty-three generations of branching bronchi between the trachea and the depths of the lungs, the tubules becoming smaller with each division. Stiff rings of cartilage offer support, and muscle cells that spiral around the cylindrical walls constrict and dilate. Two types of cells form most of the inside surface of bronchi. One type produces mucus, which forms a protective blanket that absorbs dust particles and invading microbes. The other group of cells have microscopic hairs called cilia that act like brooms to sweep mucus and foreign particles from the lungs to the throat, where they can be coughed out. When they become swollen, as happens during inflammation, the airways obstruct flow of air.

In addition, over a period of years or decades, the inflammation leads to destruction of the lung substance itself, so that empty spaces replace the millions of minute air sacs. Moving air in and out becomes even more difficult, and stale gas becomes trapped. The adjacent blood vessels become distorted or obliterated. Carbon dioxide builds up, and respiratory failure ensues. That is the natural history of chronic obstructive pulmonary disease, COPD for short, and that was Ray's predicament.

Before it finally suffocates its victims, COPD grinds them down. Every breath becomes a struggle. Flesh melts away. Work is impossible. Travel and social life withdraw beyond reach. Libido becomes a distant memory. Even intellect shrinks as the disease advances, inexorably, year by year. It's easy to understand how life can seem empty, its meaning and significance lost in minute-by-minute gasping for air.

Until recently, treatment for COPD has been aimed at managing acute flare-ups of bronchitis. Ray, like most COPD patients, received bronchodilators, long-acting adrenaline derivatives, plus antibiotics and steroids to mitigate flares of acute bronchitis that aggravate scarring and destroy lung tissue. He received immunizations against influenza and pneumonia to reduce the respiratory infections that are the archenemies of COPD patients. And of course, he received supplementary oxygen and breathing exercises to help rehabilitate his respiratory muscles.

Recently, imaginative methods of collapsing emphysematous lung segments have become available and offer promise of increasing breathing capacity in COPD. Tiny valves and thin wire coils can be inserted into the lung through a bronchoscope, and surgical trimming of emphysematous lung blisters allows for expansion of functioning pulmonary tissue. So, in the future, emphysema may not be as irreversible as it has been in the past.

COPD has another dimension. Patients can be difficult to care for. Constantly out of breath, often lacking oxygen, they become irritable and demanding. Treatment controls flare-ups but does little to add productive longevity. Physicians have to be satisfied with helping COPD patients through life's crises because medical science has no cures. But occasionally, patients become friends, like Ray was to me.

COPD is a constellation of pathologies. Chronic bronchitis, meaning "inflammation of the airways," and emphysema, meaning "overdistention and destruction of the air sacs," occur together and comprise most cases of COPD. They occur later in life, affect 12 million people, and kill 135,000 a year in this country.[4] Asthma is technically a form of chronic bronchitis; however, because of its reversibility, its connection with allergy, and its prevalence among children, it is usually considered separately from COPD. Bronchiectasis, whose most frequent cause is cystic fibrosis, also leads to airway obstruction, but it is much rarer, affecting 100,000 people in this country, and is discussed later.[5]

Despite its importance, COPD is often misdiagnosed and underdiagnosed. It lacks the perverse glamour of the high-powered executive having a heart attack. It doesn't create fear in the public mind like cancer, with dreaded implications of wasting and suffering. COPD traditionally occurs in working-class people. It kills slowly and insidiously, and treatment cannot reverse its inexorable path of lung destruction. In addition, because cigarette smoking is the most notable factor leading to COPD, patients carry the stigma they have contributed to their own predicament, like alcoholics with liver cirrhosis or the morbidly obese with diabetes. Of the most prevalent serious diseases affecting Americans, COPD research is the least well-funded by the federal government relative to its public burden.[6]

The final call came on a Monday afternoon. Ray couldn't breathe. I told Gayle, my medical assistant, to call 911 for him. When I arrived at the intensive care unit, the staff had inserted a tube into his trachea and had begun mechanical ventilation. The interns and residents were at his bedside. Without his hairpiece, he looked shrunken and desiccated. He stared at me through eyes that showed panic and terror.

I discussed strategy with the interns and residents. "This is his first bout of respiratory failure. Let's ventilate him overnight and see what happens." In Ray's room, I held his hand and said, "Hang in there. Give us a few hours to see if we can turn this around. I know the tube hurts, but the ventilator is doing the work your lungs can't do right now."

I slept poorly that night. Ray's eyes haunted me. Statistically, if we kept Ray on a ventilator, he had a 75 percent chance of stabilizing, maybe living another year or two. But Ray wasn't a statistic. He was my friend. He hadn't wanted to talk about what to do when he couldn't make decisions on his own behalf. He had no relatives. I should have been more forceful in pushing him to make a plan. It would be cruel to commit my friend to perhaps weeks of discomfort on a breathing machine so that he might spend his last days languishing in that apartment or a nursing home. Yet, who was I to decide what constituted a life worth living?

When the next morning arrived, I had decided what to do. Ray was stable, and I used that to justify disconnecting the ventilator. "We're going to take the tube out," I said. "We'll continue oxygen and the breathing treatments, but no more machines." I held his hand as the respiratory therapist removed the tube from his throat. But he remained unresponsive.

"Remember, no CPR; no code if he stops breathing," I told the nurses and house staff. "I'll be up on the floor. Call me for any changes." That afternoon, Ray died. He was seventy-two.

Ray's last hours struggling with end-stage COPD made me think about what comprises extraordinary care and how best to look after patients at the end of life. Ray's COPD led me to establish a bioethics committee at the hospital to help doctors, patients, and families struggling with these kinds of decisions. Though I never said it to anyone, I thought of the bioethics committee as my memorial to Ray.

Ray had typical COPD, with elements of both bronchitis and emphysema, so he illustrated how most cases evolve. But some individuals have almost pure bronchitis without much emphysema, and some have emphysema without much bronchitis. Their symptoms are different, but their outcome is the same.

Rosemary was referred because of sleepiness. An attorney who specialized in representing children, she was nodding off during trials and conferences, which interfered with her work. When I introduced myself, I was struck by the firmness of her handshake. She was stocky, with gray-brown hair coiffed simply and earrings but no makeup. She wore a dark-skirted power suit over a plain white blouse. Only puffy skin and swollen ankles above flat-heeled shoes belied her medical problem.

Rosemary had been coughing for years. Once a heavy smoker, she quit when she noticed herself becoming tired when she climbed stairs. The fatigue progressed slowly, and she endured it until she started to feel drowsy at work. Her internist diagnosed COPD and recommended using supplemental oxygen, but she refused, choosing instead to tough it out.

Physical findings were significant: bluish fingernail beds, quiet breath sounds, and noticeable ankle edema. Chest X-rays and pulmonary function tests pointed to severe obstructive lung disease. Her blood oxygen level was markedly reduced and her carbon dioxide elevated. Rosemary's oxygen was so low she was like someone living in the Andes, where the altitude reduces the amount of oxygen in the air. Without oxygen, her blood lost its redness, and her heart couldn't pump, causing fluid to engorge her tissues. Rosemary had the bronchitic version of COPD with respiratory failure.

When I also suggested supplemental oxygen, she balked. She was already on bronchodilators and was up to date on her immunizations. She was amenable to learning exercises to strengthen her breathing muscles and increase her overall endurance—but oxygen, no.

Her internist had briefed me this would be the sticking point. He told me her life was dedicated to her work. Never married, she had fought her way to the top rank in her profession, jousting on behalf of women and children in the male-dominated arena of the courtroom. A friend who was a judge later told me Rosemary enjoyed the highest respect in local legal circles.

I asked her why no oxygen. She shook her head, a definitive gesture, and explained in language to this effect: "You don't understand. I can't appear in court or at the conference table showing any hint of weakness." I countered with the observation that studies showed COPD patients' cognitive abilities improve when they begin using oxygen, which was true but not why she felt distress. Her head again shook, no. I respected her choice, but oxygen was the most important therapy I had to offer her.

COPD patients with predominant chronic bronchitis have great difficulty oxygenating their blood and retain carbon dioxide much more than those with predominantly emphysema. They don't appear to be working as hard to breathe as those with emphysema, but the oxygen deficiency causes the pulmonary blood vessels to constrict, which leads to hypertension in the lungs. This, in turn, creates increased back pressure in the veins leading to the lungs, which makes the legs swell. The low amount of oxygen supplied to the brain causes them to be drowsy and their skin to be blue, while the high venous pressure causes edema. Pulmonologists have nicknamed these patients "blue bloaters." They make up 10 to 20 percent of COPD patients.

Rosemary soldiered on for several more years. She received most of her care from her internist but regularly came to see me as well, and awareness of her dilemma heightened my admiration. I don't think she ever did use oxygen, not even while at home. My last recollection of her was the lengthy obituary when she finally died. Sometimes serious disease begets courage, a lesson the Rosemaries in our midst teach the rest of us.

In contrast, some COPD patients have pure emphysema with minimal indications of bronchitis and present a much different picture. Sam was sixty years old and had been short of breath for years but was worsening. Japanese American by birth, he grew up in Los Angeles and contracted tuberculosis when he was in his early twenties. After several months in a sanatorium, his lungs healed, but he became a two-pack-a-day smoker. Sam worked as a delivery truck driver, but by the time he reached fifty, he could no longer perform his job and had to quit, subsisting thereafter on social security disability payments. Never married, without friends or relatives, Sam lived alone in a small apartment in central San Diego. He rode the bus to my office.

As his breathing worsened, Sam lost what muscle mass he had, and by the time he came to see me, he weighed less than 130 pounds. When he breathed, he tensed his neck muscles and pursed his lips. He leaned forward while seated, and with his shirt off, his clavicles, scapulae, and most of his ribs were visible; he looked starved. Sam's breath sounds were so quiet they were barely audible, even with a stethoscope on his chest.

Chest X-rays showed his lungs to be overinflated, with the diaphragm pushed down and flat, and hardly any blood vessels visible in the lung substance. Pulmonary function tests confirmed severe obstruction to airflow and trapping of air in the lungs during exhalation. Despite this advanced impairment, Sam's blood oxygen was only minimally reduced, and carbon dioxide levels were normal. These were the characteristics of emphysema without bronchitis.

The emphysematous form of COPD destroys the tiny lung air sacs, so they become replaced by large inelastic bubbles. Each lung normally contains a million of these sacs. If flattened out, their area would be almost the size of a tennis court.[7] The disease reduces surface area and, because of inelasticity, causes air to be trapped during exhalation. Emphysematous lungs are flabby, like an overstretched balloon. René Laennec, the nineteenth-century French physician, first described the pathology of emphysema.[8] He commented that, during an autopsy, the first thing he noticed on opening the chest of someone with emphysema was that the lungs did not collapse as they normally would when air entered the pleural space. This indicated they were overinflated and were trapping air.

Pathologists now know that, in severe cases of emphysema, the air bubbles can become as large as golf balls and crowd normal or less affected areas. An emphysematous lung sliced in half looks like spongy Swiss cheese.

Individuals with pure emphysema work tremendously hard to breathe and maintain ventilation at near-normal levels until the end of life. This requires so much energy they lose weight and become emaciated. Among physicians, they are known as "pink puffers." Whereas a normal person uses less than 3 percent of their energy to breathe, someone with emphysema may expend a third of all caloric intake just to force air in and out of the lungs.

Over the next ten years, I saw Sam on a regular basis in the office. Isolation and depression dogged him like a black cloud. I referred him for pulmonary rehabilitation at UC San Diego and added antidepressant medications to his inhalers, but these achieved little for him. Indeed, I felt that the office staff and I helped Sam the most simply by accepting him and seeing him regularly.

Unfortunately, Sam's end was tragic. He developed acute distress, similar to what happened to Ray, and called 911. Paramedics took him to a small hospital near where he lived, and there he was treated with mechanical ventilation in the intensive care unit. No one in my office knew what happened until several weeks later, when we learned he had been moved to a nursing facility in El Cajon, east of San Diego.

The next Friday, I drove out to visit Sam. It was a warm October afternoon, and I passed a high school where a football team was scrimmaging. The nursing home was one story high, with white stucco walls and surrounded by eucalyptus trees. Inside, the atmosphere was dark. Patients in wheelchairs lined the halls, some asleep, some silently watching me find my way to Sam's room.

When I saw him, I felt like my stomach was loaded with lead weights. He was tied down, attached to a ventilator, with a tracheostomy in his neck, receiving liquid feedings by means of a tube in his stomach. I saw no sign he recognized me, no squeeze of my hand when I held his. He rolled his eyes and looked around the room aimlessly. I asked his nurse if he seemed uncomfortable, and she said she didn't think so.

I wrestled with what I should do. I knew Sam had no hope of recovery and no advocate. I didn't know the doctor attending Sam. Why were they prolonging his dying? Should I intervene and try to have him transferred to my care near Scripps Mercy Hospital? Knowing that would be virtually impossible to achieve, I mumbled a few words of encouragement to Sam and drove home, sad and empty-hearted. The high school football team was still practicing. This was not how I wished Sam could finish his life. Sam died quietly several weeks later. I never learned details of the end, maybe because I didn't want to face how the medical system let him down.

Sometimes emphysema is due to a genetic defect. During infection, the lungs are inflamed, and tissues are swollen and reddened. For healing to occur, nature must slow down the inflammatory reaction, like applying brakes in a car to prevent runaway. The liver makes a substance called AAT (alpha-1 antitrypsin) that inactivates inflammatory enzymes in the lungs. Individuals lacking AAT are prone to developing emphysema.

AAT deficiency is responsible for only a small fraction of the 12 million cases of emphysema in the United States but is significant because it shows a mechanism by which lung destruction occurs in COPD. The few patients I saw with AAT deficiency developed emphysema in their forties and were a challenge to treat. Concentrated plasma rich in AAT is available to stave off the inexorable degeneration that otherwise causes premature respiratory failure. This is a major area of respiratory research and portends a better life to come for those lacking this essential protection.

Most people with COPD have both bronchitis and emphysema, like Ray, though some, like Rosemary and Sam, have minimal amounts of one and much of the other. Furthermore, often asthma and COPD overlap. Both are common, and there may be some interconnected inflammatory process. In the majority of patients, repeated infection and irritation gradually cause irreversible damage to the bronchi and in time destroy the air sacs, as well. But both groups eventually develop respiratory failure, so being bronchitic versus emphysematous makes little difference in long-term outlook.

Patients like Ray, Rosemary, and Sam illustrate the spectrum of ways COPD manifests but also demonstrate the dilemmas the disease creates for caregivers. COPD challenges not only the technical skills of physicians but their ethical views, as well. More on this later.

COPD is the most frequent reason patients need mechanical assistance to breathing for more than a few hours. (Surgical patients frequently need postanesthetic breathing support but rarely longer than overnight.) In 2012, the most recent year for which figures are available, COPD killed three million people globally, which makes it one of the most prevalent causes of death worldwide.[9]

Furthermore, among the big killers of adults—cardiovascular disease, cancer, and respiratory disorders—lung diseases are on the upswing.[10] With cigarette smoking declining in prevalence, epidemiologists aren't sure why this is the trend. It may relate to aging of the population or atmospheric pollution or that breathing disorders are diagnosed later in their course. These grim statistics tell us we need to recognize the threat COPD entails and devote sufficient resources toward its eradication. Then, Ray, Rosemary, and Sam won't have died in vain.

16

THE GREAT MASQUERADER

"All men live enveloped in whale-lines. All are born with halters round their necks; but it is only when caught in the swift, sudden turn of death, that mortals realize the silent, subtle, ever-present perils of life."

—Herman Melville[1]

Marlene was a thirty-year-old deputy sheriff referred from the hospital emergency room because of asthma. For several months, she had been experiencing attacks of shortness of breath and wheezing. These would come on without warning, sometimes during activity, sometimes at rest. The episodes made her feel anxious and fearful but would subside in an hour or so, only to recur a few days later. They were not associated with any coughing, chest pain, or excess mucus.

Marlene had enjoyed good health, with no prior history of asthma, allergies, or any sort of breathing problems. She had never smoked. She had been in the Navy for four years, then with the sheriff's office for six years, and was deployed as a matron at the county jail. Of note was that she had recently broken up with a long-standing boyfriend and was trying to establish a new place for herself in the singles' world.

Except for carrying 150 pounds on a 5'4" frame, which was slightly overweight, her physical exam was normal. Her lung sounds were clear, and her chest X-ray and pulmonary function tests were normal. I was unsure of her diagnosis but prescribed a long-acting bronchodilator by inhalation and asked that she return in two weeks. At the second visit, she was unimproved, and so

I added a steroid inhaler and asked her to let me check her again in two weeks, after I returned from vacation.

While I was away, Marlene experienced a more severe spell of wheezing that frightened her enough to send her to the emergency room, where nothing wrong was found. She followed up in the office with one of my associates, who also could see no abnormalities and told her to see me when I returned.

I had been back on the job only a few days when the call came from the emergency room. Marlene had been brought in by paramedics and was in shock. "I think she's had a pulmonary embolus," said the ER physician.

Clots in the lungs, called emboli, originate in the deep veins of the legs, from where they break off, enter the stream of blood flowing toward the heart, and lodge in the pulmonary blood vessels. The term emboli comes from a Greek word meaning "things hurled." Occasionally, emboli may start in pelvic blood vessels after surgery or injury to the lower torso. On rare occasions, clots begin in the arms (associated with intravenous catheters) but hardly ever arise on their own in the lung.

Small clots cause no symptoms because they obstruct only tiny vessels, but large ones cause shortness of breath, cough, expectoration of blood, and sometimes immediate death. When a clot blocks flow of blood through a branch of the pulmonary artery, a reflex constricts both vessels and airways nearby. Blood coming afterward is diverted in order to keep pressure from increasing, thus it has no contact with the alveoli and so does not pick up oxygen. As the oxygen level in the lung falls, vascular constriction worsens, creating a vicious cycle of low oxygen, constriction, and further oxygen lowering.

The right ventricle of the heart pumps furiously to compensate, but if the embolus is large enough to block a major pulmonary artery, the heart can't keep up. Deprived of oxygenated blood, the left ventricle also fails. The heart then goes wild, beating rapidly and irregularly. Shock and death follow, often within a few minutes.

Precise figures are unknown, but almost a million people each year in the United States develop blood clots in their legs.[2] More than a third of these migrate to the lungs as silent pulmonary emboli, or PEs, and untreated, almost a third of these are lethal.[3] Between 60,000 and 100,000 people die of PE every year.[4] In a quarter of these fatal cases, no warning symptoms occur, and death is sudden and immediate. This makes PE among the most frightening conditions encountered in clinical medicine.

Medical science was slow to recognize a connection between blood clots in the veins of the legs and in the arteries of the lung. In the early eighteenth century, the Italian physician Giovanni Morgagni reported observing clots in the lungs at autopsy in patients who died suddenly but confessed he couldn't figure out where they came from.[5] A century later, Jean Cruveilhier, a French pathologist, called blood clots in the lungs pulmonary apoplexy, likening them to strokes in the brain, an apt comparison. But he postulated they were due to blood vessel inflammation, overlooking the possibility they reached the lungs from the legs. Even his brilliant contemporary, René Laennec, the inventor of the stethoscope, who first described the pathology of pulmonary emphysema, likewise appeared unable to connect clots in the lungs and clots in the legs.

It fell to Rudolph Virchow at the University of Berlin, the father of modern pathology, in the mid-nineteenth century to finally explain what happens. Virchow described venous thrombosis, the medical term for clot formation, and pulmonary embolism. He postulated blood clots formed in the legs and gradually enlarged, snowball-like, as red blood cells and sticky proteins congealed. Eventually the clots broke off, traveled through the bloodstream, and finally lodged in the lung. Virchow established three conditions that led to venous thrombosis. These are still used today. Virchow's triad consists of blood vessel injury, blood flow slowing, and blood hypercoagulability.

Injury to blood vessels can occur from trauma or surgery. Wounded tissues release proteins and enzymes that initiate clotting as part of nature's efforts at repair and healing. Extensive procedures, like total hip and knee replacement, are especially risky, which accounts for the orthopedic focus on postop walking and moving to prevent clotting.

Blood flow can slow and clotting can start under many situations. Surgery need not be grave. I received a call one night from a neighbor recuperating from a hernia repair who became short of breath. He had pulmonary emboli without evidence of leg vein clots. There was no way to be certain whether he developed clots from the surgery or the enforced postoperative immobility.

Completely normal situations may slow the flow of blood and facilitate fatal clots. Pregnancy is associated with stratospherically high levels of estrogens and progesterone, and as the uterus enlarges, it imposes resistance to blood flow from the lower body. Even prolonged sitting is risky. I took care of an air force sergeant who drove twelve hours without stopping to avoid being AWOL after a weekend leave. He arrived on base at 11 PM and an hour later came to the base hospital because he was unable to breathe. He had a PE. In 1940, during the German Blitz, several Londoners died of pulmonary emboli that occurred after they sat on deck chairs for prolonged periods in air-raid shelters.[6] Some have speculated that leg blood clots may be present without symptoms in as many as 10 percent of long-flight air passengers.[7]

In 2003, New Zealand researchers coined the term eThrombosis when they reported the case of a thirty-two-year-old man who worked at a computer terminal all day long and experienced life-threatening pulmonary emboli.[8] And there are victims of "couch potato clots." Japanese researchers recently reported an increase in fatal pulmonary embolism among people who watch television more than five hours a day.[9] These anecdotes are twenty-first century manifestations of this silent, frightening killer.

Before I could get to the ER, Marlene had a cardiac arrest and died. Autopsy showed a massive PE. I couldn't sleep for several nights. I reviewed her medical records, trying to figure out how I missed the diagnosis. Tucked away in her history, I found the answer. She had been taking birth control pills. Oral contraceptives contain estrogen and progesterone, hormones known to facilitate blood clotting. Ever after, I was hypervigilant about PE. I am sure I spent thousands of dollars unnecessarily ordering lung scans looking for clots in young women with obscure breathing problems. But I was determined never again to overlook the diagnosis of pulmonary embolism.

Had Marlene experienced more symptoms or had I been more alert, her story would have been different. If she had been short of breath or had chest pains or pleurisy (chest pain with deep breathing) or coughed up blood, these would have flashed a red light she had something other than asthma, and that might have saved her life.

Her blood oxygen level would have been measured, an ultrasound probe would have scanned her legs to look for venous clots, and she would have undergone a radioisotope lung scan. A CT scan of the blood vessels would have identified clots lodged in the lungs. These would have diagnosed the lung emboli.

Marlene would have been rested and received oxygen. Most important, she would have received anticoagulants until existing clots solidified and ceased to threaten her. Initial anticoagulation would have been with intravenous heparin, which works immediately. Then Coumadin, which is given orally but works slowly, would have been substituted. That would have been continued at least three months, until it was certain no more clots were lurking in her leg veins to kill her.

I would have advised Marlene to stop oral contraceptives and use some other form of pregnancy prevention, plus urged her to lose that extra weight that may have been making blood flow through her leg veins more sluggish. I would have warned her about the possibility of recurrence and how important it was she not sit immobile for prolonged periods of time, like during an airplane flight or automobile ride.

If anticlotting medications weren't sufficient and emboli continued to reach her lungs, I would have offered Marlene a filter, a miniature umbrella inserted into the vena cava, the main vein that conveys blood to the heart from the lower body. The filter would have blocked large emboli from obstructing the blood flow in her lungs.

With these approaches, she probably would have survived, regained normal pulmonary function, and been alive today, though there was no guarantee. Some people continue to have difficulty breathing afterward and suffer recurrent deep vein thrombosis. And for a few unlucky patients, the clots never resolve.

Trish was a forty-eight-year-old woman referred because she was short of breath. She had a past history of blood clots in her legs. When she started to feel tired with normal exercise, her internist suspected recurring leg clots with emboli to the lungs. But she had no sign of clots in the legs or in the pulmonary circulation. Nevertheless, he started Trish on Coumadin in case silent clots were hiding deep in the venous system. However, Trish's situation was not only mysterious but also risky.

Trish was highly resistant to Coumadin. She had a genetic quirk that metabolized anticoagulants rapidly. She required doses fifteen times higher than usual to maintain a satisfactory level of anticoagulation. Her doctor feared she would hemorrhage and bleed to death. In addition, Trish lived a turbocharged existence. If people were cars, she would be a Porsche. She was married, without children, and was a partner in a high-powered business consulting firm that sent her all over the country, tackling complicated projects. Her hobby was skydiving. I liked her and admired her enthusiasm and her spirit of adventure, though I wondered about her judgment in jumping out of airplanes 10,000 feet above ground while on whale-sized doses of a potent anticoagulant.

I worried she had pulmonary hypertension due to a continuing stream of hundreds of small clots plugging the tiny end branches of her lung arteries. But she could have pulmonary hypertension from some other cause, such as thickening of the pulmonary blood vessels. Plus, sometimes patients develop pulmonary hypertension for reasons medical science can't fathom at all.

These questions mattered a lot because, for her, prolonged anticoagulation was difficult and risky. So, I was in a quandary. By good luck, at the University of California, San Diego, (UCSD) only a mile away from my office, was a center for research on pulmonary vascular diseases. Maybe they could help.

Kenneth Moser was head of the pulmonary division at UCSD. For Trish's difficult diagnostic problem, he was definitely the go-to guy. In 1973, he and cardiac surgeon Nina Braunwald had reported the case of a sixty-seven-year-old man with gradually worsening shortness of breath, a story that in many ways resembled that of Trish. Studies showed he had blood clots in his lungs blocking flow and raising pressure throughout the pulmonary circulation.

The man underwent successful surgical removal of the blood clots. But the unusual feature of his case was that blood vessels in areas of his lungs affected by clots appeared thickened and fibrotic, while vessels in lung areas not involved with clots were normal.[10] Moser was not sure why. He speculated that perhaps microscopic hemorrhages into the vessels around the clots had damaged the surface of the artery walls. This could produce scars in the small vessels, a process sometimes seen in coronary arteries after a heart attack.

When blood vessels are injured, their walls become tougher and less elastic, like how a rubber garden hose that sits in the sun eventually loses its flexibility. In a garden hose, this leads to cracks and leaks. In lung and heart tissue, it leads to poor blood flow.

Moser gradually accumulated other patients with this unusual problem, and the UCSD thoracic surgeons developed expertise in removing clots and stripping out the fibrotic tissue lining the adjacent pulmonary arteries. This is time-consuming, technically challenging surgery, and only a few centers around the country had enough experience to achieve good results. But the pulmonary vascular team slowly came to realize the defect was not a problem in persisting clots; it was a problem in the blood vessels reacting to the clots. The fibrotic tissue in the pulmonary artery branches represented an aberrant response: scar formation instead of clot dissolution.

At UCSD, X-rays probed the architecture of Trish's pulmonary arteries, and pressure sensors measured the pressures and flows of blood in her lungs. Her vascular pressure was indeed high, but no clots were found. Even the UCSD team seemed unsure whether she suffered from chronic emboli but recommended she continue on Coumadin and agreed to follow her progress with her internist and me, thereby spreading the worry and, I hoped, increasing the chances of spotting trouble early. Trish was able to breathe well enough to continue working and, if memory serves me correctly, did agree to retire from skydiving.

Unfortunately, Trish was lost to follow-up, and her outcome is a mystery. Her best chance for improvement was to undergo surgical removal of residual clots, with stripping away the scar tissue inside the pulmonary vessels, the technique pioneered by Moser. This would reduce the load on her heart and permit her right ventricle to regain its strength. The UCSD surgeons have now performed more than three thousand of these procedures. Other centers around the country have also developed programs to offer this lifesaving operation to this perplexing group of patients.

Pulmonary embolism is a great masquerader. It can look like pneumonia, pleurisy, asthma, or tuberculosis. It can occur unexpectedly, like a heart attack, and cause instantaneous death, as happened to Marlene. Or it can resolve unobtrusively, leaving not more than a few microscopic scars in the lungs as footprints. Or it can bring on slow damage to the lungs, with pulmonary hypertension, like Trish experienced. It is as though emboli enjoy donning a disguise when they attack patients and confuse doctors. Because of this, pulmonary embolism is one of the most fearsome problems clinical medicine confronts: a stealthy, silent killer, who may attack suddenly or slowly, violently or subtly, to cripple breathing temporarily or permanently end it.

Venous clots and pulmonary emboli represent yet another of the curious paradoxes that permeate medicine. There is a good and a bad, a yin and a yang, a Jekyll and a Hyde. Blood clotting is essential to survive injury, yet reparative processes can morph into major killers without an inkling of warning. Nature is generous, mysterious, and capricious. She gives and takes away, and we have to adapt to her vagaries. We ought never to think of ourselves as being in charge, even when we feel at our most confident and sophisticated.

17

CELLS LIKE ELONGATED CRESCENTS

"The problem, Dear Brutus, lies not in the stars / But in ourselves, that we are underlings."

—William Shakespeare[1]

"He accepted each day as a gift he wasn't going to waste."

—Todd Steck[2]

December 26, 1904, the Monday after Christmas, was chilly and cloudy in Chicago, with snow forecast for later in the day. *The Tribune*, the city's biggest newspaper, reported on how President Theodore Roosevelt and his family had spent the holiday at the White House, and international news covered the Japanese siege of Russian fortifications in Port Arthur, Manchuria. The paper featured a cartoon showing Santa Claus empty-handed, saying he had given away his entire inventory of presents. Wasn't that enough to make everyone happy?

At Presbyterian Hospital, on the near-west wide, in the heart of the medical district of the city, Dr. Ernest Irons, a senior intern, was going about his tasks, when he was called to see a twenty-year-old black man named Walter Clement Noel, who'd come to the hospital with a two-day history of chills, fever, and cough. As he went to examine the patient, Irons may have enjoyed a chuckle at a patient named Noel showing up the day after Christmas but could not have realized Santa Claus was belatedly bringing a medical puzzle that would make Irons part of medical history.

Walter Clement Noel was born on the island of Grenada, in the eastern Caribbean, of African ancestry. In September 1904, he came to Chicago to enroll at the Chicago College of Dental Surgery. Noel came from a wealthy land-holding family who was able to pay for his education.[3] Race relations had begun to change at the turn of the twentieth century. Emancipated black people, many rural and impoverished, moved north after the Civil War to find a better life. They needed medical care, and the call for black health professionals grew loud. Chicago drew its share of southern immigrants, and its black professional population grew as well, partly because local white professional schools accepted black students. It was this chance for a first-rate education that drew Noel from his tropical home to the cold Windy City on the shores of Lake Michigan.

Noel had grown up healthy except for a bout of yaws, an infectious skin disorder common in warm climates. This left him with ulcers over his legs that slowly formed scars though did not impair his physical activity. In the year prior to his coming to Chicago, he had been short of breath and had spells when his eyes turned yellow. In late November, he began to cough, and on Christmas Eve, his cough grew worse, and he felt a chill.

Irons recorded a temperature of 101°F and described Noel as a bright and intelligent young man, with a tinge of yellow in the sclera of his eyes. Irons noted dullness at the lung bases during percussion, as well as crackling sounds over both sides of the chest. These findings indicated lung consolidation, likely due to pneumonia. In addition, Irons observed that Noel's heart was enlarged but couldn't connect that finding to the rest of the case.

The blood examination was markedly abnormal, with a hemoglobin level only 40 percent of normal, denoting a severe anemia. Most striking was the microscopic appearance of Noel's red blood cells, which showed extreme variation in size and color. Many were abnormally shaped, forming elongated crescents, like a new moon, or sickle-shaped, as Irons called them, using an image from his childhood in Iowa.[4]

Irons alerted his attending physician, James B. Herrick, about the curious findings, and Herrick was also at a loss to "account for this peculiar complexus [sic] of symptoms."[5] Herrick was one of the most prominent physicians in Chicago at that time, and a leader in the emerging field of internal medicine. Besides his role as attending physician at Presbyterian, he was a senior physician at Cook County Hospital and professor of medicine at Rush Medical College.

The two physicians were mystified. What was causing this strange anemia? Why was Noel's heart enlarged? Consumed with curiosity, they wracked their brains to come up with some plausible diagnosis. Maybe the blood abnormalities somehow related to the previous yaws infection—but they couldn't find any sign of yaws being active. The organism that causes yaws is in the same family as the spirochete that causes syphilis. Was this as a strange manifestation of that most-feared infection? They couldn't confirm that diagnosis either. Noel came from the tropics, and so they speculated on some exotic parasitic infection—but had to abandon that explanation as well for lack of evidence. They hypothesized whether Noel had ingested some drug or toxin that was poisoning his bone marrow—but blood and urine tests were negative, so that also was a blind alley.

Herrick and Irons treated their patient with "rest, nourishing food, and syrup of the iodid [sic] of iron."[6] Noel's fever abated, the crackling sounds in his lungs disappeared, and his red blood cell count improved, though the peculiar elongated cells persisted in blood film exams. After four weeks, he felt well and left the hospital without a diagnosis.

Noel remained under medical care. A year later Irons readmitted him to Presbyterian with a bout of bronchitis. The sickle-shaped cells were still there. In May 1906, Noel developed a swollen knee after wrenching it accidentally. Irons withdrew fluid from the joint but found nothing to aid in determining the root cause of the young man's recurring difficulties.

Herrick couldn't get the case out of his mind. He consulted Professor Ludwig Hektoen, a prominent local pathologist, for help. Together, they tried to make red blood cells turn sickle-shaped by experiments, like dissolving them in diluted sugar solution, but failed, and the strange sickling phenomenon remained undecipherable.

In April 1907, Noel reported to Herrick he had been hospitalized elsewhere the previous February with muscular rheumatism, consisting of fever, back pain, and aching arms and legs. He was still short of breath, as well. Herrick remained frustrated at his inability to unravel the mystery. Soon after, Noel graduated from dental school and returned to Grenada, never to be seen again by Herrick nor Irons.

But Herrick didn't forget Noel. In 1910, Herrick presented the case to the Association of American Physicians and published a case report, though the cause of the abnormal red blood cells remained a mystery. The medical establishment received the report with hardly a ho-hum, which disappointed Herrick so much he began to channel his energies into a new interest, cardiac diseases.[7]

Soon afterward, however, several cases similar to Noel made their way into the medical literature, and over the next four decades, medical science learned about sickle-cell anemia, as it was called. The disease ran in families and was caused by a genetic mutation that produced an abnormal form of hemoglobin in the victim's red blood cells. Any condition in which body oxygen levels fell, like an infection, could trigger a crisis, with red blood cells lumping into miniature clots and causing death of adjacent tissues.

Sickle-cell disease is a blood, not a respiratory, abnormality, but pulmonary complications are the most frequent cause of death in sickle-cell patients. Sickle-cell disease causes three types of respiratory problems: an acute chest syndrome resembling pneumonia, aggravation of coexisting asthma, and hypertension of the pulmonary blood vessels.

The acute chest syndrome occurs when aggregates of red blood cells block pulmonary blood vessels, causing lung tissue to consolidate and acquire the consistency of liver. Patients cough, wheeze, and have chest pain and difficulty breathing. Affected areas resemble pneumonia on X-ray, and indeed, infection is often a component. Walter Clement Noel likely had an acute chest syndrome when he went to the hospital in 1904.

One published series that followed a group of sickle-cell sufferers over two years suggests 30 percent of patients experience acute chest syndrome during that time. Usually these episodes are self-limited but can progress to acute respiratory failure and death.[8] Treatment relies on analgesics, which may include narcotics for pain, plus oxygen and IV fluids because these patients often become dehydrated. In addition, blood transfusions for severe anemia and hydroxyurea, a drug that reduces red blood cell clumping, are standard therapy. However, over the years, patients who survive multiple episodes of acute chest syndrome develop lung scarring, leading to respiratory insufficiency and premature death.

Sickle-cell disease also aggravates asthma, its second respiratory effect. Asthma is prevalent among African Americans, especially children. Thus, a number of youngsters have both conditions. Sickle-cell patients with asthma are more vulnerable to attacks of wheezing than the general population and are at greater risk of death.

The third major respiratory complication of sickle-cell disease is hypertension of the pulmonary circulation.[9] When sickle cells mass together in the lung capillaries, oxygen can't cross from inhaled air to the blood. Thus, the oxygen level in the lung falls. This sets in motion a vicious circle of low oxygen, sickle-cell aggregation, vessel obstruction, and further lowering of oxygen. The heart pumps harder, but eventually, as more pulmonary capillaries become obstructed, it can't keep up. Blood backs up in the lungs, pressure within the lungs rises, and eventually heart failure and death occur. This is probably why Walter Clement Noel's heart was enlarged and why he had been short of breath during the year before he went to Presbyterian Hospital for help.

Sickle-cell disease is one of the most prevalent genetic disorders in the world.[10] It has existed in Africa for thousands of years.[11] More than 200 million individuals worldwide carry the sickle-cell gene. In the United States, 100,000 African Americans suffer from sickle-cell disease, and 3 million have the sickle-cell trait, meaning they carry one abnormal gene.[12]

After he returned to his native Grenada, Walter Clement Noel opened a dental office in St. George and became a successful practitioner. He never married and died in 1916 at the age of thirty-two. His death certificate indicated asthenia due to pneumonia as the cause of his demise. Noel apparently never knew that Herrick had published his case history or that he was the first case of sickle-cell anemia reported in the annals of western medicine.[13]

Herrick remained in Chicago and achieved national prominence as a cardiologist. He is still honored today by the American Heart Association, which annually makes an award in his name for outstanding contributions in clinical cardiology. Herrick died in 1954.

Irons also became a leader in Chicago medicine and for many years headed the Board of the Municipal Tuberculosis Sanatorium. In 1949, he was president of the American Medical Association. Irons died in 1959.[14]

If you were to name the defining trait of James Herrick and Ernest Irons, you might choose curiosity, which has been called the hallmark of a caring physician.[15] It is the urge to investigate, to understand, and to make strangers into people we can empathize with. Curiosity rewards patients because, when they know the doctor is interested in them, healing begins. And it rewards physicians by giving them experiences and memories that enrich their own lives.

If Herrick and Irons hadn't identified sickle-cell disease, sooner or later, someone would have, but they are due the credit, and their observations set in motion studies that have helped thousands of patients since that chilly Chicago day after Christmas in 1904.

Besides sickle-cell disease, the other most prevalent inherited breathing disorder is cystic fibrosis (CF). Whereas the sickle-cell mutation affects those of African descent, the genetic mutation responsible for CF affects mostly white populations. Both are lethal.

Josh Stokell was a microbiologist at the University of North Carolina, Charlotte. Born in 1979, he was diagnosed with CF when two weeks old.[16] This began a lifetime of infections, difficulty breathing, and hospitalizations. There was never a time when he was in good pulmonary health.

A typical crisis would begin with coughing up blood. Stokell would be rushed by ambulance to the hospital. He said no matter how many times it happened, it never stopped terrifying him. Frequently, he would remain in the hospital as long as two weeks, receiving antibiotics to control the infections that were destroying his lungs. Determined to fight back, Stokell exercised as much as he could, ate the proper foods, followed the prescribed medications, and tried to stay positive when even the best medical efforts couldn't hold his disease in check.[17]

Despite his struggle to breathe and the never-ending hospitalizations, Stokell enrolled at the University of North Carolina, Charlotte, and in 2008 received a bachelor's degree in biology. He then embarked on a graduate program in microbiology and chose to study cystic fibrosis, using his own lungs as the source of material.

Every week for three years, Stokell and colleagues cultured his sputum and performed DNA studies on the bacteria growing in his lungs. They showed how his microbial population waxed and waned and how a spurt in bacterial growth predicted a clinical flare-up of infection.[18] This longitudinal study of bacteriology in CF turned out to be a unique contribution to the understanding of what happens in this frightening breathing disorder.

In 2013, Stokell earned his PhD and received a research grant that enabled him to remain at UNC Charlotte as a postdoctoral fellow. But his health continued to decline. His breathing capacity dropped to 24 percent of normal, barely enough to sustain him at rest, let alone allow him to work full time. His spare frame wasting away, his breathing muscles straining, an oxygen cannula in his nose, Stokell waited for the inevitable respiratory death he knew lay ahead.[19]

As breath slowly left him, Stokell decided to gamble on a double-lung transplant. This was one of the most demanding procedures in the arsenal of thoracic surgery, and only a few institutions around the country possessed expertise even to attempt bilateral lung transplantation. Fortunately, Duke University, not far from Charlotte, was one of them, and Stokell joined the patients waiting for this last, desperate way to save their lives. If the wait was too long, he knew he could die.

CF is a common disorder that affects mucus-producing glands throughout the body.[20] It is caused by a defect in a gene that controls how the body transports chloride ions in and out of cells. This transport deficiency leads to thick, cheesy mucus which clogs the lungs as well as digestive and sweat glands. Attacking both males and females, CF is most common in individuals of European descent but occurs throughout the world. In the United States, about 30,000 individuals suffer from the disease.

The first clues to diagnosis are usually multiple respiratory infections during infancy. Due to abnormal amounts of sodium and chloride in sweat, babies with the disease often have salty skin, which can also be the tip-off to diagnosis. Testing for the concentration of chloride in sweat confirms the diagnosis in most instances.

CF treatment requires the skills of multiple specialists. The first goal is to clear secretions and keep the airways open. Aided by respiratory therapists, affected children inhale saline and enzymes that break down the thick mucus. With the help of physical therapists, they and their parents learn how to massage and vibrate the chest to jar mucus plugs loose from the blocked bronchi. Guided by nutritionists, they ingest supplements of pancreatic enzymes, calcium, and vitamins to maintain weight.

Because respiratory infections in CF are severe, patients require frequent antibiotics and need to keep up to date on immunizations. Due to these complexities, regional centers have emerged, most often associated with children's hospitals or universities, to assemble the many talents required to manage this hydra-like disease.[21]

For CF patients, life is a never-ending medical saga. But for many, treatment works. Expected lifespan has climbed over the past decades, and whereas a generation ago, most CF patients died before reaching adulthood, now many live into their fifth and sixth decades.

In 2012, a major step forward occurred when the Food and Drug Administration released ivacaftor, a drug that facilitates water and chloride movement in lung cells. This was the first medicine that actually attacked the basic defect in CF. Plus, gene therapy is just over the horizon, so the future appears brighter than the past for CF patients. Unfortunately, none of these treatments could reverse the end-stage scarring in Josh Stokell's lungs.

When asked what he wanted from the lung transplant, Stokell responded, "I want to be able to say four words in a row without feeling out of breath. I want to be able to run more than five feet. I want to be unattached to an oxygen tank that limits the time I can spend outdoors. I want to spend quality time with family and friends. I want to wake up in the morning and not feel as if I'm drowning from the inside. Most of all, I want to breathe freely."[22]

It was not to be. On June 8, 2015, a few weeks after his thirty-sixth birthday, Stokell died from pulmonary failure.

If you wanted to name the distinguishing traits of Josh Stokell, you might pick courage and good humor. These sustained him in the face of a fatal illness that he refused to let cripple his spirit, though he couldn't stop it from ravaging his body.

It's too soon to know how significant Stokell's studies of CF bacteriology will turn out to be. Surely, recognition of the pulmonary microbiome, the population of organisms that normally live in the lungs, is one of the important advances in respiratory medicine this decade, and Stokell helped shed light on its role in CF. So, Josh Stokell's shortened life span, like that of Walter Clement Noel a century earlier, was not wasted. Both their lives were gifts to the rest of us.

⑱

THE PUMP AND THE BELLOWS

"The body is one and yet has many members, and all the members of the body, though they are many, are one body."

—1 Corinthians 12:12–31[1]

"All that wheezes is not asthma."

—Chevalier Jackson[2]

Juanita was thirty-five years old when I first saw her. She was an adult "blue baby," born with a hole in the wall between the left and right ventricles of her heart. This diverted blood from one side of her heart to the other without it passing through the lungs to pick up oxygen. She had undergone several operations to close the defect that had alleviated but not cured the problem. As she matured into adulthood, the pressure in her right ventricle became so high it damaged the blood vessels in her lungs.

Juanita was breathless with any exertion, needed oxygen continuously, and was able to walk only short distances. Unmarried, she lived with her brother and accepted her predicament without complaining, relying on friends or family to drive her to run errands or to come to the doctor's office. When she was at her best, she could ride the bus, pulling her oxygen cylinder like a small grocery cart. Juanita was bright and managed to hold down a part-time position as a bookkeeper for a small company. She frequently missed work when her heart tired and she needed hospitalization, but her employer kept her on the payroll.

In addition, Juanita also had long-standing asthma, not by itself severe but it placed an added strain on her already-weak heart. Whenever she got a cold, she wheezed, became severely short of breath, and had to be brought to the office or hospital. How many times did she arrive in a wheelchair or by ambulance, gasping for air, her fingers and lips blue, her lungs sounding like an out-of-tune pipe organ? This made her prone to frequent bouts of pulmonary edema, in which her heart muscles, struggling with fatigue, caused fluid to back up in her lungs, making them boggy, like wet sponges.

During these crises, Juanita's cardiologist and I had a running debate about which abnormality was causing the most difficulty. Was it heart failure or airway obstruction? Most of the time, we couldn't be sure, so we treated for both and hoped she would improve. We did agree that her having both heart and lung disease made her life precarious and our jobs more difficult.

As time passed and pressure in her right ventricle rose, unoxygenated blood flowed directly to the left side of the heart through the gap in the partition between the right and left sides. That meant Juanita's organs received less and less oxygen. Her brain, kidneys, and liver, all starved for oxygen, lost their capacity to function. She struggled to breathe, she struggled to eat, she struggled to think. Navigating a path between the Scylla and Charybdis of cardiac and respiratory failure challenged the skills of all of us who treated her. Juanita's plight illustrated the downhill spiral of patients with combined heart and lung disease.

The pump and the bellows, the heart and the lungs: These two major systems have to work together, minute by minute, to deliver life-giving oxygen. If either fails, the other immediately feels the stress. The lungs in an adult move five liters of air in and out every minute, while the heart pumps five liters of blood around the body during that time; nature matches oxygen supply and demand.

Normally, the heart adjusts the rate and strength of its contractions in response to signals from the brain, muscles, and kidneys. At the same time, the lungs dilate and constrict the bronchi, secrete chemicals to keep the alveoli open, and break down hormones circulating around the body. With miles of airways and blood vessels, the two organs collaborate to extract life-giving oxygen from 7,000 liters of air inhaled every day—all within a space the size of two single-gallon milk cartons.

When the heart fails, the lungs become boggy, like wet sponges. It's easy to understand why the breathing muscles have to work extra hard to move air in and out. On occasions when I have bronchoscoped patients with pulmonary edema due to heart failure, I have been struck by the frothy, bloody fluid that wells up in the airways, striking evidence of the congestion deep in the lungs.

Five million people in the United States have heart failure, and the number is increasing. Heart failure is a contributing cause to nearly 10 percent of deaths among the elderly, and half the patients with heart failure die within five years of the diagnosis. Thus, heart failure portends a worse outlook than many cancers. In addition, heart failure costs society more than $30 billion each year, including the cost of services, medicines to treat the condition, and missed days of work.

For many centuries, the interplay between the heart and the lungs to sustain life was a mystery to science. Then, in the mid-sixteenth century, anatomist Andreas Vesalius, court physician to the Spanish king Philip V, had an unusual experience. While performing an autopsy on the body of a nobleman who had been executed during the Inquisition, he inflated the lungs by blowing air into the trachea, and the man's heart began to beat. We don't know how much time had elapsed between the man's "death" and the autopsy or if his heart truly regained the capacity to beat or only quivered for an instant. Possibly, air forced into his lungs squeezed some oxygenated blood from the pulmonary veins and stimulated the man's dying cardiac muscles to contract a few times. But the occurrence surprised Vesalius enough that he reported it to his medical colleagues.

Vesalius's insistence that only dissecting the human body could lead to understanding how organs work had already made him suspicious in the eyes of the church. The episode of the heart beating after lung inflation really landed him in hot water with the ecclesiastical authorities, who condemned him for desecrating the human body. Forced to make a pilgrimage to the Holy Land to atone for his sin, Vesalius died on the journey in a shipwreck.[3] However, his observation demonstrated the connection between breathing and life and showed a connection between respiratory and cardiac action.

Soon after, Michael Servetus, a Spanish colleague of Vesalius, claimed that blood courses through the lungs and mixes with inspired air, which cleanses it of its "sooty vapors" and makes it change color (oxygenated blood is a brighter red than unoxygenated), thus producing the "vital spirit" that flows into the heart.[4] Servetus was correct but ahead of his time. For another infraction (he challenged the doctrine of the Trinity of God), he was branded a heretic and in 1553 was burned at the stake.[5]

After the Renaissance, scientists knew that the lungs expanded and contracted so that air moved in and out but were ignorant of the exchange of oxygen and carbon dioxide that occurred as blood and air flowed by each other. (Carbon dioxide wasn't discovered until 1754, and oxygen wasn't discovered until 1774.) Physicians used artificial ventilation in animal experiments but not in humans, possibly because of concerns about contagiousness—the Black Death had ravaged Europe only a century earlier—as well as religious scruples.

Yet no one grasped how blood flowed through the body. Most physicians either thought the lungs somehow propelled blood or ignored the question.[6] In modern times, this appears strange. Surely, when an artery was severed, by accident or during battle, physicians would have noticed how bright red blood pulsated from the wound and might have wondered why the blood kept time with the throbbing heartbeat.

Then, in 1628, William Harvey published *De Motu Cordis*, "Regarding Movement of the Heart," which showed that blood circulated because the heart pumped it throughout the body. It was a radical idea that revolutionized medical science.

Born in Kent, England, Harvey studied medicine at the University of Padua in Italy, where one of his teachers was Fabricius, the anatomist who discovered that veins have valves. Harvey returned to England, where he was a fellow of the College of Physicians and "physician extraordinary" to King James I. Harvey studied the heart in living animals and was able to see its muscular contractions pumping blood into the aorta. He observed the amount of blood pumped was far too much to be absorbed into the tissues and so reasoned blood flowed in a circular route throughout the body, moving forward from the left side of the heart, from arteries to veins, until it returned to the right side of the heart. From there, it flowed through the lungs, then reached the left ventricle to start the cycle again. Harvey did not have access to a microscope (it hadn't been invented yet), but he postulated that small vascular connections must exist between arteries and veins. Thirty years later, in 1661, Marcello Malpighi discovered these tiny conduits, called capillaries, from the Latin word meaning "hair," and confirmed Harvey's theory.

Experiments on ventilation and circulation continued for the next two hundred years, and by the end of the eighteenth century, scientists were beginning to understand cardiac and respiratory interactions, as well as how failure of each organ system affected the other. When William Osler compiled his famous textbook, *Principles and Practice of Medicine*, in the 1890s, a pivot point between Victorian and modern medicine, he explained congestion and edema in the lungs as results of blood backing up from obstruction to the return of blood to the left side of the heart. Most often this was inability of the heart to pump the blood flowing into it. So, Osler understood the effect of heart disease on the lungs.[7]

In addition, medical science slowly came to understand the concept of damage to the lungs from heart weakness and damage to the heart from lung disease. Coronary artery disease and hypertension are the most frequent injuries to the left ventricle, causing blood to back up in the lungs. COPD, lung fibrosis, and pulmonary emboli are the most frequent lung disorders that strain the heart, mainly the right ventricle. All cause difficulty breathing and eventually combined heart and lung failure.

In Osler's day, the only treatment for heart failure was rest and blood-letting, or venesection, drawing off blood to lower the volume circulating through the lungs. (The body compensates for reduced cardiac output by increasing blood volume.) By the time I entered medicine fifty years later, we had oxygen to alleviate breathlessness, plus diuretics to cause the kidneys to excrete the excess fluid. We also injected morphine to relieve the terrible anxiety that accompanies the breathlessness these patients experience and applied tourniquets to the arms and legs to retard blood flow to the lungs. These helped but, compared to what medicine can do now, are like a Model T Ford versus a Ferrari.

Nowadays, physicians have high-tech diagnostic tools to discern the weak links in the process. Cardiac and pulmonary artery catheterization allows for precise measurements of pressures and flows throughout both systems. Ultrasound probes, angiograms, and radionuclide scans fill in the diagnostic gaps. Drugs that dilate blood vessels reduce the load on the heart, and others increase heart muscle strength. Ventilators can take over breathing; pumps connected to the aorta can propel blood forward; and in drastic situations, total bypass of both the heart and lungs, as in cardiac surgery, is lifesaving.

But sometimes, alertness is the greatest need. Clem was an eighty-five-year-old man who developed asthma in his ninth decade of life. It came on gradually over several months, with wheezing and breathlessness that prevented him from exercising, and woke him up at night, forcing him to sit upright to alleviate his distress. Except for high blood pressure, his health had been good. He had no prior history of lung disease or allergies and had never smoked. His chest was clear, and his chest X-ray showed only minimal cardiac enlargement, consistent with chronic hypertension. Pulmonary function tests indicated nothing unusual.

I was perplexed because, while asthma can first manifest itself in old age, it is uncommon. When Clem failed to improve with bronchodilators, I considered adding steroids but, with no sign of obstruction on pulmonary-function tests, decided to refer him for allergy evaluation first. Imagine my chagrin when the allergist called me to say he didn't t think it was asthma, rather that the wheezing was due to heart failure. He thought Clem's lungs were normal, and he was recommending a diuretic as additional therapy. With a red face, I wrote the prescription but could feel a little better when I watched Clem's "asthma" disappear.

Heart failure can cause wheezing and difficulty breathing, though lung function itself is normal. When the heart is weak, like in long-standing hypertension or after multiple heart attacks, even a small amount of exercise raises the pressure in the pulmonary veins, so that fluid seeps into the walls of the bronchi, making them swollen and edematous. This obstructs airflow and leads to wheezing. This is cardiac asthma, the problem affecting Clem.

Juanita and Clem illustrate a general biological phenomenon: Organ systems support one another, like members of a team. If short on home-run hitters, a baseball manager can build a strong offense with singles hitters and fast runners. So, a vigorous heart can prolong life in patients with chronic lung disease, and a weak heart will decrease longevity. A well-working respiratory system won't by itself protect a patient with a weak heart, but without good lungs, a failing heart causes worse trouble and an earlier death.

Nature compensates wherever she can. Scientists call this homeostasis, an almost-miraculous ability of the body to maintain a steady internal environment in the face of constantly changing external conditions. Homeostasis is a fundamental natural process. It enables complex biological organisms, including humans, to move throughout the world, explore the environment, flourish, and evolve. When cardiac and respiratory diseases occur, unless other organs compensate, vital functions weaken and deteriorate. The lungs and heart, the bellows and the pump, star players in the contest of life, can no longer maintain homeostasis, and when breathing fails, death follows.

⑲

THAT SLEEP OF DEATH

"Each night, when I go to sleep, I die. And the next morning, when I wake up, I am reborn."

—Mahatma Gandhi[1]

"To die, to sleep— / To sleep—perchance to dream. Ay, there's the rub! / For in that sleep of death what dreams may come, / When we have shuffled off this mortal coil, / Must give us pause"

—William Shakespeare[2]

Sophie was a sixty-year-old woman I saw because she was drowsy all the time. For years, she had been falling asleep whenever she sat down to watch television, and her family nagged her because she even dozed off during conversations. Sophie slept alone and couldn't relate what happened to her at night while she was in bed, but she knew she woke up tired and stayed that way all day.

Sophie had never smoked nor had asthma nor any other respiratory disorder. She had high blood pressure and diabetes, both managed with oral drugs, plus had struggled with weight all her life. Steadfastly refusing to step on a scale at the office, Sophie forced me to estimate her height and weight, which I placed at less than five feet and over two hundred pounds. Retired from work in retail sales, she lived by herself in a small house and neither owned nor drove a car but rode the bus or depended on relatives to bring her to the office. Walking more than a short distance was out of the question.

Sophie dressed plainly, affected no makeup, and spoke softly but directly, using few words to respond to questions. Occasionally she cracked a little smile that told me she understood me quite well, though her tight-lipped demeanor suggested she was suspicious of me. She remained fully alert while I took her history, and indeed, when she questioned why I wanted to do some test or procedure, I could see beneath her taciturn manner was quite an intelligent mind.

Sophie's physical exam was normal except for her body shape. She had no visible neck, and a diminutive chin that rested on her sternum. Her arms and legs were thick, like hams, while her hands and feet were tiny. Indeed, she resembled a toy doll wrapped inside a mass of flesh.

Routine blood studies and X-rays were normal, except her blood sugar was mildly elevated. I felt Sophie had sleep apnea related to her obesity, and I recommended an overnight sleep study to confirm the diagnosis. The test, called a polysomnogram, monitors the EEG, eye movements, pulse, oxygen saturation, chest movements, and airflow through the nose and mouth during sleep by means of wires and electrodes attached to the head and chest. Like many patients, Sophie found the test uncomfortable. I often wondered how any patient was able to sleep with all the paraphernalia attached, but thousands of studies have proved its acceptance and reliability.

The study demonstrated that, during sleep, Sophie's breathing drastically decreased. Multiple times every hour while she slept, she stopped breathing entirely, the criterion for apnea. (The word means "not breathing" in Greek.) Furthermore, her blood oxygen level dropped to dangerously low levels during these spells. No wonder when she awoke she felt drowsy and nodded off during the daytime.

Sophie had severe sleep apnea with respiratory failure. She was going to die soon if nothing changed.

Normal processes that go awry can lead to respiratory difficulties. Even a universal human function like sleep carries risks for abnormal breathing that can be catastrophic. Disordered breathing during sleep affects at least 25 million adults, and the problem is worsening.[3] More than a quarter of adults in the United States have some form of sleep-breathing disturbance, whether it is snoring or apnea. Sleep-disordered breathing is also a major threat to infants, especially those born prematurely. Sleep apnea occurs in obesity, in those whose throat narrows during sleep, and when the brain fails to signal the lungs to breathe—or combinations of all three.

Normally, the brain controls breathing. It responds to any fall in oxygen or rise in carbon dioxide by increasing the drive for the lungs to inhale more deeply. But, 30 percent of obese patients don't respond to this increased drive; their breathing muscles become fatigued and they underbreathe. Plus, fat tissue itself produces a hormone called leptin, which acts on centers in the brain to stimulate ventilation.[4] Research suggests some obese people may be deficient in leptin and thus don't breathe normally.

Whatever the exact mechanism, certain obese individuals stop breathing while asleep. This drops their blood oxygen level, leads to awakening from sleep, and initiates a vicious cycle of underbreathing, drop in oxygen, fragmented sleep, and drowsiness during wakeful hours. Obese patients with sleep apnea develop high blood pressure, cardiac rhythm abnormalities, and diabetes. Pulmonary artery pressure rises in response to decreased oxygen, and eventually the right ventricle of the heart fails, with shortness of breath, edema, and death.

In addition, the body responds to low oxygen tension by increasing red blood cell production, which makes circulating blood more viscous. Blood clots form and may break loose to migrate to the lungs. Obese, sleep-deprived individuals feel fatigued, can't exercise, gain more weight, and so restart the lethal cycle. Impaired breathing and disordered sleep in obesity doubles the mortality rate. So, it's easy to see why Sophie worried me. She was at high risk of dying.

Medical science has only recently recognized disordered sleep and breathing due to obesity as a serious medical problem, though historians have described the picture since antiquity. In the fourth century BCE, during the time of Alexander the Great, Dionysius ruled Heracleia, a region on the south coast of the Black Sea. Claudius Aelianus, a Greek military historian, said, "I am informed that Dionysius, through daily gluttony and intemperance, increased to an extraordinary degree of corpulence and fatness, by reason whereof he had much adoe to take breath." Dionysius would fall into a deep sleep, and to prevent him from suffocating, his physicians pushed a long, thin needle through the layers of fat until "it came to the firm flesh, he felt it and awakened." Drastic as it sounds, observers testified this unusual treatment worked, noting "up to a certain point under the flesh . . . the needle caused no sensation; but if the needle went through so far as to touch the region which was free of fat, then he would be thoroughly aroused."[5] History offers no record that the needle in the belly approach endured as therapy for obesity, shallow breathing, and sleepiness, which shouldn't surprise us.

References to obesity, drowsiness, and disordered breathing were scarce in historical records for nearly twenty centuries afterward, perhaps because food was scarce; malnutrition was common; and, except for royalty and a few extravagantly rich, no one could afford to eat more than required to sustain life.

Then in the nineteenth century, the medical profession began to recognize the connection of sleepiness with obesity and shallow breathing. In 1816,

William Wadd, a British surgeon, published a monograph on obesity as a disease. He noted how "accumulation of fat . . . cannot fail to impede the free exercise of the animal functions. Respiration is performed imperfectly, or with difficulty." Wadd was also aware that obese people may become sleepy. He described a patient who "became at length so lethargic, that he frequently fell asleep in the act of eating, even in company."[6]

The best-known commentary on obesity and sleep came not from a medical but from a literary source. In 1836, the novelist Charles Dickens wrote the *Posthumous Papers of the Pickwick Club*. A sharp observer of human behavior, Dickens is generally recognized as the first person to offer a detailed description of obesity-related sleep apnea. One character in the *Pickwick Papers* was the fat boy called Joe, who constantly fell asleep. Dickens mentioned Joe had a voracious appetite, snored loudly, and was difficult to arouse. The accuracy of the description suggests Joe was more than a product of Dickens's imagination and was likely based on a real person from Dickens's life.

The advent of the twentieth century saw increasing awareness of the pathologic connection between sleep and obesity but still did not make much of the role of breathing. In 1918, William Osler, in the eighth edition of *Principles and Practice of Medicine*, coined the term *Pickwickian* to refer to severe obesity with sleepiness, still no acknowledgment of the crucial role of breathing.

Finally, in 1956, Burwell and Robin reported the case history of an obese, sleepy patient who resembled Dickens's character Joe and dubbed the problem Pickwickian Syndrome. Readers liked the literary allusion, and this article put obesity with abnormal sleep on the medical radar screen. Burwell's report stimulated interest in sleep research, and investigators soon described what happens to breathing in severe obesity.[7] When these individuals go to sleep, especially reclining, their respiratory systems are forced to work extra hard. Pushed up toward the head by the weight of the abdomen, the diaphragm has a difficult time contracting, and so the chest does not expand. This results in shallow breaths that don't allow sufficient oxygen and carbon dioxide to be exchanged in the lungs.

Apnea also occurs without obesity when the tongue falls back and obstructs airflow during sleep. This obstruction tends to occur mostly in males, often in individuals with large tongues, thick necks, or small lower jaws. Anyone who takes a shirt collar size seventeen inches or higher is suspect. (Perhaps sleep researchers should canvass men's clothing stores for patients to study.)

Normally, when people sleep, the muscles of the throat relax. If the throat is small, as occurs with a thick neck, the tongue may fall back and block the airway. Snoring results. Oxygen is unable to reach the brain. Affected individuals awaken, often without being aware, and take a few deep breaths, which partially corrects the problem. They go back to sleep, but in a while, the process starts over again. This pattern may occur dozens of times an hour, hundreds of times during a night, so that, the next morning, the victims arise deprived of sleep and drowse off as the day goes on. Any sedating drugs, especially alcohol, aggravate the problem, and just as with obesity-related underventilation, these people develop hypertension and heart rhythm abnormalities.

Research continued on the physiology of sleep, but scientists couldn't understand why certain people had daytime sleepiness. Nor did they fathom the relation to abnormal breathing, though articles like Burwell's in 1956 nudged thinking forward.

In 1965, with development of new techniques to study the nervous and respiratory systems during repose, researchers worked out the abnormal process in what we now call obstructive sleep apnea—airway obstruction, cessation of breathing, and arousal. The pattern repeated, sometimes hundreds of times a night, and the ineffective sleep culminated in drowsiness the following day. This milestone in understanding the biology of sleep brought sleep disorders into the realm of pulmonary as well as neurological physiology.[8]

But mainstream medicine was slow to accept the findings. Polysomnography (even the name is complex) consisted of all-night recording of EEG waves, eye movements, oxygen levels, electrocardiograms, chest movements, and airflows. The studies were costly, time-consuming, and complicated. Most doctors remained in the dark about sleep apnea. As late as 1972, one study reported the average patient waited fifteen years and consulted five physicians before symptoms of excessive daytime sleepiness were recognized as abnormal.[9] Eventually, diagnostic standards for the various sleep disorders emerged, and laboratories arose to study sleep disorders. These shone a light on the role of breathing and stimulated ways to manage sleep apnea.

Initially, physicians overcame obstruction to airflow in the throat by inserting a tube into the windpipe below the vocal cords, bypassing the obstruction. This required a tracheostomy, a surgical procedure that left patients unable to talk unless the tube was plugged. In addition, the tube was an irritant, increasing mucus and saliva, as well as posing a danger of infection in the airway.

Otolaryngologists developed surgical procedures to trim away tissue in the throat. These helped many patients and were less drastic than a permanent tracheostomy but necessitated surgery. Dentists created appliances that prevented the tongue from falling back during sleep, which also helped though were cumbersome for some users.

In 1980, Australian physician Colin Sullivan reported reversing obstructive sleep apnea by placing a pressurized mask over the nose and mouth to prevent the tongue from falling backward and the airway from collapsing during sleep. While not comfortable, patients woke up in the morning refreshed, and this offered enough incentive for patients to put up with the apparatus.

Today the CPAP (constant positive airway pressure) mask is the most widely used form of treatment for sleep apnea, and several large companies have been built around manufacturing the devices. But some individuals, neither obese nor exhibiting obstruction to airflow, simply seemed to stop breathing while sleeping.

In 1962, Severinghaus and Mitchell reported three patients with a remarkable breathing disorder. After the nerves in their spinal cords were surgically cut to alleviate intractable pain, they could breathe on command while awake, but when they went to sleep, they stopped breathing. One died from asphyxiation, and the other two required permanent artificial ventilation during sleep. The authors entitled their paper "Ondine's Curse: Failure of Respiratory Center Automaticity."[10] *Ondine's curse* alluded to a medieval legend of a sea nymph who broke the pact between water spirits and humans that requires eternal separation when she fell in love with a man, married him, and bore his child. She was turned into a spring of water, and he was cursed by having to consciously command his body to perform all its functions, including breathing. When he fell asleep, exhausted by efforts not to drowse off, he suffocated to death. Ondine's curse came to be applied to almost every medical entity in which brain malfunction impairs breathing during sleep.

Nerves in the base of the brain send rhythmic impulses down the spinal cord to the diaphragm and other breathing muscles to activate inhalation. Under normal circumstances, breathing becomes shallow during sleep, but nature controls the system tightly, and even a tiny rise in carbon dioxide or drop in oxygen causes the brain to stimulate the respiratory system to breathe more deeply and rapidly. It is like a finely tuned thermostat that turns up the furnace should the temperature fall and turns it down promptly when the proper degree of warmth is reached.

When the brain doesn't stimulate the lungs to breathe, this is called central apnea. It is rare, accounting for less than 10 percent of sleep disorders, and is most often secondary to some other pathology, such as heart failure, a brain tumor, or narcotic overdose. Sometimes doctors can't find a cause and so call the disorder primary or idiopathic. Central sleep apnea also occurs in children, especially in premature babies, where it is called congenital central hypoventilation and is a major cause of infant death. More than two thousand babies die each year from sudden infant death syndrome, and most relate to impaired breathing.[11]

Like those with obesity-related or obstructive sleep apnea, these individuals are constantly fatigued and drowse during waking hours. They develop hypertension and suffer strokes. And, they may die during sleep.

Treating central apnea is difficult because it depends on the underlying cause, such as heart failure, brain tumor, or narcotic abuse. Supplementary oxygen and drugs that stimulate breathing may help, as may adding pressure during inspiration with CPAP.

Sleep-disordered breathing has major impact on people's lives and may be lethal. A traveling salesman was referred after he fell asleep while driving and plowed into a telephone pole. I was told of another man who snored and tossed and turned so badly his wife moved into another bedroom and threatened to leave him if he didn't seek help.

An elderly physician with a failing heart was stopping breathing during sleep. I went to see him in consultation at the hospital and knocked on the door of his room; when he didn't answer, I opened the door a crack to see if he was OK. He was asleep, and I watched him from the entryway. His breaths became more shallow until he completely stopped. For nearly thirty seconds he didn't breathe at all. Then the pattern reversed, and each breath became larger, until he was gulping in huge amounts of air. And after this, his breathing decreased and the cycle started over. He had Cheyne-Stokes breathing, a form of central apnea first described in the nineteenth century and seen often in heart failure. Lack of oxygen from a heart that can't pump adequately makes the brain create waves of overbreathing and underbreathing. Cheyne-Stokes portends a bad prognosis, and he died a few weeks later.

Sophie had obesity, obstructive, and central apnea and was in trouble. She couldn't tolerate the CPAP mask. Surgical trimming of the tongue and palate was unproven enough I was not willing to recommend it. She continued to deteriorate, sleeping poorly at night and drowsing during the day. Constant headaches from high blood pressure made her miserable. She was so short of breath she was barely able to move around at all. I recommended consultation at Stanford, the mecca for sleep-related problems in the western United States. Her family drove her to Palo Alto, where she underwent evaluation. Eventually a decision emerged to perform a tracheostomy.[12]

The procedure didn't work. The surgeon had a difficult time dissecting through the three inches of fatty tissue in her neck. In the middle of the case, he called me to the operating room. (More than a call, it was an order: "Get your ass down here right now before she chokes to death.")

Sophie's airway was so small and so far beneath the skin of her neck the surgeon had commandeered a pediatric endotracheal tube from the anesthesia department to reach the trachea. But after he cut into it, he was not able to thread the tube through the incision into the windpipe itself. Fortunately, through a bronchoscope, I was able to find the cut and maneuver the curved plastic trach tube into her airway.

Postop, Sophie was still miserable. A plastic tube protruded from her neck, irritated her trachea, and prevented her from talking. Even switching to a custom-made pediatric tracheostomy tube was unsuccessful. Mucus and saliva accumulated. She coughed incessantly. Within a few weeks, we had to admit failure, and I removed the tracheal tube. Afterward, she refused any more procedures and was treated with supplemental oxygen by nasal prongs and attempts at weight loss. Her exercise capacity was severely limited, and her diabetes and high blood pressure continued to take their toll. She lived a couple of more years and finally died of heart failure without ever experiencing relief from the sleepiness and struggle to breathe that constantly plagued her.

Sophie's course troubles me to this day. She was a difficult case but a lovely person. I liked her and respected her. I felt we gave her the best care we could but made her suffering worse. Yet, were I to see her for the first time now, twenty-five years later, I would probably recommend the same course of treatment.

People like Sophie challenge us. And Dionysius, Dickens's fat boy Joe, and Ondine, whether they be historical figures, literary characters, or fantasies, fascinate us because they tell us something about our own nature, how it works, and how it goes awry.

Sleeping and breathing are metaphors for dying and living. A sleeping person looks dead, except breath remains as a sign of life. Breathing signifies the human spirit, its hopes and dreams. When death occurs, the spirit leaves, and with it, aspirations for the future disappear: Psalm 146 says it poetically: "When his breath departs, he returns to the earth; on that very day his plans perish."[13]

20

THE FIRST BREATHS

"When we are born, we cry that we are come / To this great stage of fools."

—William Shakespeare[1]

"In the fields of observation, chance favors only the prepared mind."

—Louis Pasteur[2]

Virginia Apgar faced a dilemma. Should she choose a career in surgery or anesthesia? The twenty-six-year-old had no way to know that her decision would influence the lives of thousands of children for the next forty years.

Born in New Jersey in 1909, Apgar decided while in high school she wanted to be a medical doctor. She attended Mt. Holyoke College in Massachusetts and graduated in 1929, just before the stock market crashed. She began medical school that fall at Columbia University College of Physicians in New York, assisted by scholarships to finance her education. Only nine women were among the ninety members of her class, and Apgar excelled. She graduated in 1933, fourth in her class, and was accepted at the prestigious Presbyterian Hospital for an internship and residency in surgery.

Over the next two years, in a highly competitive specialty dominated by men, Apgar continued to shine. But Dr. Allen Whipple, chief of surgery and her mentor, was concerned about her. He wanted her to succeed, and the previous female surgical residents he had trained had experienced great hardships getting established. Even male surgeons were finding it difficult to make a living during those hard times. Then Whipple had an idea. He felt that, to advance his department of surgery, he needed to improve anesthesia, and Apgar might be the person to carry the banner for this endeavor.

In the United States at that time, nurses administered most of the surgical anesthetics. Surgeons did not consider anesthesiologists their equals, which discouraged medical graduates from entering the field. However, Whipple thought a woman director might work well with the nurses. So, he suggested that Apgar concentrate in anesthesia.

After weighing the pros and cons, Apgar decided to follow his advice and switch from surgery to anesthesia. But only a handful of institutions in the United States had academic anesthesia programs for physicians. One was at the University of Wisconsin in Madison, and Apgar moved there in 1937. She returned to New York after six months and spent an additional six months at Bellevue Hospital, where the director of anesthesia was a Wisconsin alumnus. In 1938, Apgar became director of the Anesthesia Division in the Department of Surgery at Columbia.[3]

She had a difficult start: a huge clinical workload, trouble recruiting other physicians, and no way to bill for her services. Surgeons, who felt they should be in charge, clashed with her over intraoperative management of patients. But she persisted and slowly gained their respect by working long hours, producing successful outcomes, and even establishing a modest research program. She succeeded, and in 1949, Virginia Apgar became the first woman to achieve status as a full professor at Columbia University Medical School.

Apgar then decided to concentrate on obstetric anesthesia. She instituted the practice of visiting mothers before and after anesthesia. She changed the anesthetic gases used in delivery to agents with less tendency to suppress breathing. This reduced the incidence of respiratory depression in both mothers and newborns. Known to carry a laryngoscope and tracheal tube at all times in case she needed to perform emergency intubation, Apgar's motto was "Nobody, but nobody, is going to stop breathing on me."[4]

Meanwhile, forward-looking pediatricians began to focus on newborn care. During the early twentieth century, obstetricians concentrated on the mother, and pediatricians oversaw newborn nurseries. But immediately after birth, while still in the delivery room, newborns were caught in a transitional state and needed support. In the early 1920s, Julius Hess, a Chicago pediatrician, established a center at Michael Reese Hospital to help preemies breathe. Hess added an oxygen source to incubators and developed an ambulance system to transport premature babies to centers where they could receive up-to-date care. Most importantly, he established a training program to teach nurses how to care for premature babies. Hess's method became a model of neonatal nursing. Other progressive pediatricians in major medical centers around the country created similar systems and started a new specialty, neonatology, care of newborns.

For the next thirty years, treatment of respiratory distress in newborns, especially preemies, centered on developing centers that could keep babies warm, supply oxygen, suction mucus, and stimulate coughing. In the 1950s, assisted mechanical ventilation for infants began to take hold. Engineers adapted pressure valves designed for military aviation for medical use. Manufacturers came up with infant ventilators that allowed for small-sized breaths and rapid rates needed by tiny infants. Anesthesiologists skilled in surgical breathing support, like Apgar, began to work with pediatricians to care for newborns with respiratory problems.

Apgar began to look for some way to assess newborns at risk. She wrote down five ways to evaluate newborns: overall appearance, breathing, pulse, activity, and reflexes. Over the next three years, she tested her idea and in 1953 published a paper describing a scale based on these five observations. This became known as the Apgar score. It became the standard in delivery suites all over the country and eventually all over the world.

When I rotated through obstetrics as a medical student in 1959, we calculated the Apgar score on babies as soon as they were delivered. A robust response in each category received two points, a borderline response earned one point, and absence earned no points. Thus, a healthy baby had ten points, and any score less than five meant immediate action was needed.

The common denominator of the Apgar measurements was breathing. If the lungs didn't supply the brain and heart with oxygen, the result was a lethargic baby with sluggish reflexes; rapid, shallow breaths; and a fast pulse. Those babies needed immediate oxygen and mechanical ventilation. The Apgar score gave physicians a guide to know when to resuscitate newborns with breathing difficulties but did not answer the gnawing, persisting questions. What caused respiratory distress of newborns? And what could be done to treat it?

The first few minutes after birth are among the most dangerous in all of life. While in the uterus, the developing baby inhales and exhales but receives oxygen from the placenta—the lungs are full of amniotic fluid. So, immediately after birth, when the umbilical cord is cut and the baby is on its own, breathing is crucial. Stimulated by the cold environment outside their mother's body, most babies take a big gulp and let out a cry within a few seconds.

However, not all babies breathe right away as they should. They pant and grunt. Their nostrils flare as they gasp for air. If these babies can be helped through the first few days by suctioning mucus, stimulating cough, and administering enough oxygen, the problem usually subsides, and they survive normally.

For babies born prematurely, it's a different story. The lungs are one of the last organs to develop. Infants born with underdeveloped lungs can't bring in life-giving oxygen, and so they struggle to breathe and often suffocate. After thirty-five weeks' gestation, the lungs become mature enough for most babies to survive, but for those delivered earlier, inability to breathe is a killer.[5] And in the 1950s, medicine had little to offer.

Scientists recognized for a long time that preemies' lungs did not expand normally. Those babies who died were said to have succumbed to congenital atelectasis, lung collapse present at birth. Microscopic examination of the lungs of these infants showed a glassy, pink-staining substance coated the air sacs. Pathologists postulated this was causing the babies to suffocate and named it hyaline membrane disease. (*Hyaline* means "glassy" in Greek.) This obscure disease with a strange name was the number-one cause of death in preterm infants, yet most people had never heard of it. Nor did medical science understand what caused hyaline membranes to form. Some speculated they resulted from babies breathing amniotic fluid. Others thought the membranes came from aspirating mother's milk. But all agreed respiratory distress in preemies was lethal.

In the early 1960s, 25,000 premature babies a year died of hyaline membrane disease.[6] It struck all segments of society. Even the son of the president of the United States was vulnerable.

In August 1963, the First Family decided to vacation on Cape Cod. The First Lady was pregnant, and though she had experienced difficulties with premature delivery in previous pregnancies, the president and she were optimistic enough to travel from Washington to Massachusetts. Then, disaster struck. Six weeks before her due date, the First Lady went into labor. She was rushed to Otis AFB, where she delivered a four-pound-ten-ounce boy named Patrick Bouvier Kennedy.

His Apgar score isn't public knowledge, but accounts discuss how the baby grunted and breathed rapidly, with flaring nostrils[7]. These indicate Patrick Kennedy's lungs were underdeveloped. He quickly developed respiratory distress and was transferred to Boston Children's Hospital. There he was kept warm and treated with oxygen in a hyperbaric chamber, but thirty-nine hours after delivery, he died of respiratory exhaustion brought on by hyaline membrane disease. The death of the Kennedy baby awakened the public to the tragedy of respiratory distress of newborns and stimulated Congress to allocate funds for research into the syndrome.

Though researchers were confused about the cause of hyaline membranes, bedside physicians still had to treat respiratory distress in newborns. Their efforts were only partially successful, and hyaline membrane disease continued to take its toll on newborns well into the 1960s, as the tragic death of Patrick Kennedy illustrated. The ingenuity of clinical caregivers couldn't go any further until the scientists unraveled the mystery of hyaline membranes. But the

Sherlock Holmes of infant respiratory distress syndrome was about to appear on the scene.

Mary Ellen Avery was a pediatrician. Soon after graduating from medical school in 1952, she developed tuberculosis and went to Trudeau's sanatorium in Saranac Lake to be treated.[8] While recuperating, she became interested in lung diseases, and when she finished her pediatric training at Johns Hopkins, she moved to Harvard to study with Jere Mead, an authority on the mechanics of lung function. Because she was a pediatrician, Avery thought a lot about infants dying of hyaline membrane disease. She noticed their lungs didn't show the foamy fluid seen in babies dying from other causes. This made her curious. Why did the lungs of those infants collapse? Why didn't they form bubbles? What was going wrong? So she began sleuthing.

Avery's investigations into bubble behavior led her to consider surface tension. Surface tension is an esoteric physical process simply defined as the tendency of molecules to squeeze as close together as they can. It is what causes drops of water to be perfectly spherical.[9] It's also why soap bubbles float through the air without collapsing. Soap reduces the surface tension on the inside of bubbles, lessening their tendency to collapse and disappear. Soap is what scientists call a surfactant.

Avery learned of John Clements, an American physician at the US Army Chemical Center in Maryland. Clements had noted that, when poison gases killed experimental animals, a foamy fluid formed in their lungs. The bubbles in the fluid were remarkably stable and often persisted for several hours. By coincidence, Richard Pattle, a physicist working for the British Ministry of Defense, independently observed the same phenomenon. Both scientists figured that some substance in the lung must coat the bubbles to make them resist popping. Clements called it antiatelectasis factor, indicating it protected against lung collapse. Pattle speculated that absence of this chemical, a surfactant, might be involved in the respiratory difficulties experienced by premature babies.

Pattle and Clements were actually plowing ground turned over earlier by a German physiologist, Kurt Von Neergard. In 1929, Von Neergard studied surface tension in the lungs. He conceived the air sacs as tiny bubbles covered by blood vessels. He envisioned a soap-like substance coating their inner surface and lowering the surface tension inside the air sacs, thus preventing collapse; this substance was a surfactant.

Von Neergaard wondered if the reason preemies were unable to expand their lungs was due to inadequate amounts of surfactant.[10] But he never followed up on the question, and little more was learned until 1947, when pathologist Peter Gruenwald, working with lungs of babies who had died of respiratory failure, made observations that supported those of Von Neergard.

But most doctors weren't aware of these findings and continued to focus on hyaline membranes as the crucial factor in newborn respiratory distress.

In 1957, when Avery heard about Clements's work, she made a trip to Maryland to visit him. Clements had devised a crude instrument to measure surface tension, and upon her return to Harvard, Avery made a copy to use in her own research. She examined the lungs of babies dying of various causes and found those succumbing to hyaline membrane disease had a higher surface tension in their lungs than babies dying from other causes.

Avery reasoned these babies were deficient in surfactant. This was her "lightbulb" moment: Hyaline membranes weren't the cause of the disease; they were the result. The babies couldn't expand their lungs. Within a couple of days, a glassy layer of proteins formed inside the lung air sacs, preventing oxygen from reaching the blood. In 1959, Avery and Mead published their studies and revolutionized the understanding of what caused premature babies to suffocate.[11] But knowing the pathology didn't immediately lead to a solution. Effective treatment was still years away.

Once Avery's insights reached the medical world, physicians realized why their therapy for hyaline membrane disease didn't work better. They had been using ventilators to inflate preemies' lungs, but ventilators didn't prevent collapse during exhalation. Doctors had been focusing on the wrong phase of breathing. If they were going to counteract the lack of surfactant in underdeveloped lungs, they had to devise a way to keep the air sacs open.

In 1971, George Gregory, a pediatric anesthesiologist at the University of California, San Francisco, tried adding airway pressure to the ventilator during exhalation to keep the air sacs from collapsing.[12] This reduced mortality rates in respiratory distress syndrome at UCSF from 75 percent to 20 percent. Neonatal centers all over the country soon adopted Gregory's technique and gave preemies unable to breathe a new chance for those first crucial breaths.

Neonatologists ventilated babies with tiny face masks, like pilots used at high altitudes. These didn't even have to cover the whole face. Air delivered by nasal prongs or a miniature dome over the nostrils inflated the airways satisfactorily. If you visit the neonatal ICU in many medical centers today, you will see these tiny babies, their noses covered by a plastic appliance, breathing quietly as they sleep.

If premature babies couldn't make surfactant in the lungs, was there some way to speed up lung development? Animal studies suggested steroids stimulated the lungs to make surfactant. In 1966, neonatologist Louis Gluck developed a technique to measure the levels of surfactant precursors in amniotic fluid.[13] This helped to spot endangered pregnancies and guide therapy.

New Zealand obstetrician Graham Liggins showed that treating mothers at high risk for premature birth with cortisone before delivery lowered the incidence of neonatal respiratory distress from 25 percent to 9 percent, almost a threefold drop.[14] So, steroids emerged as another promising way to reduce the mortality in this tragic disease.

These successes notwithstanding, what premature babies really needed to breathe after delivery was surfactant. But surfactant was a complex chemical combination of fats and proteins synthesized in the lungs. Researchers initially collected the soapy substance by washing the foamy liquid out of the airways of animals, such as sheep, cattle, or swine. Sometimes they minced lung tissue or even filtered amniotic fluid to obtain the precious liquid. When they instilled surfactant into the airways of preterm experimental animals, they increased survival rates after delivery. But other problems arose. The foreign proteins induced an immune reaction in the lungs. And the risk of infection was a constant threat.

In 1980, another breakthrough occurred. Tetsuro Fujiwara, a Japanese pediatrician, showed that bovine surfactant improved survival in human premature infants as well as in experimental animals.[15] Because replacing surfactant was the most direct way to manage respiratory distress in preemies, physiologists and biochemists all over the world scrambled to develop ways to extract the beneficial compound from animal lungs and make it safe and nonallergenic. Within a few years, animal surfactant became commercially available, and the survival rate of preemies increased. Infants of smaller and smaller weight could get through those crucial first hours and days after birth.

The success with animal surfactant stimulated efforts to perfect a synthetic version. Researchers hoped such a substance would not cause immune reactions and would be safe. By 1990, synthetic surfactants came on the market, and today both types offer comparable effectiveness and safety. And fewer than one in a hundred newborn babies develops infant respiratory distress syndrome.

If Patrick Kennedy were born today, his mother would have received steroid injections as soon as she appeared at risk for preterm labor, days or weeks before delivery. Once delivered, in addition to being warmed in an incubator, he would receive oxygen, combined with mechanical ventilation and expiratory airway pressure. He would receive surfactant dripped into his airways, and he would inhale nitric oxide, which dilates blood vessels and promotes oxygenation. A team of specialists would pay scrupulous attention to his nutrition, fluid requirements, blood count, and need for antibiotics. Today, the Kennedy baby, born in the thirty-fifth week, would have greater than a 90 percent chance of making it through those harrowing days after delivery. Indeed, with these combined approaches, babies born as early as the twenty-second week can now survive, and those born after the twenty-eighth week have nearly an 80 percent chance of being able to breathe.[16]

Can we prevent premature births? That would further reduce the incidence of infant respiratory distress, but the solution will have to be more than medical. High blood pressure, diabetes, and drug abuse certainly cause mothers to be at increased risk of early delivery. However, social and economic factors, like poverty, malnutrition, and not having access to prenatal care, contribute as well. So, newborn respiratory health is as much a social challenge as a medical problem.

Four million babies are born each year in the United States. Four hundred thousand are preterm. Twenty-three thousand die, just under six per thousand deliveries. Since the advent of neonatal intensive care, mortality rates from respiratory distress syndrome have fallen to levels not thought possible a generation ago. Birth defects and chromosomal abnormalities have now replaced breathing disorders at the top of the list of infant killers in this country. Respiratory distress syndrome hasn't disappeared. It remains a major neonatal concern but not the hopeless tragedy of earlier times. In the sixty years since Virginia Apgar devised her scoring system and Mary Ellen Avery identified surfactant deficiency, that first breath has become a lot easier for the vast majority of preemies.

Eventually Apgar left Columbia to study public health and later joined the March of Dimes as head of its division on birth defects. She spent the rest of her career traveling, speaking, and writing about the importance of good prenatal and obstetrical care in lowering infant mortality. She warned about the risks of teen pregnancy in an era when that kind of discussion was controversial. Apgar never had children of her own. But she was a surrogate mother to millions of babies everywhere in the world. She died in 1973 at the age of sixty-five.

Mary Ellen Avery had a productive career in academic pediatrics. She advanced to become professor at Harvard and chief pediatrician at Boston Children's Hospital. In 1991, President George Bush presented her with the National Medal of Science for her work on infant respiratory distress syndrome. Toward the end of her life, she became a spokesperson in the fight against polio and an advocate for women's health. Avery died in 2011 at the age of eighty-four.

What if Apgar had continued as a surgeon instead of switching to anesthesia? How many more babies would have died? What if Avery hadn't developed tuberculosis? Would she have become interested in breathing problems of newborns? What if she hadn't been curious about why the lungs of infants dying of respiratory distress were collapsed? How long would it have been before someone discovered the role of surfactant? How many more babies would have died?

IV
BREATHING DEFENDS

㉑

AROUND THE WORLD ON OXYGEN

"Laughing is also good for your respiratory system."

—Allen Klein[1]

"People say you can't live without love. . . . I think oxygen is more important."

—Anonymous[2]

In 1918, newly graduated from medical school and interning in New York City, Alvan Barach watched patients suffocate to death from pneumonia brought on by the Spanish flu.[3] Sometimes he and his colleagues had to sign as many as five death certificates a day, young lives ended as fast and capriciously as a lit candle snuffed by a puff of wind. As patients lay gasping for their last breath of air, the interns placed a funnel over their faces and flushed oxygen from a bedside tank into their lungs in a desperate effort to keep them alive. The treatment rarely worked, but the experience stimulated Barach's curiosity about the effect of oxygen in pneumonia. It would turn into a lifelong passion.

Oxygen was first recognized as a separate element of atmospheric air in 1774. (Air is 21 percent oxygen.) Ever since that time, physicians have explored medical uses of the life-supporting gas, but it wasn't until 1885 that a Pennsylvania doctor reported administering oxygen via rubber tubing to a young man dying of pneumonia. After several hours of oxygen blowing across his face, the man's crisis passed, and he recovered.[4] Though medical science didn't understand exactly how it helped, enriching the inhaled air with oxygen appeared beneficial for patients with respiratory distress.

Soon inventive physicians fashioned rubber face masks or catheters that streamed oxygen into the nostrils or mouths of patients with respiratory distress. But these were uncomfortable, and innovators looked for better ways to deliver oxygen. In the early 1900s, small tents containing oxygen mixed with air appeared on the market. These supplied extra oxygen to patients whose lungs were unable to extract the gas from inhaled air. However, whenever anyone opened the tent flaps, the oxygen diffused into the environment, and its benefit literally blew away.

Barach set out to improve on this. He devised a system using a mouthpiece to deliver 50 percent oxygen to patients. Their skin turned from blue to pink and their breathing became less labored. Barach was so enthused he dashed down the halls announcing his results to his colleagues. How much they shared his exuberance is not known. Barach later tried oxygen for heart failure and observed similar results, so that his fascination for the invisible gas intensified.

Barach wanted both to control the level of oxygen administered and to make patients comfortable, while allowing caregivers to do their jobs. In 1926, he published a paper describing his modification of the oxygen tent. His ingenuity showed in every detail. Smaller and more portable than previous versions, Barach's tent covered only the head and chest of the patient. The walls of the tent consisted of rubberized silk with a celluloid roof and windows that allowed the patient to see out and nursing staff to see in. A motorized fan circulated cool air inside the tent, and a finely tuned valve system controlled the concentration of oxygen flowing in, while accumulating carbon dioxide was eliminated.[5] With the entire apparatus mounted on a four-wheeled cart, one person could transport it wherever it was needed.

Barach's tent became standard treatment for patients with pneumonia and heart attacks and endured for the next forty years. When I was an intern in 1961, I cared for many patients with pneumonia and heart attacks who were placed in the O_2 tent. It worked fine and made patients more comfortable, even if the canopy made nursing care more difficult. Eventually the cumbersomeness of the tent led to its replacement by nasal cannulas, but Alvan Barach deserves credit for inventing the first practical way of delivering controlled amounts of oxygen to suffocating patients.

Barach had to overcome widespread professional resistance to his ideas about oxygen therapy, so he became a salesman. Toting his portable tent, he traveled the eastern United States, administering oxygen to lung and heart patients. Once he went to Ann Arbor to treat Dr. Cyrus Sturgis, the redoubtable chief of medicine at the University of Michigan, when the famous professor came down with pneumonia. Barach recalled that, after a few minutes of oxygen therapy, Sturgis exclaimed, "Take it off," however a short time later asked that it be restarted. Barach was unclear about whether this was an endorsement of oxygen, but Sturgis did recover from the pneumonia. At another prominent medical school, a skeptical professor quipped the only benefit of oxygen was to make the patients die pink instead of blue.[6] An irony of medicine, like all of life, is that a great idea is often a hard sell.

The medical establishment also fought Barach's recommendation to use industrial-grade oxygen tanks on patients. At that time, pure, filtered gas was difficult to acquire, but pragmatic Barach felt industrial-grade gas was clean enough to work satisfactorily in sick patients. Later, as manufacturers learned how to filter gases and compress them in steel cylinders under high pressure, medical-grade oxygen became available, and the heavy green tanks grew to be commonplace in hospitals everywhere.

Barach crusaded on behalf of oxygen therapy for the next five decades, writing and speaking to persuade his reluctant and skeptical colleagues. Meanwhile, he continued innovating. In 1934, he conceived the idea of mixing oxygen with helium to assist suffocating asthma patients. Helium is less dense than air and therefore should be easier to inhale and exhale. Though the literature debates its value, Heliox, the commercial name, is still widely used today as an adjunct in treating asthmatics in respiratory distress.[7]

In 1948, Barach publicly advocated using continuous supplementary oxygen for COPD, which was drastic but prescient. He again faced concerns by the medical establishment that oxygen would suppress breathing in these patients. Normally, nature maintains very tight control of the rate and depth of breathing, so that oxygen and carbon dioxide levels fluctuate very little. If blood oxygen falls or carbon dioxide level rises, the brain senses this and stimulates breathing, like a thermostat driving a furnace.

However, respiratory patients become adapted to living with low oxygen levels, like high-altitude residents. As their diseases worsen and they can't eliminate carbon dioxide, they adjust to living with elevated levels of that gas, as well. But, they may lose the breathing stimulus carbon dioxide normally provides. That means their drive to breathe depends entirely on the amount of oxygen reaching the brain. A fall in oxygen increases breathing; a rise in oxygen decreases breathing.

If respiratory patients inhale enough supplementary oxygen to bring the level in their bodies to normal, their stimulus to breathe decreases or disappears. Breathing becomes shallow or even stops entirely. So, the goal in treating severe COPD patients with oxygen is to administer just enough oxygen to avoid oxygen deprivation but not enough to reduce breathing.

Knowing this, Barach placed emphysema patients in hospital rooms enriched with oxygen, where they remained full time, which he defined as more than sixteen hours a day. Some essentially lived in the hospital for months. One patient reportedly stayed in the hospital for three years. While the chamber kept these patients alive, it must have been like being in a prison. Barach must have felt it helped them because he continued using oxygen, but reports about how patients tolerated these conditions give us no details about their day-by-day lives.

Barach also experimented with small oxygen cylinders that patients could push on a cart, thus enabling them to exercise. In the 1950s, the idea of exercising respiratory patients was radical. Conventional wisdom preached that patients with breathing disorders required rest so they could conserve their meager energy. Of course, their muscles atrophied, and they quickly became bedbound. Recognizing this, Barach again found himself bucking the medical establishment. He advocated treating emphysema patients like athletes in training, albeit with very low exercise levels. This approach benefited patients and later became a mainstay in pulmonary rehabilitation.

Fortunately, Barach did not have to fight the oxygen battle alone forever. Briton Moran Campbell was one of the foremost respiratory physiologists of his generation.[8] In the late 1950s, he became interested in respiratory failure, whose most frequent cause is COPD. Campbell saw the dilemma these patients presented: They were asphyxiating from lack of oxygen but could stop breathing if supplied with too much oxygen.

In 1968, Campbell relocated to Hamilton, Ontario, Canada, and became known among pulmonary physicians for advocating precision dosing of supplementary oxygen for COPD patients. He devised a face mask with a nozzle carefully milled so that a thin jet of oxygen bathed the patient's nose and mouth, increasing the inspired oxygen only a few percent more than atmospheric levels. He called it a Ventimask. The device worked well and greatly reduced the number of COPD patients who required mechanical ventilation to survive respiratory failure.

But the overarching question persisted: Did supplementary oxygen prolong life or improve its quality for respiratory patients? If exercise with oxygen helped COPD patients to improve, why not use oxygen intermittently, say an hour on and an hour off? Sad to say, that turned out to worsen their predicament and prompted Campbell to quote the British physiologist J. S. Haldane, who had said, "[I]ntermittent oxygen therapy is like bringing a drowning man to the surface—occasionally."[9] Unable to store oxygen, the body immediately felt its lack. If oxygen was administered, the patient improved, but if it was stopped, within a few minutes the patient began to suffocate, with dizziness, shortness of breath, and air hunger.

Before the Ventimask, we tested the optimum oxygen flow rate for COPD patients, monitoring the blood saturation as we adjusted valves, observing pulse and respiratory rates, seeing if patients perked up or said they felt more comfortable. One colleague called it the Goldilocks approach: not too little, not too much, but just right.

With Campbell and Barach advocating controlled oxygen therapy for COPD, pulmonologists on both sides of the Atlantic came to agree that exercise with oxygen could help emphysema patients. In 1958, Barach developed a small refillable oxygen cylinder suitable for use during exercise. Soon other investigators showed that ambulatory oxygen increased how long and how far emphysema patients could walk. But at a flow rate of three liters per minute, a tank small enough to be pulled, which contained six hundred liters of compressed gas, ran out of oxygen in less than four hours. Depletion of oxygen from the cylinders was a major practical obstacle for respiratory patients who wanted to exercise.

During the early 1960s, while a resident, I cared for patients with advanced lung disease and felt frustrated because they could exercise while they were hospitalized, but at home they were limited. Imagine someone who required thirty cylinders of oxygen each week. That person would need a supply delivered almost every day and would spend hundreds of dollars a month on oxygen alone.

However, medicine was about to benefit from industrial ingenuity dating to the previous century. In 1895, German physicist Carl von Linde had developed a method to liquefy gases, including oxygen. This spawned a host of products for welding and cutting steel that the construction and shipbuilding industries quickly put to use. In time, engineers experimented with liquid oxygen for medical use. As it evaporates, one liter of liquid oxygen expands into hundreds of liters of gas. Also, liquid oxygen requires less pressure to store than compressed gas, which meant that liquid tanks could be smaller and lighter than compressed gas cylinders.

The medical breakthrough came in 1965 when the Linde walker came on the market. It consisted of a barrel of liquid oxygen, nicknamed a "cow," that remained stationary in the patient's home, plus a small reservoir weighing eight pounds, about the size of a briefcase, with a strap that hung over the patients' shoulders. A port on the reservoir connected to a plastic tube that ran oxygen to the users' nostrils. With the Linde walker, patients could fill the reservoir with liquid oxygen whenever they needed and enjoy several hours of sauntering and strolling.

Soon other companies made further modifications, such as substituting an oxygen concentrator for the liquid cow. The concentrator removed nitrogen from air, increasing the amount of inspired oxygen. Also, thin catheters, threaded directly into the trachea through a puncture wound in the neck, allowed for very low oxygen flows that enabled reservoirs to last even longer. Today it's commonplace to see people in theaters, airports, and stores with tubes in their nostrils, breathing life-giving oxygen while they participate in living.

Portable oxygen for home use was a major advance. But respiratory physicians faced other problems, such as how to help patients to inhale deeply enough to clear secretions and expand collapsed lung segments. In addition, doctors sought ways to deliver life-saving medications, like adrenaline, to the lungs of those with asthma and bronchitis. Because the interior surface of the respiratory tract absorbs gases and liquids well, it was possible to inhale drugs, as well as oxygen, under pressure, to treat respiratory difficulties.

Humans have been breathing in substances for medicinal, religious, or pleasure-seeking purposes since the earliest times. Asians and Africans inhaled hashish and opium to produce euphoria. Native Americans smoked peyote and tobacco as part of social rituals. Science entered the picture in 1738, when the Dutch-Swiss mathematician Bernoulli showed that forcing a liquid or gas through a small opening increased its speed of flow, and Italian physicist Giovanni Venturi later used this principle to create jets of air or water in glass vessels. Armed with this knowledge, by the nineteenth century, doctors and pharmacists invented pipes, atomizers, and nebulizers that enabled inhalation of drugs as therapy for asthma and bronchitis.[10]

Earlier, I described my first visit in 1946 to the hospital emergency department for an asthma attack and how I received an injection of adrenaline that I felt saved my life. At home, I had a nebulizer, an egg-shaped glass device with a rubber bulb that looked like a miniature football with a spout. My parents would put a few drops of adrenaline solution into the glass egg and squeeze the bulb, generating a fine mist of drug particles that supposedly were absorbed into the lungs when I inhaled. I didn't feel it helped much. Based on what I now know, they used too little medication and synchronizing their squeezes with my breathing depended on pure luck. But, just as liquid oxygen, originally invented for industry, benefited medicine, in the mid-twentieth century, aviation also gave breathing a helpful thrust in its quest for oxygen.

When airplanes first flew higher than 12,000 feet, many pilots were sensitive to the decrease in atmospheric oxygen pressure and became dizzy or lost consciousness. During World War I, military aviators needed to fly above 15,000 feet to escape antiaircraft fire and so required oxygen supplementation to avoid blacking out.[11]

At first, pilots carried small canisters of oxygen and, holding a hose between their teeth, adjusted flow by means of simple needle valves. These proved unreliable, and during the 1920s, pressure regulators and liquid oxygen sources came into use, as well as tight-fitting facemasks that directed the life-saving gas to the nose and mouth. But problems remained. Water vapor from exhaled air accumulated in tubing. Ice formed at high altitudes and blocked flow. Also, fighter pilots had to breathe oxygen while climbing, rolling, and diving. During the 1930s, researchers in the growing field of aerospace medicine designed devices to solve these important problems.

By the time World War II broke out, planners in the US War Department realized that planes would need to fly over 30,000 feet high to avoid flak. Long-distance bombers required large amounts of oxygen delivered under pressure for these flights. Aeronautical engineer V. Ray Bennett designed a pressure-activated valve used by the US Army Air Corps to supply oxygen.

After the war ended, he adapted his valve for medical use, and by the 1950s, the Bennett machine became a fixture in hospitals all over the country. One popular model was a metal box mounted on an oxygen cylinder. It featured flexible corrugated tubes and two dials that stared out like the eyes of a space alien. Forrest Bird, another World War II aeronautical engineer and inventor, designed a similar device to help a friend of his with emphysema to breathe better. His Bird respirator, which looked like a green plastic portable radio, also delivered oxygen under pressure and competed with Bennett's devices. The Bird casing was translucent, so that the valves and clutches inside were visible as they moved and clicked with each breath.[12] These early pressure devices were finicky and difficult for nonexperts to use, problems that eventually led to the birth of a whole new field of respiratory care, as I found out firsthand.

In 1960, in my third year at Northwestern University Medical School, I spent three months on surgery as a subintern, a medical student who functioned as a junior intern. Living in the hospital and being on call every other night, I was the first person the nurses contacted when patients got in trouble. Respiratory problems were common after surgery. Postop pain prevented patients from breathing, and many needed extra oxygen. Anesthetic gases left the lungs dry and irritated. Many patients were elderly, overweight, or had asthma and COPD, which made them vulnerable to pneumonia. A typical patient would be a smoker who had undergone upper-abdominal surgery. Forty-eight hours postop, he or she would spike a fever and complain of being short of breath. Exam would show rapid, shallow breathing, with breath sounds decreased at the bases of the lungs. Suspecting portions of the lungs were collapsed, the attending surgeon would order the nurses to perform deep breathing exercises, plus IPPB (intermittent positive-pressure breathing) with oxygen every four hours to nebulize medications into the lungs.

The hospital where I was subintern used Bennetts to create the pressure to inflate collapsed lung segments. But the valves were temperamental and difficult to use. They would often stick. Sick patients would become confused and exhale when they were supposed to inhale. The nurses struggled to make them work and so would call the intern, who every other night was me.

I had no training in respiratory medicine, no knowledge of how Bennett valves worked, and as soon as the call came, I began to feel that itching stress that accompanies not wanting to fail but being fully aware of one's inadequacy. I dutifully went to the bedside; stared at the intimidating dials; adjusted valves, usually without success; and finally, hopelessly lost amid the mechanical maze, I would call the oxygen orderly for help. Hired because they were strong enough to hoist steel cylinders containing pressurized gases, these burly men were part of hospital maintenance and stationed in the basement. They dressed in work clothes, carried toolboxes full of wrenches and pliers, with rags in their hip pockets to wipe grease and dirt off the cylinders. They were low in the hospital hierarchy, but they were the only people who understood how to unstick valves, adjust pressures, and persuade the finicky breathing equipment to function. In fact, the nurses and doctors depended on them. These humble repairmen were the precursors of the high-tech respiratory care practitioners of today.

In the early 1920s, when Alvan Barach created a respiratory department at Presbyterian Hospital in New York to implement his ideas about oxygen and treatment of emphysema, some of his technical assistants remained with him for decades. Barach felt that, because they worked with patients and assisted the nurses and physicians, they needed training. He organized classes to teach the rudiments of physics and biology needed for their jobs and encouraged them to act as professionals, as part of the hospital care team.

Barach was not alone. In the 1940s, Edward Levine of Chicago's Michael Reese Hospital trained a cadre of technicians to manage the breathing problems of surgery patients.[13] He called this service inhalation therapy. Whether Levine was in contact with Barach is unknown, but in 1946, Levine convened a group at the University of Chicago and formed a nationwide Inhalation Therapy Organization.

In time, programs to train oxygen orderlies to become inhalation therapists arose in community colleges all over the country. Some universities even offered bachelor's degrees in the field. Textbooks and journals on respiratory care were published. Certification examinations and licensure helped ensure the public that those who helped them breathe were competent professionals.

Levine's Inhalation Therapy Organization became the American Association of Respiratory Care and has grown to more than 100,000 members today. The field attracts individuals who want to work directly with patients but enjoy the technical aspects of mechanical and electronic instruments. With advances in bioelectronics and fluidic engineering coming at warp speed, respiratory care is a major battlement defending breathing against the ravages of lung diseases.

By the time I finished training in 1969, intermittent positive-pressure breathing treatments with Bennetts and Birds were becoming suspect. Studies showed IPPB helped patients for a short time, perhaps a few minutes, but they soon lost their effect and seemed to be a waste of energy and money.

However, the Bennett and Bird devices themselves were very helpful when used continuously. They turned out to be the Model T Fords of mechanical ventilators, early versions of what are today the workhorses of intensive care units all over the world. (More on this later.)

By the late 1960s, most of medicine accepted Barach's work that oxygen helped COPD patients to feel better. But no one knew if pulmonary patients could, like those with strokes or trauma, be rehabilitated, brought back to previous levels of function. It was at that point Dr. Thomas Petty of Colorado, the evangelist of pulmonary rehabilitation, appeared on the scene.[14]

Patients with respiratory diseases had been moving to the mountains for centuries to breathe the clean, pure air. It was not an accident that Denver became home to several major pulmonary centers, such as National Jewish Hospital, Fitzsimons Army Medical Center, and the University of Colorado. It was also ironic that breathing the rarified atmosphere of the Mile-High City made respiratory patients, especially those with COPD and pulmonary fibrosis, more vulnerable to the adverse effects of oxygen deprivation than those at sea level.

Petty was high-energy. Naturally upbeat and sociable, he was easy to like. A native of Boulder, he joined the faculty at Colorado in 1963, just as liquid oxygen delivery systems were adapted to medical use.[15] Recognizing that lightweight canisters might enable patients to receive oxygen in their homes, Petty was the right man at the right time in the right place for respiratory care.

In 1968, Petty and his associates reported a study of twenty advanced COPD patients who, by using liquid oxygen twenty-four hours each day for eighteen months, not only had fewer hospital admissions but also actually improved their ability to exercise and lived longer. This was the first solid evidence that medical treatment could prolong life for those with this distressing disease.

Encouraged by this success, Petty developed a multidisciplinary respiratory rehabilitation program at the University of Colorado. It included physicians, nurses, respiratory and occupational therapists, exercise physiologists, and vocational counselors on its staff. The pillars of the project were oxygen and exercise, including both walking and training the diaphragm, the main breathing muscle. With his bow tie and informal style, Petty was a popular feature at meetings, preaching the benefits of pulmonary rehabilitation to all who would listen.

Petty soon inspired other institutions to follow his example. During the 1970s, several medical centers around the country established pulmonary rehabilitation programs. Under the guidance of the late Ken Moser and Andy Ries, the University of California, San Diego, was one of the earliest. Not only was it a resource for the region's clinical pulmonologists, like me, but it was also one of the institutions that showed the world how oxygen and exercise could make life better for respiratory patients.

In 1976, Petty interviewed Barach.[16] The older physician was eighty-one at the time and would die the next year. He spoke in the raspy voice of an octogenarian but showed the imagination and curiosity that made him a leader in respiratory medicine in the mid-twentieth century. Barach said, "It may seem unusual perhaps to suggest exercise to these breathless people, but in fact it is one of the ways by which they can restore physical fitness. These patients can begin walking 50 to 100 steps the first day and gradually extend the . . . walking distance to half a mile twice a day."[17]

Petty became Barach's successor. Like Barach, he had to fight the skepticism of the medical profession, but he also had to surmount insurance industry resistance. Payers supported only programs modeled after cardiac rehabilitation. After a heart attack, patients were motivated to change diet, stop smoking, and control blood pressure and diabetes. They could begin walking and, in a month or two, increase endurance to normal levels. Thus treadmills, nurse coaches, and nutritionists formed the backbone of a cardiac rehab center. In contrast, pulmonary patients generally had been impaired for years, were unable to engage in any strenuous activity, had been in and out of the hospital, and were malnourished and depressed. Their rehabilitative needs were more complex, and their results more modest. They required oxygen, physical therapy, vocational counseling, and often psychotherapy. They needed many months to improve and were prone to becoming discouraged.

Petty needed the skills of a political lobbyist as well as those of a physician to overcome medical skeptics and cost-conscious insurance companies. In the late 1970s, he orchestrated a series of trials for the federal government that would establish the proper role of oxygen therapy and pulmonary rehabilitation in medical care. Experts debated how many hours a day respiratory patients needed to breathe oxygen in order to benefit. Was twenty-four hours of extra oxygen better than twelve or fifteen? British investigators showed increased survival from fifteen hours daily in a group of emphysema patients. Because oxygen therapy was, even at its best, expensive and cumbersome, knowing the optimum schedule was of practical importance. Petty continued writing papers and preaching at meetings, a tireless advocate for the benefits of pulmonary rehabilitation.

It took until nearly 1990 before enough evidence accumulated to satisfy doubters that pulmonary rehabilitation with oxygen and exercise could improve and prolong life for respiratory patients, plus was cost-effective. Two major studies, the fruits of Petty's vision and effort, showed that using supplementary oxygen more than twelve hours a day prolonged life in respiratory insufficiency and that some patients required continuous treatment, twenty-four hours each day, to survive.

Ed, a sixty-something-year-old man, resided in an upscale coastal community near San Diego, where he owned a travel office and was a great success booking tours and arranging cruises. But, Ed was so short of breath he was having difficulty running his business. The least bit of activity tired him, which, because he was accustomed to being active, greatly frustrated him. His doctor suspected emphysema and requested pulmonary consultation.

Ed was outgoing and chatty and always made sure he offered me a firm handshake whenever I entered the examining room. Spare to the point of being skinny, he dressed in a natty sport coat, brightly colored, with well-creased slacks and a matching rep tie. A breast-pocket handkerchief and loafers, often tasseled, completed his ensemble. Endowed with mental wheels that whirred continuously, Ed was not ready for life as an invalid. He had quit smoking, was on a well-crafted schedule of medications, and was up to date with relevant immunizations. But Ed wanted to do more.

Pulmonary function tests confirmed the presence of severe obstruction to airflow and increase in the work of breathing, which confirmed Ed indeed had advanced emphysema. An exercise study demonstrated his blood oxygen level plummeted with exercise, coming to resemble that of someone on a mountaintop. So, I began him on supplementary oxygen and recommended he enroll in pulmonary rehabilitation at nearby UC San Diego Medical Center, which he did with enthusiasm. Within a few months, aided by a portable oxygen system, Ed was working full time and was more active, and his mood was as bright as his wardrobe. He was a poster child for the benefits of pulmonary rehabilitation, an unknowing beneficiary of the efforts of Alvan Barach and Thomas Petty. Then, one day in the office, as we were discussing his situation, Ed said, "I have an idea."

Emphysema destroys lung tissue and causes two major problems: increase in the work of breathing and maldistribution of inhaled air and blood flowing through the pulmonary capillaries. Normally, inhalation and exhalation require minimal effort, except during extreme exercise. When emphysema is present, the inelastic lungs require extreme force to pull air in and push it out, meaning the sufferer continuously labors to breathe.

Also, nature normally disperses inhaled air and blood flow evenly in the lungs, so that the air sacs, the business portion of the lungs, are surrounded by capillaries for efficient exchange of oxygen and carbon dioxide.[18] But when emphysema is present, some portions of the lungs receive air but little blood flow, and other regions, blood flow but little air. The result is that blood reaching the various organs of the body is deficient in oxygen, especially during exercise and sleep. Eventually, carbon dioxide accumulates as well, leading to respiratory failure and death. However, pulmonary rehabilitation can forestall these events by teaching patients to breathe efficiently, stay active, and use oxygen supplementation.

Ed's idea was to broker cruises for COPD patients like those he had met at UC San Diego. He was confident he could negotiate with airlines and shipping lines to arrange for oxygen refills at various ports of call. He even thought of bringing respiratory therapists along to work with the globe-trotting COPD patients. I thought it was a great idea and encouraged him to go for it. He advertised in the newsletter of the Better Breathers' Club, a program for respiratory patients sponsored by the local chapter of the American Lung Association, and customers soon began signing on.

Ed loved to travel and the payoff for him was free passage on the excursions. He occasionally called the office to ask about some subject, like the safety of taking an oxygen reservoir onto a plane (safe but unnecessary; airlines supply extra oxygen when needed) and even suggested I come along on the cruises and give medical lectures. Unfortunately, I was too busy and had to decline the offer.

Ed's idea was a great success. Not only did he help fellow patients participate in one of the pleasures of living, but he also enjoyed what he was doing. Ed also demonstrated the progress of respiratory care. His COPD cruises would never have been possible had not portable oxygen therapy and pulmonary rehabilitation existed.

The growth of respiratory care didn't occur spontaneously. It followed the evolution of pulmonary medicine during the mid-twentieth century, from an arcane specialty that concentrated on tuberculosis to a dynamic branch of internal medicine based on applying pulmonary physiology to bedside care of patients unable to breathe. That progression depended on the vision and energy of many pioneers, leaders venerated today as founders of modern pulmonology, like Barach and Petty. As pulmonologist Richard Casaburi said, "If Tom Petty was the father of pulmonary rehabilitation, Alvan Barach was certainly the grandfather."[19]

Barach lived to be eighty-two and remained active right up to the end. In his last year of life, he managed to publish six papers. He is remembered as a pioneer in pulmonary rehabilitation and in establishing respiratory care as a professional specialty.

Petty remained a leader in pulmonary medicine through the turn of the twenty-first century. He wrote about the importance of screening patients with pulmonary function tests to detect lung diseases, campaigned against tobacco smoking, and remained a champion of long-term oxygen therapy. In another of those ironies of medicine, he became an oxygen patient himself and, for the last four years of his life, learned firsthand what his patients of the previous forty years had been experiencing. In 2008, at the age of seventy-six, Petty died of pulmonary hypertension following several cardiac surgical procedures. His influence continues, and his memory inspires the new generation of pulmonologists.

And how distant and primitive seem those midnights fifty years ago, when I staggered bleary-eyed to the wards to face postop patients with lung collapse or pneumonia and breathed a sigh of relief when the elevator door opened and the oxygen orderly appeared, to rescue both the patients and me.

22

THANK YOU FOR MY LIFE

"Mechanical ventilation is ubiquitous to intensive care. In fact, the modern day intensive care unit (ICU) owes its origins to the need to care for patients on ventilators in a common location."

—Neil Macintyre and Richard Branson[1]

In 1960, our medical school class was introduced to various subspecialties of medicine and surgery. Only a few graduates would enter these fields, but the faculty wanted all of us to be acquainted with them. Part of the exposure to anesthesiology was a field trip to Cook County Hospital, the sprawling institution at which Chicago's poor received care. One of the largest hospitals in the country, County had three thousand beds, with operating rooms in use around the clock, wards full of knife and gunshot victims and alcoholics with liver failure, and babies born in hallways for lack of delivery room space. It was chaotic; colorful; and, for newcomers, an exciting exposure to the real clinical world.

Dr. Ernst Trier Mørch was chief of anesthesiology at County. Known for having invented one of the first positive-pressure mechanical ventilators, which replaced the iron lung as the preferred way to inflate the lungs of patients unable to breathe on their own, Mørch was born in Denmark in 1908 and graduated from the University of Copenhagen Medical School in 1935.[2] He embarked on a career in surgery but, having undergone a tonsillectomy without anesthesia when he was five years old, decided to study anesthesiology.

When the Germans occupied Denmark in 1942, they were initially lenient toward physicians, and Mørch received permission to study anesthesia at the famous Karolinska Institute in Stockholm, Sweden. When he returned to Copenhagen, he was so expert that the other surgeons asked him to anesthetize their patients. In Sweden, he had learned to use a small mechanical respirator called a spiropulsator but was unable to import one to Denmark. Thwarted but not defeated, he cobbled together the first mechanical ventilator in his country from sections of sewer pipe, bicycle pump parts, and a small electric motor discarded by the Nazis.[3]

Mørch was not just a medical innovator; he was also a patriot and a hero. As the war progressed, the Nazis put ever-increasing restrictions on Danish citizens, and Mørch joined the resistance. They smuggled Jews to Sweden in fishing boats, and when the Gestapo deployed bloodhounds to detect fugitives hidden below false-bottomed decks, Mørch and a pharmacist mixed rabbit blood with cocaine, which they sprinkled on the deck planks to anesthetize the dogs' noses. They also used barbiturate suppositories to quiet hidden children and arranged for sympathetic Swedish physicians to meet the boats and attend the deeply sedated infants.

In 1946, after World War II ended, Mørch received a scholarship to study anesthesiology at Oxford, where he worked under the renowned Sir Robert Macintosh. Mørch was particularly concerned about the danger of inadequate breathing during anesthesia. Anesthetic gases depressed the central nervous system. This meant they could suppress breathing. Further, when curare-like drugs were used to relax patients' muscles during surgery, artificial breathing became even more important.

At that time, anesthetists assisted breathing by placing a tight-fitting mask over the patient's face and manually inflating the lungs by squeezing a rubber bag attached to the anesthesia circuit, a procedure called bagging. If the anesthetist should let up, the patient began to suffocate. As late as 1961, when I was an intern on surgery at Northwestern, I remember the surgeon would often look toward the head of the operating table and comment, "Blood's looking a little blue. Better give it some more bagging." A better system was needed.

In 1947, Mørch presented a paper to the Royal Society of Medicine in London that advocated mechanical control of ventilation during surgical anesthesia, but many of his colleagues in the audience were skeptical about the feasibility of machines replacing human hands for breathing support during surgery. Mørch became discouraged and in 1949 emigrated with his family to the United States, settling in Kansas City, Missouri, where a new medical school was opening. There he redesigned his artificial ventilator, which he felt was far superior to the iron lung. Mørch's ventilator had several unique features, such as a bellows to measure the volume of each breath. He later claimed, "It was so simple even a doctor could operate it."[4]

In 1953, Mørch became the director of anesthesia at Billings Hospital of the University of Chicago and in 1958 moved across town to Cook County, where I first saw him and his breathing machine. It was a clear plastic box the size of a suitcase, on rollers, so that it could be placed under a hospital bed. A motor turned a wheel attached to a rod and piston that forced air into the patient's trachea and thereby inflated the patient's lungs. The main problem was that, if the patient's lungs were stiff or boggy from pneumonia or edema, the inflating pressures could become high enough to tear the spongy lung tissue. Despite that, Mørch's device was one of the first workable ventilators built on the principle of inflating the lungs rather than expanding the chest, like the iron lung, the alternative method to treat respiratory failure.

Mammals inhale by expanding their chests, creating negative pressure in the lungs, so that air rushes in from the atmosphere. The iron lung and devices like it mimic nature in this regard but are not strong enough to expand lungs that are inflamed or scarred or soggy with fluid. In these circumstances, applying positive pressure works better. However, it took a long time for medical science to realize this.

Claudius Galen, who lived in the second century CE, was the most famous medical scientist of his time.[5] Galen believed that the lungs transported some substance from the air into the body and that the lungs discharged "fuliginous wastes" from the body.[6] (The Latin word *fuliginosus* means "sooty or dusty.") He noticed, when he opened the chest of an animal, its lungs collapsed and it died. In time, he learned to blow air through a reed into the animal's windpipe, which distended the lungs and kept the animal temporarily alive. Galen so strongly influenced western thought throughout the middle ages that no one dared challenge his beliefs for more than a thousand years, until the rebirth of science during the Renaissance.

In 1543, Andreas Vesalius, mentioned earlier, published his masterpiece, *On the Fabric of the Human Body*. Vesalius felt that only by examining the human body directly could one understand how it worked.[7] He based his anatomic studies on dissections of human corpses, and when he repeated Galen's experiments, he reached different conclusions, many of which challenged Galen's teachings. Among these was the notion of mechanically inflating the lungs.

After Vesalius's time, artificial ventilation was used in animal experiments but not in humans, possibly because of concerns about contagiousness—the Black Death had decimated Europe only a century earlier—as well as religious scruples. But two centuries later, in 1740, the prestigious Academie des Sciences in Paris was advising mouth-to-mouth resuscitation of drowning victims.

In 1776, British surgeon John Hunter invented a double-bellows ventilator that pumped air into the lungs and then sucked it out. In 1780, French physician Francois Chaussier devised a simple bag and face mask for artificial ventilation to protect the rescuer from breathing exhaled air.[8] However, bellows ventilation could blow a hole in the delicate lung tissue, permitting air to rush into the space between the lungs and chest wall, which made the lungs collapse. Both the French Academy and the British Royal Humane Society withdrew support for the bellows technique, and by the mid-nineteenth century, physicians abandoned positive-pressure ventilation.

Nevertheless, in the physiology laboratory, scientists relied on positive-pressure ventilation in animal experiments. In 1878, French physiologist Paul Bert wrote of ventilating experimental animals by means of a tracheostomy tube and a bellows,[9] and by 1879, ventilators were standard equipment for animal studies in science labs at Harvard University.[10]

During the nineteenth century, lung surgery was limited to aspirating lung abscesses and tuberculous cavities. These disorders caused the surface of the lung to adhere to the inside of the chest wall, so surgical drainage could be accomplished without causing the lungs to collapse. Though surgeons wanted to operate inside the chest, they were stymied by the difficulty of maintaining breathing. Thus, the mortality rate of thoracic surgery was high, and lung procedures were rare.

As early as 1915, the Scandinavians were experimenting with use of positive-pressure ventilation during anesthesia, but the rest of the medical world was unaware of that. By 1930, anesthetists purposely gave enough anesthetic gas to suppress patient breathing, which eliminated the patient partially awakening and coughing or moving during surgery.

When I was an intern in 1961, the surgeon would often become angry at the anesthesiologist if the patient bucked just as he was about to perform some delicate part of the procedure. In addition, as mentioned earlier, paralyzing agents like curare were administered to relax the patients' muscles. These certainly rendered the surgical field quiet but made the need for ventilation during surgery even more important.

In 1940, Swedish surgeon Carl Gunnar Engstrom invented a constant-volume ventilator similar to Mørch's, which was used at hospitals in his home country to support critically ill patients.[11] But because the Scandinavians published in Danish or Swedish journals, as E. T. Mørch later quipped, "they might as well have been writing in water."[12] Thus, much of the medical world, particularly the western hemisphere, was unaware of their progressive ideas.

In the United States, after World War II, innovation in mechanical breathing assistance came from aeronautical engineers. As mentioned earlier, V. Ray Bennett and Forrest Bird adapted for medical use valves designed to deliver oxygen to pilots. These valves converted continuous to intermittent pressure, so they could enhance breathing during inspiration but let expiration occur naturally.[13]

The Communicable Disease Service at Los Angeles County Hospital became the proving ground for Bennett's innovations. During 1946 and 1947, nearly 75 percent of the Los Angeles polio patients with respiratory paralysis died, despite the widespread use of negative-pressure ventilators like the Drinker and Emerson iron lungs.[14] The high mortality rate troubled Dr. Albert Bower, chief of communicable diseases, and he and his team concluded that buildup of carbon dioxide was the cause.

Beginning in September 1948, Bennett attached his intermittent positive-pressure valve to a tracheostomy tube. (The patient's neck, with the tracheostomy, was outside the iron lung.) By combining positive lung pressure with the negative pressure of the iron lung, Bennett was able to increase the volume of each breath by 30 percent, a significant improvement. The next year, Bower and Bennett showed that this lowered the mortality rate in polio-related respiratory paralysis from 75 percent to 16 percent. Their work marked the first large-scale success for intermittent positive-pressure ventilation in poliomyelitis.

Around the same time, Hurley Motley at the University of Pennsylvania showed positive pressure could be used in treating patients with asphyxiation, asthma, and postoperative breathing insufficiency as well.[15] Unfortunately, the initial studies of Bower, Bennett, and Motley were published locally or in journals directed toward aviation medicine, and the medical community at large remained unaware of their work. But the practice of breathing assistance would soon change forever.

In the summer of 1952, a severe polio epidemic hit both Europe and America, and Denmark was the epicenter in Scandinavia.[16] Cases of respiratory paralysis overwhelmed the Blegsdamhospital, Copenhagen's communicable disease hospital. From July to December, 2,722 polio patients were admitted, and 315, just more than 10 percent, needed respiratory support. Fifty to sixty patients were coming in daily, and five or six of them would develop respiratory failure. Results were tragic. In the first month of the epidemic, 80 percent of those with respiratory paralysis died within three days.[17]

Dr. Henry Lassen, the chief physician, faced a major crisis. Later he said, "Although we thought we knew something about the management of bulbar and respiratory poliomyelitis it soon became clear that only very little of what we did know at the beginning of the epidemic was really worth knowing."[18] Some held that little could be done because the virus was so powerful it had overwhelmed the patient's nervous system and death was inevitable. Besides, the hospital had only one Emerson iron lung and six vacuum vests to augment breathing.

On August 25, four patients died in one day, and Lassen called an emergency staff meeting to discuss what to do. Lassen invited Bjorn Ibsen, a young staff anesthesiologist who had trained for a while in Boston and knew of the success at Los Angeles County Hospital with positive-pressure breathing.[19] Ibsen had also been involved earlier that year in treating a child with tetanus by paralyzing her with curare and ventilating through a tracheostomy.

In addition, Ibsen observed in many surgical patients that exhaled carbon dioxide levels fluctuated markedly and could be controlled by vigorously squeezing the bag through which anesthetic gas was pumped. He noted that, when patients in the operating room did not eliminate carbon dioxide, their skin became clammy and their blood pressure rose, like paralytic polio patients just before they died. Ibsen reviewed the records of patients who had died, and like Bower, Ibsen concluded they were dying from carbon dioxide retention.

Based on these observations, Ibsen recommended that polio patients with respiratory failure undergo tracheostomy and be ventilated manually by squeezing bags containing oxygen, as was done during surgery.[20] Lassen was reluctant. The iron lung had sufficed in the past. Ibsen countered by citing the reports from Bower's group at Los Angeles County Hospital that positive pressure could augment breathing in patients with polio-related respiratory paralysis. Lassen finally agreed to let Ibsen try his method.

Ibsen's first patient was a twelve-year-old girl with paralysis of all four extremities. She was sweating, gasping for air, and drowning in her own secretions.[21] A surgeon made a tracheotomy incision under local anesthesia, and Ibsen put a cuffed tube into her trachea. He was unable to ventilate her, and she lost consciousness. He figured her airways were full of mucus and suctioned her through the tracheostomy, without success. She was dying. The situation was desperate. Ibsen decided to paralyze her with curare, like the child with tetanus a year earlier. Her muscles immediately relaxed, and he was able to ventilate her. She improved quickly.

Ibsen's success gave hope to everyone in the Blegsdamhospital. However, it created logistical problems. Each patient had to be ventilated by hand, using an anesthetic bag to inflate the lungs. There were five hundred patients already in the hospital, and sixty new cases were arriving daily. All staff felt overwhelmed, but Lassen and Ibsen created an organization to meet the demand. They recruited nurses and medical students to bag the patients continuously. Ibsen calculated that, in each twenty-four-hour period, they needed 260 extra nurses and 250 medical students, which allowed them to handle as many as 75 patients each day, enough to keep abreast of the admissions.

The medical school in Copenhagen closed temporarily so that its students could volunteer as ventilators. The students worked six- to eight-hour shifts around the clock. The need for student volunteers became so great that Lassen recruited dental students as well. These students, many of whom had only graduated from high school a year or two before, had to rely on the patient's appearance to adjust the rate of bagging. The students and the patients worked out systems whereby the patients could signal when they felt the discomfort of insufficient breathing, and their team could adjust the rate of bagging accordingly. One account mentioned a patient rolling her eyes up to signal when she needed more ventilation.

Both patients and students were under intense pressure: One group had their lives at stake; the other group needed the courage to proceed and the endurance to keep bagging. Young patients struggling to breathe underwent tracheostomy and then met the team of nineteen-year-old students who were supposed to keep them alive by squeezing the bag every few seconds for an indefinite time. Each patient had the same team of baggers every day. If the patient was a young child, the students read to them or tried to play games.

Technical and equipment problems were constant threats. Tanks ran out of oxygen, tubes kinked, and ventilating bags sprung leaks. Tracheostomy tubes slipped down too far and occluded the trachea. In addition, when patients died, especially at night, heartbreak followed. The students for the next day shift arrived only to learn their patient had expired. But, results with positive-pressure ventilation were superior to those of the iron lung. The mortality rate dropped from 90 percent to 25 percent, a heroic achievement. Fifteen hundred students took part in the effort and logged 165,000 hours of volunteer bagging until the epidemic passed.

Years later, at a conference held in his honor, Professor Ibsen was sitting in the front row, when a sixty-plus-year-old woman approached him and kissed him on the cheek. She said, "Thank you for my life." In 1952, she was the twelve-year-old girl he had first saved through a tracheostomy and positive-pressure ventilation.[22]

By the mid-1950s, the Scandinavians were using positive-pressure ventilation for other conditions besides polio. Physicians in the United States gradually came to see its value, as well. Thoracic surgeons noticed they got better results if they ventilated patients with positive pressure for several hours after lung and heart surgery. Positive pressure worked better than the iron lung for pneumonia or COPD with respiratory failure. By the time I graduated in 1961, positive pressure had made the iron lung a relic of the polio era.

Armed with more powerful ventilators, surgeons removed lungs and parts of lungs to extirpate lung cancer and tuberculosis. When cardiac surgery became commonplace, the need for postoperative ventilator support skyrocketed. These very ill patients needed doctors with specialized medical skills—rapid treatment of cardiac rhythm disorders, fluid infusions, kidney dialysis, and especially mechanical ventilation. Physicians with these competencies began to converge in these nascent intensive care units. They often came from surgery or anesthesiology, like Mørch and Ibsen, or from cardiology. Anesthesiologists and surgeons were temperamentally well-suited for the fast pace and quick decision-making required in critical care, and some left the operating room to work in these units.

As the western world faced an epidemic of heart attacks and surgeons introduced coronary artery bypass, cardiologists concentrated their efforts in cardiac catheterization laboratories. Special cardiac care units, often adjacent to intensive care units, came into existence in many hospitals. But, because the common denominator of the ICU patients was their need for respiratory care, specialists in pulmonary medicine emerged as well to oversee intensive care units.

Major obstacles confronted those caring for patients undergoing mechanical ventilation. First was managing the airway. When I was a medical student, it was thought that, if a patient could not safely come off a ventilator in twenty-four hours, a surgical tracheostomy should be performed to prevent damage to the vocal cords. (A tracheostomy is located below the larynx.) However, tracheostomy carries risks. The procedure requires a separate surgical operation, and the wound can become infected. As they accumulated experience, physicians learned they could safely leave a tube in the trachea for longer amounts of time. By the end of the 1960s, a tracheostomy wouldn't be done unless the patient required ventilation for longer than a week.

In 1967, the Puritan Gas Corporation, which had acquired Bennett's company, introduced the MA-1, a volume ventilator like Mørch's and Engstrom's, powerful enough to inflate the lungs even in the presence of pneumonia or pulmonary edema. The MA-1 became the workhorse for the era that followed. Quickly, other manufacturers produced similar instruments, and more and more patients throughout the world received mechanical ventilation.[23]

But problems persisted. For example, infants of low birth weight developed respiratory distress syndrome. The lungs of these babies collapsed and filled with fluid. Despite mechanical ventilation at high pressures, many of these babies died. In addition, high concentrations of oxygen damaged the eyes and caused blindness in many of the babies who did survive. Pediatricians soon realized that oxygen, while essential to life, is toxic in high concentrations.

During the Vietnam War, military physicians also recognized that battlefield wounds could release toxic substances that caused the lungs to become inflamed and swollen. This went under different names like shock lung, wet lung, and Da Nang lung.[24] Despite much research and heroic treatments, the mortality rate from acute lung injury reached nearly 50 percent. In 1967, David Ashbaugh and Thomas Petty of the University of Colorado reported they could reduce the injurious effect of lung edema by adding pressure to the ventilator during expiration, which was a major improvement, used to this day to treat lung edema.[25]

But with these successes, intensive care physicians faced another previously nonexistent problem: how to wean ventilator patients. Mechanical ventilation helped do the work of breathing and allowed patients' breathing muscles to become weak from disuse. Initial strategies relied on stopping the ventilator for short periods of time, say five minutes every hour, with gradual increases as tolerated until the patients regained enough muscle strength to breathe entirely on their own. This often took days to accomplish and produced discomfort for patients, anxiety for physicians, frustration for nurses, and extra costs for hospitals.

In 1971, Robert Kirby and John Downs introduced a technique in which the ventilator was set to cycle less frequently than the patient breathed, so that it augmented only a fraction of patient breaths.[26] But often the patient initiated a breath just as the mandatory breath was at its peak, which caused overinflation. So, engineers adapted ventilators to synchronize with the patient's own breathing. Patients learned to train their breathing muscles and thus came off the ventilator faster and more comfortably.

Modern ventilators contain few moving mechanical parts. Instead, their power comes from compressed air, with valves and jets set to control flow, volume, and pressure. Since the 1980s, ventilators have used compressed air rather than electric motors as their source of power. When microprocessors arrived in the 1990s, engineers designed ventilators that generated complex patterns of flow rates and pressure changes, which offered physicians a broader menu of ventilator settings.

For example, normal humans at rest breathe approximately twelve times a minute. That means each breath is five seconds long. Inhaling lasts 1.5 seconds, and exhaling, 3.5 seconds. But if a patient can't get enough oxygen, it's possible to adjust the ventilator to make inspiration longer than expiration. Or if the patient needs extra pressure in the airways only during expiration, the respiratory therapist can adjust expiratory pressure accordingly. Or if the lung is maximally distended and added pressure is dangerous, it is possible to inject tiny jets of oxygen hundreds of times a minute with minimum pressure change during each breath.

Nowadays, ventilators contain digital controls to achieve all these goals, just as contemporary automobiles contain microchips that control fuel injection, power steering, and power brakes. These controls go under a myriad of names so specialized they confuse everyone except experts: pressure-support ventilation, pressure-control inverse-ratio ventilation, airway pressure-release ventilation. Or dual-control, breath-to-breath, pressure-limited, time-cycled ventilation. Just saying it is a test of lung function.

Modern ventilators have solved many difficult breathing problems confronted in critical care medicine; for example, how to avoid toxic oxygen concentrations, how to ventilate one lung only (necessary if the other lung has a hole in it), and how to manage air leaks in the lungs and obstructions of the trachea. And even more versatile instruments will surely soon follow.

In addition, it's now possible to use positive-pressure breathing on patients who are awake and whose respiratory impairment is less threatening without having to insert a tube in the trachea. So-called noninvasive ventilation, or NIV, emerged in the 1980s to assist patients with sleep-related breathing disorders.[27] NIV relies on a tight-fitting face mask and the ventilator's ability to deliver variable pressures, flow rates, and volumes. These ventilators are small and compact enough that they aren't much larger than a laptop computer and can be adapted for home care.

Though ventilators do the work of breathing for patients unable to inhale and exhale on their own, they don't by themselves directly replace the other major function of the respiratory system: the transfer of gases into blood to be pumped throughout the body. However, cardiac bypass machines used for heart surgery collect venous blood, oxygenate it, and pump it into the aorta. These extracorporeal membrane oxygenators (called ECMO) work in desperate cases where the patient would otherwise die.

What does the future hold for machines that breathe? Microprocessors and fluidics (the science of using gas and liquid to perform mechanical functions) are growing more sophisticated. Ventilators are becoming tiny, self-adjusting machines and soon will be implantable, electronically connected with remote monitoring systems to permit patients to move about freely while being ventilated.

Science has come a long way from the time when Galen blew air into the trachea of animals to resuscitate them. Even E. T. Mørch's piston ventilator fifty years ago is ancient history. We can be proud of the progress made during the past generation but should remain humble because, with respiratory disorders continuing to increase in prevalence, the challenges won't let up. We can look forward to the innovative genius of physicians and engineers yet to come that will make our efforts today look as primitive as those of John Hunter in 1776 trying to revive drowning victims by inserting a bellows into their throats.

V
BREATHING ADAPTS

23

I WOULDN'T WANT
THAT FOR MYSELF

"When you want wisdom and insight as badly as you want to breathe, it is
then you shall have it."

—Socrates[1]

"Life is not measured by the number of breaths we take, but by the moments that take our breath away."

—Maya Angelou[2]

I first met Gertrude after an urgent phone call from her internist. He raced to
get out his words, panting, "I have a seventy-year-old woman here in the office
who can't breathe. She smokes, misses appointments, skips her medications,
only shows up when she's in trouble. I've had it. Maybe a specialist can help
her. I can't."

He was a good doctor—and a steady source of referrals—so I answered,
"Send her to the ER. Tell them to page me when she gets there."

Gertrude was sitting upright on the gurney, sweating, her eyes bulging, her
lips pursed, every available muscle recruited to aid in exhalation. The odor of
stale tobacco permeated the air around her. Gray hair curled in an unkempt
marcel above a sallow face conspicuous for its plainness. A shapeless gray
blouse and a black skirt speckled with lint completed a picture of shabby drab-
ness. She grabbed my sleeve and gasped, "Do something. I can't breathe."

"Let me listen to your chest," I said and lifted her blouse. All I heard were a few tight, forced wheezes. Her heart was beating rapidly, its tones barely audible. I added, "Let's feel your liver, OK?" When I started to unzip her skirt, she pushed my hands away.

"No, don't do that." She let me do a superficial exam, but her hands remained on her abdomen, poised to resist any intrusive probing.

I admitted her and treated her with oxygen, steroids, and antibiotics for an acute flare-up of chronic obstructive lung disease. The next morning, she was still short of breath but improved enough for a hoarse bark: "Get me out of here."

A wave of annoyance hit me. "Yesterday you couldn't breathe and wanted me to do something. Now you're better and you want me to send you home. At least give the medicines time to work."

And so it went for the next five days. Whenever I asked a question, she repeated her mantra: "Please, just let me go home." I did learn she was never married and had worked as an administrative clerk for an insurance company. She had shared an apartment with a sister who recently died. Otherwise she seemed to have no family, no friends, and no hobbies except smoking.

She went home with a prescription for oxygen and home health visits. I also asked her to make an appointment to follow up in the office. Two days later, the home health nurse called me. "She's tough. I can't get through to her. Wouldn't even let me listen to her chest."

"Did she get the O_2?"

"Turned it down. Sent the driver back to the warehouse."

I didn't see Gertrude again until five months later, when I received another frantic call from her internist informing me she was in trouble, and he was calling 911.

I caught up with her in the ICU. She had a tube in her trachea and was unresponsive, a mechanical ventilator controlling her respirations. Blood oxygen and carbon dioxide levels indicated severe respiratory failure. I sat down at the nursing station with the interns and residents to discuss our plans.

Meanwhile, Gertrude's nurse went through her checklist of tasks—attaching ECG leads and an oximeter, passing a stomach tube and a bladder catheter, the usual monitoring for a patient receiving mechanical ventilation. A few minutes later, the nurse came dashing out of her room. "Dr. Glynn, come quick. I have to show you something."

I immediately went to the bedside, with the house officers, interns, and residents at my elbows. The nurse said, "I was putting in the catheter and . . ." She pointed toward Gertrude's pelvis.

We lifted the sheet and stared. Gertrude's legs were spread, and from beneath the labia protruded a stubby penis. I felt a stab of sadness for her. I thought to myself, no wonder she wouldn't let anyone examine her; she was intersex. No wonder she spent her life as a recluse. I motioned the team back to the nursing station. "We ventilate her, keep going with steroids and antibiotics," I said. "And respect her privacy." I looked at the nurse. "Go ahead and put in the catheter. Inform the charge nurse, but don't say anything about this outside the ICU."

Over the next few days, Gertrude remained unresponsive, her eyes closed, the ventilator controlling her breathing. When we approached the one-week mark, I faced a dilemma. Should we perform a tracheostomy? It could take weeks to get her off the ventilator. Trying to be a good teacher, I asked the interns and residents what they thought.

"If we trach her, we can take our time weaning her from the vent," the resident said.

I nodded. "We can do that. She'll go to a rehab hospital, then to a long-term nursing facility. She has no one to care for her. She'll be in an institution forever. How long do you think she'll live?"

He shrugged. "Maybe a year."

"At best." To myself, I thought, "A year with everybody sneaking in to peek at her secret." I answered, "What if we take her off the vent?"

"But if we stop, she'll die," they all came back at me.

"I think that's what she would choose if she could decide for herself."

"I'm not comfortable with that," said the resident.

I arched my eyebrows. "Sounds like we need to convene the biomedical ethics committee."

In the past half-century, medical technology has advanced so fast that law and public attitudes have had difficulty keeping up. Society has been forced to grapple with problems posed by futile treatments, withdrawal of life support, and end-of-life care. Ventilators and respiratory assistance have been at the eye of the storm in many of these debates. How far should we go to treat those unable to breathe? When should we stop a mechanical ventilator? Must we always use respiratory support if it is available? These ethical questions go to the heart of what it means to be alive and how we define ourselves as civilized human beings. Furthermore, disputes over breathing support moved from the bedside and the consultation room into the courts, further complicating already-complex questions.

In April 1975, twenty-one-year-old Karen Ann Quinlan attended a party near her home in suburban New Jersey. After an evening that involved lots of alcohol and tranquilizers, she passed out and stopped breathing.[3] Paramedics resuscitated her and took her to the hospital where she was placed on a ventilator. She remained in a coma, however, with no sign of recovery. After several months, her parents felt the situation was hopeless and requested that she be removed from the ventilator. But the physicians and the hospital authorities refused, claiming they were afraid of being prosecuted if she died.

Unable to gain assistance from the medical and hospital establishment, Quinlan's parents sued, requesting a court to order the ventilator removed. The case gathered national attention and became the focus of intense debate over the right to die. The Superior Court in Morristown, New Jersey, denied the parents' request, but on appeal, the New Jersey Supreme Court reversed the decision in March 1976. The court held that, if medical authorities saw no reasonable possibility Quinlan would recover, the state's interest in preserving life did not apply, and the ventilator could be discontinued.

The court also ruled that her father, not her doctors, had the legal authority to decide on her behalf. This decision provided for substituted judgment, a legal term that means allowing someone else to take over for a person legally incompetent due to a medical problem.

But when the doctors removed Karen Quinlan from the ventilator, she breathed on her own. During the year while her family's lawsuit wended its way through the courts, surprisingly, no one had tried disconnecting the ventilator for a short period to determine if she would breathe.

Nevertheless, Karen Quinlan remained in coma and was transferred to a nursing facility, where she was fed via a stomach tube. In 1985, ten years after her catastrophe, her weight had dropped from 115 pounds before the accident to 65 pounds, and she finally died from respiratory failure brought on by pneumonia. Her family continued to visit her to the end.

The Quinlan court held that removing the life-support systems, especially the mechanical ventilator, was not a criminal act. Her death was not homicide but rather "expiration from existing natural causes." The court also encouraged the medical profession to adopt this line of reasoning in future similar cases. The crux of the matter was to ascertain what the patient would want and, if that was not possible, consider what a reasonable person would want. This seemed to me to illustrate the same questions and problems we faced as we struggled to decide what to do on behalf of Gertrude.

The ICU conference room was full. Nurses lined one wall, doctors the other, chaplains and social workers in between. I presented my case. "This lady has lived in the shadows all her life. She grew up in the 1930s, when her condition wasn't as well understood as it is today. She's lived with shame. It's defined her existence. I believe if she could speak to us, she would say no to chronic ventilator care."

"If you remove the ventilator, it will kill her," one intern said.

"If we remove the ventilator, her terminal lung disease will kill her," I countered. "Not absence of a ventilator. If her lungs were normal, she wouldn't need a machine to breathe for her."

"What does her family doctor say?" a social worker asked.

"Her internist said I should do whatever I think is best."

After a few rounds of debate, everyone agreed that, in the absence of relatives or friends to speak for her, the legal decision fell to me, the senior attending physician. I felt I had the obligation as well as the authority. But the interns and residents remained reluctant.

I didn't want to make this a power struggle, but I pressed the issue. "I think it would be torturing her to do a trach and keep her on the ventilator. She won't be able to talk; she'll need to be restrained. She'll be isolated and alone. I wouldn't want that for myself." That turned the tide of the discussion. The residents finally agreed, and the committee consensus was that I should do what I thought best.

That night, as I lay in the darkness waiting for sleep to come, I began to question myself, going through my own internal checklist. Did I have a right to claim to know what was best for Gertrude? Was I being selfish? She was a difficult patient. I didn't want to have to deal with her every day for the next year until she died from some overwhelming infection. I had passed off her resistance as a straightforward antisocial personality. What if I had tried harder to understand her? Would it have mattered? Nothing I pondered changed my mind.

When morning came, I was sure of my decision, and so we went through a speed wean—lowering the rate of the ventilator hour by hour—and twenty-four hours later, we removed the tube from her trachea. I had no intention of reinserting it.

One can never knew if a spark of consciousness flickers in the mind of comatose ventilator patients, and so early on in practice, I adopted the habit of talking as though they could hear me. As the tube came out, I said to Gertrude, "Your voice is going to be hoarse. You may not be able to talk for a little while. We're going to continue the oxygen and the other treatments. If you want anything different, tell us. I promise I'll honor your wishes."

She lay there with her eyes closed. I held her limp hand but received no squeeze, no sign of recognition, no help with what to do. Gertrude continued on oxygen and steroids and antibiotics and died that evening.

The next morning, the ICU chaplain, one of the Sisters of Mercy, caught me in the hallway and said, "I think you did the right thing."

"Thanks," I said. "Someone had to be her advocate."

Dilemmas like the one Gertrude posed were rare before the era of intensive care units, ventilators, and life-support systems. They were also rare when health care was only a small part of the gross domestic product and the government's role was restricted to ensuring professional standards and public safety. They were rare when people died at home and everyone witnessed their grandparents, parents, and relatives pass on.

Physicians' roles were simpler, too. They did what they could and deferred to nature. An unspoken ethic calibrated what was overly heroic. But now, the extraordinary has become the ordinary, and medical ethics has had to adapt as well. Fortunately, philosophers and jurists helped their medical colleagues learn how to analyze these difficult cases and communicate.

The advent of hospital biomedical ethics committees, hospices, and palliative care all followed in the wake of the Quinlan case and other court decisions that addressed conflicts created by breathing support. Also, articles and books by bioethicists codified the philosophy underpinning biomedical ethics. For example, in 1992, Albert Jonsen, an ethics professor, and Mark Siegler, a physician, with William Winslade, another ethicist, published *Clinical Ethics*, a short book that offered bedside physicians a practical way to approach these dilemmas. *Clinical Ethics* focused on four factors for determining whether a particular course of action was morally acceptable. What are the medical factors? Will the treatment help the patient to have a better life? What does or would the patient want? Is the treatment just and fair, relative to the interests of others and society as a whole?

These became my checklist in difficult cases and offered a helpful system for making moral decisions and recommendations. Overuse of the ventilator symbolized medicine's obsession with technology. I had to learn to ignore the medical imperative to employ technology whenever possible. The ventilator might be mandatory at one stage of a disease but vetoed at another. This awareness freed me to focus on the person, not the disease. It wasn't about oxygen and carbon dioxide; it was about the fellow humans entrusted to my care. I was a physician, not a body engineer.

Breathing is surely a vital sign, a symbol of life. Yet, we breathe to live, not live to breathe. Resolving moral dilemmas in breathing depends on putting ventilators, respiratory care, and all medical therapies into perspective. They are tools, sometimes wondrous ones, but they are not ends in themselves. They are most useful when they assist nature, but for everyone, a time arrives when breathing has to cease. In any battle with nature, she will ultimately win. Good medicine understands and respects this.

24

A SCIENCE OF UNCERTAINTY

"Medicine is a science of uncertainty and an art of probability."

—William Osler[1]

"Illness is the night side of life, a more onerous citizenship."

—Susan Sontag[2]

The year 2019 will mark the centennial of the death of William Osler, the father of modern medicine. Osler's career straddled the turn of the twentieth century, a pivot point between the old and the new eras of the profession. In 1901, recounting for the Johns Hopkins Historical Club what he considered the important medical advances of the nineteenth century, he cited the growth of scientific medicine, professional nursing care, and the importance of instilling confidence in the mind of patients.[3] Osler was looking back, but from our view more than a century later, we can see how his thoughts were prescient, pointing forward, and how, though intended as general comments, they especially related to breathing disorders.

Osler praised the growth of bacteriology, which demystified the "fevers" of ancient times. These included respiratory diseases, like influenza, pneumonia, and plague. Soon viruses would be discovered. Penicillin and sister antibiotics would revolutionize the treatment of infections. Lauding the importance of vaccination and preventive medicine, Osler stressed their importance as future tools to control infections. Widespread immunization would save thousands of lives, virtually eliminate polio, bring pertussis under control, and mitigate the effects of pneumonia and influenza. Indeed, vaccines would become the single-greatest medical achievement of the twentieth century.

In his list of the weapons of public health against the scourge of tuberculosis, Osler included education of the public, compulsory registration of all cases, and sanatorium treatment. (This was 1901. A little over a half-century later, antituberculosis drugs would close the sanatoriums of the world.). But the white plague would continue to be the "disease that medicine never cured," morphing into the contemporary threat of multi-drug-resistance, the infamous MDR-TB.

The father of modern medicine also celebrated the growth of scientific pharmacology, which led to rational use of a small number of drugs rather than shotgun prescribing for diseases poorly understood by medical practitioners. Osler would be pleased and maybe even amazed to see which pharmaceutical advances have contributed to treating respiratory diseases a century after his death.

Aware that healing is a team endeavor, Osler cited the importance of nursing care. He said, "[P]erhaps in no particular does nineteenth century practice differ . . . than in the greater attention which is given to . . . the art of nursing."[4] No one would argue that nursing, treating the effects of illness and disease, has matured into the profession most identified with helping sick people. Nursing ideals have also proliferated in fields like respiratory, physical, and occupational therapy, which have inestimably increased the impact of respiratory medicine since 1901.

Osler also highlighted the importance of instilling confidence and hope in the minds and hearts of patients, of tapping into the human capacity for faith. He said, "We have never had, and cannot expect to have a monopoly on this panacea, which is open to all, free as the sun, and which may make of everyone . . . a good physician out of Nature's grace."[5] Osler foretold the importance of the human spirit in coping with the chronic diseases that would replace acute infections and injuries as the major causes of misery and death in the twentieth century.

Yet, in another of those recurring ironies of clinical medicine, as he grieved the loss of his only son, Revere, in World War I, the revered physician himself succumbed to pneumonia during the influenza pandemic of 1918–1919. The proverb "Physician heal thyself" eventually becomes an impossible-to-fulfill admonition.[6]

At the mid-twentieth century, another pivot point in medicine occurred, and soon after, by chance, I happened to enter the profession. The rise of the modern hospital centralized and organized medical care to bring lifesaving technology to all the sick, not just the wealthy. Research went from modest undertakings in academic surroundings to giant government-sponsored efforts against scourges of the time, particularly cancer and heart disease. Better understanding of physiology made it possible for surgery on the heart and lungs to become everyday procedures. This led to intensive care units and brought respiratory support to the forefront of high-tech medicine. Pulmonology went from an esoteric specialty focused on tuberculosis and inhaled dust diseases to a dynamic field requiring a broad knowledge of immunology, physiology, pharmacology, infections, public health, and occupational medicine.

Also, costs of medical care exploded, threatening to crowd out other publicly supported functions, like education and social security. The hospital and ICU became targets for serious ethical questions about what medicine ought to do. Care for the very sick and dying thrust respiratory medicine into the vortex of both economic and moral controversies in health care.

The twenty-first century, the "age of biology," is demarcating another pivot point in medicine.[7] Genomics, informatics, the microbiome, the Internet, and bioelectronics promise to revolutionize care of the sick as strikingly as immunization did a century ago and the intensive care unit did a half-century later. Respiratory medicine will be a prominent part of these transformations.

When I learned physical diagnosis, I was taught to feel the chest for vocal vibrations; thump, or percuss, the skin overlying the ribs to hear changes in tone; and listen to breath sounds to detect pneumonia, lung collapse, or fluid in the chest. These techniques, which even predate Osler, require only a stethoscope, good ears, and sensitive fingers. But the X-ray is better and, by the mid-twentieth century, became the standard diagnostic study in pneumonia. Now, portable ultrasound has come on the scene and is replacing the X-ray in many situations. Performed at the bedside using less costly equipment, ultrasound does not expose the patient to radiation and can be repeated as often as desired. One app even connects a portable ultrasonic probe with a smartphone and shows pneumonia and fluid around the lung. Another app analyzes breath sounds to convert the ancient stethoscope into a space-age tool that complements ultrasound. Imagine: The same device I use to photograph my grandchildren's birthdays or do crossword puzzles can diagnose pneumonia. Who knows what the future will bring?

A while back, I attended a panel discussion that included Eric Topol and Abraham Verghese, two leaders in American medical thought. Topol is a cardiologist and an evangelist of technological advances. When he told us how he used a smartphone app to diagnose a heart attack on a passenger in the middle of an airplane flight, his voice became louder and faster.

Verghese is an infectious disease specialist and author of the best-selling novel *Cutting for Stone*. He sounded a counterpoint melody, speaking slowly and gently as he pleaded for us to return to our roots, as descendants of Hippocrates and Osler, to exercise the power of curious eyes, sympathetic ears, and a warm touch as tools of healing.[8] Both were right. We need technology, and we need compassion. But technology without compassion is no more than body engineering, and compassion without technology is an anachronism, incomplete and outdated. This dichotomy, to blend high-tech and high-touch, is a core challenge of this age of biology.

Furthermore, we in clinical medicine, schooled to treat each patient as unique, focus on the individual. Yet the most pressing medical problems facing us today affect large segments of the public.[9] Tens of millions of Americans suffer from such respiratory diseases as asthma, COPD, and lung cancer. We need ways to treat all these people yet maintain the personal connection that is the basis of healing. Pope Francis wrote, "All of us are linked by unseen bonds and together form a kind of universal family, a sublime communion which fills us with a sacred, affectionate and humble respect."[10]

In the summer of 2014, when I was planning which stories to use in this book, I shared a cup of coffee at Starbucks with my former patient Nancy, described in the third chapter. She nearly died of pneumonia following an influenza infection. I was her physician from 1975 until my retirement in 2002 but hadn't seen her in twelve years. Nancy had been as sick as anyone I ever cared for, yet there she was, almost forty years later, across the little table, stirring her latte, living a normal life.

I asked her what she remembered about that terrible experience, and she shared thoughts and feelings I never heard before. She could not recall much about her week on a ventilator in the ICU nor her six weeks in the hospital, though she remembered how it hurt when nurses suctioned her trachea and punctured the arteries in her arms to measure blood oxygen and carbon dioxide. She said her wrists were sore for six months afterward. She also had vague recollections of the nurses packing ice bags around her trunk and legs because of her high fever.

One time in the ICU, when Nancy's oxygen system malfunctioned, she turned blue, and a pressure bag was required for several minutes to restore her breathing. But Nancy was not afraid. She had already been to the brink. After going home, Nancy needed supplementary oxygen while she recuperated. Her sister, who was a nurse, came to care for her. Indeed, her strength slowly improved, and five months after the illness, Nancy went back to work.

Nancy is seventy-three now and works part time. Able to perform normal activities of daily living, she becomes short of breath with anything more than moderate exercise. She picks up respiratory infections easily and lives with the possibility of pneumonia recurring, which fortunately has never been a problem. But Nancy emphasizes how the experience of January 1975 irrevocably changed her, body, mind, and soul. From that time forward, she has known she has to take care of herself. Susan Sontag wrote, "Everyone holds dual citizenship in the kingdom of the well and of the sick. In addition, sooner or later, each of us has to realize we are citizens of the other place."[11] Nancy knows what Susan Sontag meant when she called illness the "night side of life."

In February 2016, as I was putting the finishing touches on the manuscript for this book, Nancy and I met again at Starbucks. When I made the allusion to Sontag, Nancy became quiet. Her voice steady, she said, "I had another experience in the ICU I never mentioned to you before." I nodded, and she resumed, "I felt like I was in the corner of the room looking at myself on the ventilator. It was a sensation of disengagement, I guess what they call an out-of-body experience. I felt compassion for that person lying in the bed and a sense of peace, of love, and of being.

"I felt I was going to survive, but if I didn't, I was sure there is another side, a life after death." Nancy took a sip of tea. "I feel differently from Susan Sontag. My illness in 1975 persuaded me there is a bright side of life, a mystique based on love."

I was silent a few seconds. Unsure just how to respond, I thanked her for divulging that profound experience. To myself, I wondered how many other very sick patients had that same reaction but never shared it. Or didn't remember it because they were so sick. I told Nancy I would include the event in the book.

A few months ago, I watched my twelve-year-old grandson play soccer. He has asthma. For an hour, he raced up and down the field, dribbled the ball, chased opponents, and even scored a goal. What a pleasure to see him leading a full, active life. Perhaps with the help of medical advances, he can avoid ever having to confront Sontag's night side of life because of asthma.

At the beginning of the book, I discussed the role asthma played in developing my character. The many days at home with attacks of wheezing made reading a way to pass the time, and the frequent visits to the doctor and hospital emergency room eventually drew me to a career in medicine and to concentrate on treating respiratory disorders. I consciously feel a bond with those who gasp for air. We are survivors of the same battles.

I've benefited from advances in asthma treatment over the past half-century. I'm eighty years old, walk five miles up and down hills playing golf, and still have nearly normal lung function. But I stay vigilant. I keep inhalers in my bathroom, get flu shots every fall, and avoid dusts and irritants. My children with asthma have fared better. They run marathons and never had to restrict activities like I did. But they also keep inhalers available; no one smokes, and they also are careful about exposure to respiratory irritants. The two grandchildren with asthma are doing even better than that. They take their medicines and enjoy their lives, hardly aware of any limitations amid their blessings. I won't live to see what happens to great-grandchildren, but I'm optimistic because science will advance further, and humans will learn and adapt.

Threats to breathing will always lie in the miasma. In Osler's time, people died of influenza and pneumonia and chronic tuberculosis. Today we die from heart attacks, cancer, and COPD. Who knows what will be the most frequent causes of death a century from now? We hope they won't be pandemic infections or massive collective suffocation from air pollution.

Nature has given us ingenuity, perseverance, and adaptability. But we have to be humble and remember we are part of nature. If we use our intelligence and act responsibly, we can be confident she will offer us the tools to survive and flourish. And as today is better than yesterday, so tomorrow can be better than today.

NOTES

EPIGRAPH

1. Barker, Kenneth, ed. *The New International Version Study Bible*. Grand Rapids, MI: Zondervan, 1995.

AUTHOR'S NOTE

1. "The Top 10 Causes of Death." World Health Organization, Fact Sheet no. 310. May 2014. http://www.who.int/mediacentre/factsheets/fs310/en.

INTRODUCTION

1. Barker, Kenneth, ed. *The New International Version Study Bible*. Grand Rapids, MI: Zondervan, 1995.
2. "Number of Candidates Certified Annually by the American Board of Internal Medicine." American Board of Internal Medicine. 2015. http://www.abim.org/~/media/ABIM%20Public/Files/pdf/statistics-data/candidates-certiified-annually.pdf.
3. American Cancer Society. *Cancer Facts and Figures 2014*. Atlanta: American Cancer Society, 2014. http://www.cancer.org/acs/groups/content/@research/documents/webcontent/acspc-042151.pdf.
4. "The Top 10 Causes of Death." World Health Organization, Fact Sheet no. 310. May 2014. http://www.who.int/mediacentre/factsheets/fs310/en.

5. Wong, Edward. "Life in a Toxic Country." *New York Times*, August 4, 2013.

6. Kuehn, Bridget M. "WHO: More Than 7 Million Air Pollution Deaths Each Year." *Journal of the American Medical Association* 311, no. 15 (April 16, 2014): 1488.

7. Wong, Edward. "China Exports Pollution to U.S., Study Finds." *New York Times*, January 20, 2014.

8. "State of the Air." American Lung Association. 2015. http://www.stateoftheair .org/2015/city-rankings/most-polluted-cities.html.

9. "Press Release: More Than 100,000 Americans Quit Smoking Due to National Media Campaign." Centers for Disease Control and Prevention. September 9, 2013. http://www.cdc.gov/media/releases/2013/p0909-tips-campaign-results.html.

10. "Paracelsus Quotes." Brainy Quote. 2017. https://www.brainyquote.com/quotes/quotes/p/paracelsus138349.html.

CHAPTER I: THE DISEASE THAT MEDICINE NEVER CURED

1. Bunyan, John. *The Life and Death of Mr. Badman*. Published by Nathaniel Ponder, 1680. Republished by the Perfect Library, 2015. https://www.amazon .com/Life-Death-Mr-Badman-ebook/dp/B00T0HCISQ?ie=UTF8&ref_=dp_kinw_ strp_1#reader_B00T0HCISQ.

2. Dickens, Charles. *The Life and Adventures of Nicholas Nickleby*. 1st American ed. New York. MacMillan, 1982, chap. 49, p. 322.

3. "Paul Farmer Biography." Academy of Achievement. Last updated October 17, 2016. http://www.achievement.org/autodoc/page/far1bio-1.

4. Dutt, Asim. "Epidemiology and Host Factors." In *Tuberculosis and Non-Tuberculous Mycobacterial Infections*. 5th ed. David Schlossberg, ed. New York: McGraw-Hill, 2006, p. 1.

5. Sontag, Susan. *Illness as Metaphor*. New York: Vintage Books, 1979, p. 5.

6. Farrell, Tom. Personal communication.

7. Wallace, Joseph. *Colleagues in Discovery: One Hundred Years of Improving Respiratory Health*. San Diego, CA: Tehabi Books, 2005, p. 26.

8. Koehler, Christopher W. "Consumption, the Great Killer." The Timeline. http://pubs.acs.org/subscribe/archive/mdd/v05/i02/html/02timeline.html.

9. "Introduction to the American Lung Association and the Fight against Tuberculosis: 'The Christmas Seal People.'" University of Virginia. 2007. www.hsl .virginia.edu/historical/medical_history/alav/tuberculosis.cfm.

10. Roberts, Charles Stewart. "Trudeau at Lake Saranac." In *Clinical Methods: The History, Physical, and Laboratory Examinations*. 3rd ed. H. Kenneth Walker, W. Dallas Hall, and J. Willis Hurst, eds. Boston: Butterworths, 1990. www.ncbi .nlm.nih.gov/books/NBK699.

11. Shampo, Marc A., Robert A. Kyle, and David P. Steensma. "Edward L. Trudeau—Founder of a Sanatorium for Treatment of Tuberculosis." *Mayo Clinic*

Proceedings 85, no. 7 (July 2010): e48. https://www.ncbi.nlm.nih.gov/pmc/articles /PMC2894729.

12. Shampo, Kyle, and Steensma, "Edward L. Trudeau."

13. Europeans used the term *sanatorium*, while in America, *sanitarium* was frequently the preferred term. I use *sanatorium*.

14. Shampo, Kyle, and Steensma, "Edward L. Trudeau."

15. Ryan, Frank. *The Forgotten Plague: How the Battle against Tuberculosis Was Won—and Lost*. Boston: Little, Brown, 1992, p. 9.

16. Koehler, "Consumption." See also Garrison, Fielding H. *An Introduction to the History of Medicine: With Medical Chronology, Suggestions for Study and Bibliographic Data*. 4th ed. Philadelphia: W. B. Saunders, 1929, p. 656.

17. Bastion, Hilda. "Down and Almost Out in Scotland: George Orwell, Tuberculosis, and Getting Streptomycin in 1948." *James Lind Library Bulletin: Commentaries on the History of Treatment Evaluation* (2004). Cited by Geffen, Nathan. "Battling the White Plague." TB Online. 2011. http://www.tbonline.info /posts/2011/6/29/battling-white-plague/#bastion.

18. Connolly, Cynthia A. "Experiments in Children's Health: The Early Twentieth-Century Tuberculosis Preventorium." *Nursing History Review* 10 (2002): 127–57.

19. Trudeau, E. L. *An Autobiography*. Lea and Febiger, 1915. Reprinted New York: Doubleday, Doran, 1936, p. 26.

20. Quoted in Ryan, *Forgotten Plague*, p. 26.

21. "History." Waksman Institute of Microbiology. 2013. www.waksman.rutgers. edu/about/history.

22. Kresge, Nicole, Robert D. Simoni, and Robert L. Hill. "Selman Waksman: The Father of Antibiotics." *Journal of Biological Chemistry* 279 (November 26, 2004): e7.

23. Catanzaro, A. Personal communication, March 2016.

24. Tiemersma, Edine W., Marieke J. van der Werf, Martien W. Borgdorff, Brian G. William, and Nico J. D. Nagelkerke. "Natural History of Tuberculosis: Duration and Fatality of Untreated Pulmonary Tuberculosis in HIV Negative Patients: A Systematic Review." *PLoS ONE* 6, no. 4 (April 4, 2011): e17601. http://journals.plos.org/ plosone/article?id=10.1371/journal.pone.0017601.

25. "Tuberculosis Fact Sheet: Trends in Tuberculosis, 2015." Centers for Disease Control and Prevention. Last updated November 29, 2016. http://www.cdc .gov/tb/publications/factsheets/statistics/TBTrends.htm.

26. Moser, Kathleen, San Diego County Department of Health. Personal communication.

27. Frieden, Thomas R., Karen F. Brudney, and Anthony D. Harries. "Global Tuberculosis: Perspectives, Prospects, and Priorities." *Journal of the American Medical Association* 312, no. 14 (October 8, 2014): 1393.

28. "Tuberculosis: Data and Statistics." Center for Disease Control and Prevention. Last updated December 9, 2016. http://www.cdc.gov/tb/statistics.

29. Journalist Tracy Kidder told Farmer's story in his best-seller, *Mountains beyond Mountains*. New York: Random House, 2003.

CHAPTER 2: CAPTAINS OF THE MEN OF DEATH

1. "William Osler Quotes." AZ Quotes. http://www.azquotes.com/quote/903120.
2. Örkqvist, Åke, Jonas Hedlund, and Mats Kalin. "Streptococcus Pneumoniae: Epidemiology, Risk Factors, and Clinical Features." *Seminars in Respiratory and Critical Care Medicine* 26, no. 6 (2005): 563–74. Cited in Medscape. http://www.medscape.com/viewarticle/521337_2.
3. Osler, William. *The Principles and Practice of Medicine*. 3rd ed. New York: Appleton, 1899, pp. 108ff.
4. "Achievements in Public Health 1900–1999: Control of Infectious Diseases." *MMWR Weekly* 48, no. 29 (July 30, 1999): 621–29. https://www.cdc.gov/mmwr/preview/mmwrhtml/mm4829a1.htm#fig2.
5. Musher, Daniel M. "Streptococcus pneumonia." In *Mandell, Douglas, and Bennett's Principles and Practice of Infectious Diseases*, Gerald L. Mandell, John E. Bennett, and Raphael Dolin, editors. 7th ed. Philadelphia: Churchill Livingstone, 2010, p. 2623.
6. Watson, David A., Daniel M. Musher, James W. Jacobson, and Jan Verhoef. "A Brief History of the Pneumococcus in Biomedical Research: A Panoply of Scientific Discovery." *Clinical Infectious Diseases* 17 (1993): 913–24.
7. Austrian, Robert. "The Pneumococcus at the Millennium: Not Down, Not Out." *Journal of Infectious Diseases* 179, supplement 2 (March 1999): S338–41.
8. Örkqvist, Hedlund, and Kalin, "Streptococcus Pneumoniae," 563.
9. Torres, Antoni, Rosario Menéndez, and Richard Wunderink. "Pyogenic Bacterial Pneumonia and Lung Abscess." In *Murray and Nadel's Textbook of Respiratory Medicine*. 5th ed. Robert J. Mason, V. Courtney Broaddus, Thomas R. Martin, Talmadge E. King Jr., Dean E. Schraufnagel, John F. Murray, and Jay A. Nadel, eds. Philadelphia: Saunders Elsivier, 2010, p. 720.
10. "William Osler Quotes."
11. Cushing, Harvey. *The Life of Sir William Osler*. Oxford: Clarendon Press, 1925, vol. 2, p. 661.
12. Cushing, *Sir William Osler*, p. 686.
13. Bean, Robert Bennett, comp., and William Bennett Bean, ed. *Sir William Osler: Aphorisms from His Bedside Teachings and Writings*. 2nd ed. Springfield, IL: Charles C. Thomas, 1961, epitome 323, p. 143.
14. "The Top 10 Causes of Death." World Health Organization, Fact Sheet no. 310. May 2014. http://www.who.int/mediacentre/factsheets/fs310/en.

CHAPTER 3: THEY STACKED CASKETS IN THE HALLS

1. Barry, John M. *The Great Influenza*. New York: Penguin Books, 2004, p. 5.
2. "Influenza." Online Etymology Dictionary. 2016. www.etymonline.com/index.php?allowed_in_frame=0&search=influenza.

3. "Covering Pandemic Flu." Nieman Foundation for Journalism at Harvard University. November 4, 2014. http://nieman.harvard.edu/wp-content/uploads/pod-assets/microsites/NiemanGuideToCoveringPandemicFlu/NiemanGuideToCoveringPandemicFlu.aspx.html.

4. "Selecting Viruses for the Seasonal Influenza Vaccine." Centers for Disease Control and Prevention. Last updated May 4, 2016. http://www.cdc.gov/flu/about/season/vaccine-selection.htm.

5. Barry, *Great Influenza*, p. 119.

6. Ballon-Landa, G. L. Personal communication, January 2016.

7. Barry, *Great Influenza*, p. 446.

8. Tumpey, Terrence M., et al. "Characterization of the Reconstructed 1918 Spanish Influenza Pandemic Virus." *Science* 310, no. 5745 (October 7, 2005): 77–80. doi:10.1126/science.1119392. Cited in "Reconstruction of the 1918 Influenza Pandemic Virus." Centers for Disease Control and Prevention. Last updated July 17, 2014. http://www.cdc.gov/flu/about/qa/1918flupandemic.htm.

9. Biondi, Eric A., and C. Andrew Aligne. "Flu Vaccine for All: A Critical Look at the Evidence." Medscape Pediatrics. December 21, 2015. http://www.medscape.com/viewarticle/855937.

10. Barry, *Great Influenza*, pp. 223ff.

CHAPTER 4: THE MAN IN THE IRON LUNG

1. Frankl, Victor. *Man's Search for Meaning*. Pocket Book ed. Boston: Beacon Press, 1959, p. 99.

2. Meyer, John A. "A Practical Mechanical Respirator, 1929: The 'Iron Lung.'" *Annals of Thoracic Surgery* 50, no. 3 (September 1990): 492.

3. Drinker, Philip, and Louis A. Shaw. "An Apparatus for the Prolonged Administration of Artificial Respiration: I. A Design for Adults and Children." *Journal of Clinical Investigation* 7, no. 2 (June 1, 1929): 229–47.

4. Mørch, E. T. "History of Mechanical Ventilation." In *Mechanical Ventilation*, Robert R. Kirby, Robert A. Smith, and David A. Desautels, eds. New York: Churchill, Livingston, 1985, p. 9.

5. Drinker, Philip, and Charles F. McKhann. "The Use of a New Apparatus for the Prolonged Administration of Artificial Respiration: I. A Fatal Case of Poliomyelitis." *Journal of the American Medical Association* 92, no. 20 (May 18, 1929): 1658–60.

6. "John 'Jack' Haven Emerson." Polio Place. 2011. www.polioplace.org/people/john-h-emerson.

7. Griscom, Stewart. "Paralysis and Profits." *The Nation*, March 1, 1933. www.disabilityhistorymuseum.org.

8. Emerson, John H. "Some Reflections on Iron Lungs and Other Inventions." *Respiratory Care* 43, no. 7 (July 1998): 573–82.

9. Emerson, "Some Reflections."

10. Emerson, "Some Reflections."

11. Emerson, "Some Reflections."

12. Griscom, "Paralysis and Profits."

13. "Respirator Fight." *Time* 21, no. 9 (February 27, 1933): 28.

14. Griscom, "Paralysis and Profits."

15. Tobin, J. "Breath by Breath." Medicine at Michigan (Spring 2010). www.medicineatmichigan.org/magazine/2010/spring/lookingback.

16. "The History of Polio: A Hypertext Timeline—1789–2000." The Polio History Pages. Last updated November 22, 2015. www.eds-resources.com/poliotimeline.htm.

17. "Polio Elimination in the United States." Centers for Disease Control and Prevention. Last revised June 21, 2016. https://www.cdc.gov/polio/us/index.html.

18. "Polio Now." Polio Global Eradication Initiative. http://polioeradication.org/polio-today/polio-now.

19. Raia, James. "Heavy Metal: Sacramento Exhibition Showcases Iron Lung." *Sacramento News and Review*. April 12, 2012. www.newsreview.com/sacramento/heavy-metal-sacramento-exhibition-showcases/content?oid=5701334.

20. "John 'Jack' Haven Emerson."

21. Emerson, "Some Reflections."

22. Hawkins, Leonard C. *The Man in the Iron Lung: The Frederick B. Snite, Jr., Story*. Garden City, NY: Doubleday, 1956, p. 17.

CHAPTER 5: PRODUCTS OF PARASITIC BEINGS

1. Quoted in English in Mazzarello, Paolo. *The Hidden Structure: A Scientific Biography of Camillo Golgi*. Henry A. Buchtel and Aldo Hadiani, trans. and ed. 1999. http://todayinsci.com/B/Bassi_Agostino/BassiAgostino-Quotations.htm.

2. Bean, Robert Bennett, comp., and William Bennett Bean, ed. *Sir William Osler: Aphorisms from His Bedside Teachings and Writings*. 2nd ed. Springfield, IL: Charles C. Thomas, 1961, aphorism 214, p. 106.

3. Hirschmann, Jan V. "The Early History of Coccidioidomycosis: 1892–1945." *Clinical Infectious Diseases* 44, no. 9 (2007): 1202–7.

4. Hirschmann, "Early History of Coccidioidomycosis."

5. Pappagianis, Demosthenes. Personal communication.

6. Pappagianis.

7. Hirschmann, "Early History of Coccicioidomycosis."

8. Hirschmann, "Early History of Coccidioidomycosis."

9. Pappagianis.

10. Pappagianis.

11. Tsang, Clarisse A., Farzaneh Tabnak, Duc J. Vugia, Kaitlin Benedict, and Benjamin J. Park. "Increase in Reported Coccidioidomycosis: United States, 1998–2011." *MMWR* 62, no. 12 (March 29, 2013): 217–21. https://www.cdc.gov/mmwr/preview/mmwrhtml/mm6212a1.htm?s_cid=mm6212a1_w.

12. "Valley Fever (Coccidioidomycosis) Statistics." Centers for Disease Control and Prevention. Last updated December 12, 2016. http://www.cdc.gov/fungal/diseases/coccidioidomycosis/statistics.html.

13. "Preventing Work-Related Valley Fever (Coccidioidomycosis)." California Department of Health. 2016. http://www.cdph.ca.gov/programs/ohb/Pages/Cocci.aspx.

14. Pappagianis.

15. "Histoplasmosis Statistics." Centers for Disease Control and Prevention. Last updated February 8, 2016. www.cdc.goc/fungal/diseases/histoplasmosis/statistics.html.

16. Wheat, L. J., T. G. Slama, H. E. Eitzen, R. B. Kohler, M. L. V. French, and J. L. Biesecker. "A Large Urban Outbreak of Histoplasmosis: Clinical Features." *Annals of Internal Medicine* 94, no. 3 (1981): 331–37.

17. Pappas, Peter G. "Blastomycosis." *Seminars in Respiratory and Critical Care Medicine* 25, no. 2 (April 2004): 113–22.

18. Craig, M., W. Davey, and R. Green. "Conjugal Blastomycosis." *American Journal of Respiratory Disease* 102 (1970): 86–90.

19. Gigliotti, Francis, and Terry W. Wright. "Pneumocystis:Where Does It Live?" *PLoS Pathogens* 8, no. 11 (November 29, 2012): e1003025. doi:10.1371/journal.ppat.1003025.

CHAPTER 6: SOME LIKE IT HOT

1. Barker, Kenneth, ed., *The New International Version Study Bible*. Grand Rapids, MI: Zondervan, 1995.

2. Popovic, Tanja, and Dixie E. Snider. "60 Years of Progress—CDC and Infectious Diseases." *Emerging Infectious Diseases* 12, no. 7 (July 2006): 1160–61. http://wwwnc.cdc.gov/eid/article/12/7/06-0531_article.

3. "Legionnaires' Disease—A History of Its Discovery." *The Hitchhiker's Guide to the Galaxy: Earth Edition*. January 16, 2003. http://h2g2.com/edited_entry/A882371.

4. Shortell, David. "Seven Dead in Legionnaire's Outbreak in New York." CNN. August 3, 2015. http://www.cnn.com/2015/08/01/health/new-york-legionnaires disease.

5. "Bacteria in Hot Tub May Hurt Lungs." WebMD Health News. May 24, 2005. http://www.webmd.com/lung/news/20050524/bacteria-in-hot-tub-may-hurt-lungs.

6. Fjallbrant, H. et al. "Hot Tub Lung: An Occupational Hazard." *European Respiratory Review* 22 (March 1, 2013): 88–90.

7. "Bacteria in Hot Tub."

8. Martin, Ralph. "Want a Creepy Kick? Check into a Deadly Hotel." NBC News. October 29, 2008. http://www.nbcnews.com/id/27297223/ns/travel-seasonal_travel/t/want-creepy-kick-check-deadly-hotel/#.WGfCUFzWdPY.

CHAPTER 7: THE VIRUS WITH NO NAME

1. "Helen Keller Quotes." Brainy Quote. 2017. https://www.brainyquote.com/quotes/quotes/h/helenkelle382259.html.

2. "Carlo Urbani Obituary." *British Medical Journal* 326 (April 12, 2003): 825.

3. Duffy, Jim. "Anatomy of an Epidemic: School Faculty Share Five Lessons from SARS." Johns Hopkins Public Health (Fall 2003). http://magazine.jhsph.edu/2003/fall/SARS.

4. Castle, Matt. "The Heroes of SARS." Damn Interesting no. 316. May 23, 2008. Last updated March 22, 2016. http://www.damninteresting.com/the-heroes-of-sars.

5. Duffy, "Anatomy of an Epidemic."

6. Duffy, "Anatomy of an Epidemic."

7. "Severe Acute Respiratory Syndrome—Singapore, 2003." *MMWR* 52, no. 18 (May 9, 2003): 405–11. https://www.cdc.gov/mmwr/preview/mmwrhtml/mm5218a1.htm.

8. "SARS: Timeline of an Outbreak." WebMD Health News. 2003. http://www.webmd.com/lung/news/20030411/sars-timeline-of-outbreak.

9. Castle, "Heroes of SARS."

10. "SARS." NHS Choices. Last reviewed October 13, 2016. www.nhs.uk/conditions/sars.

11. Duffy, "Anatomy of an Epidemic."

12. Lupkin, Sydney. "French Lab Loses SARS Vials." ABC News. April 16, 2014. http://abcnews.go.com/Health/french-lab-loses-sars-vials/story?id=23349738.

13. Zaki, Ali M., Sander van Boheemen, Theo M. Bestebroer, Albert D. M. E. Osterhaus, and Ron A. M. Fouchier. "Brief Report: Isolation of a Novel Coronavirus from a Man with Pneumonia in Saudi Arabia." *New England Journal of Medicine* 367, no. 19 (November 8, 2012):1814–20.

14. Gorney, Cynthia. "The Camels and the Contagion." *National Geographic Magazine Daily News*, May 14, 2014.

15. Gorney, "Camels and the Contagion."

16. Chu, Daniel K. W., et al. "MERS Coronaviruses in Dromedary Camels, Egypt." *Emerging Infectious Diseases* 20, no. 6 (June 2014).

17. Friedrich, M. J. "Dromedary Camels and MERS." *Journal of the American Medical Association* 311, no. 15 (April 16, 2014): 1489.

18. Gorney, "Camels and the Contagion."

19. Epstein, Jonathan H., and Kevin J. Olival. "Animal Reservoirs of Middle East Respiratory Syndrome Coronavirus." *Emerging Viral Diseases: The One Health Connection*. Forum on Microbial Threats, Institute of Medicine, Washington, DC, March 19, 2015. https://www.ncbi.nlm.nih.gov/books/NBK284994.

20. "Tracking a Mystery Disease: The Detailed Story of Hantavirus Pulmonary Syndrome (HPS)." Centers for Disease Control and Prevention. Last reviewed August 29, 2012. www.cdc.gov/hantavirus/hps/history.html.

21. "Hantavirus Pulmonary Syndrome (HPS)." Robert Siegel. https://web.stanford.edu/~siegelr/uda.html.

CHAPTER 8: SUFFOCATING WORK

1. Einstein, Albert. Speech at the California Institute of Technology, Pasadena, California, February 16, 1931. In the *New York Times*, February 17, 1931, p. 6.

2. "Asthma in the Workplace." American Lung Association. 2017. http://www.lung.org/lung-health-and-diseases/lung-disease-lookup/asthma/living-with-asthma.

3. Mayo Clinic Staff. "Occupational Asthma." Mayo Clinic. June 12, 2014. http://www.mayoclinic.org/diseases-conditions/occupational-asthma/basics/definition/con-20032379.

4. "Occupational Asthma." United States Department of Labor. https://www.osha.gov/SLTC/occupationalasthma/index.html.

5. Leigh, J. Paul, Patrick S. Romano, Marc B. Schenker, and Kathleen Kreiss. "Costs of Occupational COPD and Asthma." *Chest* 121, no. 1 (January 2002): 264–72.

6. Auger, J., D. Perrotin, and A. Sonneville. "Asthma Caused by Isocyanate Exposure." *Allergie et Immunologie* (Paris) 34, no. 8 (2002): 297–301.

7. Campbell, J. M. "Acute Symptoms Following Work with Hay." *British Medical Journal* 2 (1932): 1143–44.

8. Legiest, Barbara, and Benoit Nemery. "Management of Work-Related Asthma: Guidelines and Challenges." *European Respiratory Review* 21 (2012): 79–81.

9. "Occupational Lung Diseases." Johns Hopkins Medicine. http://www.hopkinsmedicine.org/healthlibrary/conditions/respiratory_disorders/occupational_lung_diseases_85,P01318.

10. Lucas, Ashley, and Ariadne Paxton. "About the Hawk's Nest Incident: Background for Muriel Rukeyser's *The Book of the Dead*." Modern American Poetry. http://www.english.illinois.edu/maps/poets/m_r/rukeyser/hawksnest.htm.

11. Humphrey, Craig R. "Gauley Bridge, West Virginia." Pollution Issues. http://www.pollutionissues.com/Fo-Hi/Gauley-Bridge-West-Virginia.html.

12. Cherniack, Martin. *The Hawk's Nest Incident: American's Worst Industrial Disaster*. New Haven, CT: Yale University Press, 1986, p. 3.

13. Cherniack, *Hawk's Nest Incident*.

14. Lucas and Paxton, "About the Hawk's Nest Incident."

15. Chag-Yeung, Maria, and Jean Luc Malo. "Asbestos Related Fibrosis of the Lungs." In *Murray and Nadel's Text of Respiratory Medicine*. 5th ed. Robert J. Mason, V. Courtney Broaddus, Thomas R. Martin, Talmedge E. King Jr., Dean E. Schraufnagel, John F. Murray, and Jay A. Nadel, eds. Philadelphia: Saunders Elsevier, 2010, p. 1568.

16. Morgan, W., and A. Seaton. *Occupational Lung Diseases*. 2nd ed. Philadelphia. W. B. Saunders, 1984, p. 383.

17. Blackley, David J., Cara N. Halldin, and A. Scott Laney. "Resurgence of a Debilitating and Entirely Preventable Respiratory Disease among Working Coal Miners." *American Journal of Respiratory and Critical Care Medicine* 190, no. 6 (September 15, 2014): 708–9.

18. "Coal Giants: The World's Biggest Coal Producing Countries." Mining-Technology.com. March 4, 2014. http://www.mining-technology.com/features/featurecoal-giants-the-worlds-biggest-coal-producing-countries-4186363.

19. Yap, Chun-Wei. "China's Coal Addiction Brings Scourge of Black Lung." *Wall Street Journal*. December 15, 2014. http://www.wsj.com/articles/chinas-coal-addiction-brings-scourge-of-black-lung-1418593741.

20. "Coal Miners Get Help for Occupational Lung Disease." China.org.cn. January 8, 2015. http://www.china.org.cn/china/2015-01/08/content_34515667.htm.

21. Phillips, "Black Lung Escalates."

22. Einstein, Speech.

CHAPTER 9: CODE RED

1. "Natural Disasters Quotes—Page 2." Brainy Quotes. 2017. http://www.brainyquote.com/quotes/keywords/natural_disasters_2.html.

2. "Injuries and Illnesses among New York City Fire Department Rescue Workers." *MMWR* 51 (September 11, 2002): 1–5. http://www.cdc.gov/mmwr/preview/mmwrhtml/mm51spa1.htm; "911 Health Effects." Statement of David Prezant, MD before the Appropriations Committee, US House of Representatives, March 12, 2008.

3. "Rescue and Recovery Workers: What We Know from the Research." NYC 9/11 Health. http://www1.nyc.gov/home/search/index.page?search-terms=rescue+and+responders++to+9%2F11&collection=&start-number=0.

4. Luft, Benjamin. "Doctor: 9/11 Responders' Illnesses Becoming Worse." WBUR. September 11, 2014. http://www.wbur.org/hereandnow/2014/09/11/first-responders-doctor.

5. Aldrich, Thomas K., et al. "Lung Function in Rescue Workers at the World Trade Center after 7 Years." *New England Journal of Medicine* 362, no. 14 (April 8, 2010): 1263–72.

6. Aldrich, Thomas K., et al. "Lung Function Trajectories in World Trade Center–Exposed New York City Firefighters over 13 Years: The Roles of Smoking and Smoking Cessation." *Chest* 149, no. 6 (June 2016): 1419–27.

7. "9/11 Health and Compensation Act." NYC 9/11 Health. http://www1.nyc.gov/site/911health/enrollees/9-11-health-and-compensation-act-faq.page.

8. "As 9/11 Compensation Awards Top $1 Billion, Advocates Urge Congress to Reauthorize Bill to Help 9/11 Responders and Survivors." Citizens for the Extension of the James Zadroga Act. April 8, 2015. http://www.renew911health.org/as-911-compensation-awards-top-1-billion-advocates-urge-congress-to-reauthorize-bill-to-help-911-responders-and-survivors.

9. Broughton, Edward. "The Bhopal Disaster and Its Aftermath: A Review." *Environmental Health* 4 (2005): 6.

10. "Union Carbide's Disaster." The Bhopal Medical Appeal. http://bhopal.org/what-happened/union-carbides-disaster.

11. "Union Carbide's Disaster."

12. Brooks, S. M., M. A. Weiss, and I. L. Bernstein. "Reactive Airways Dysfunction Syndrome (RADS): Persistent Asthma Syndrome after High Level Irritant Exposures." *Chest* 88, no. 3 (September 1985): 376–84.

13. "U.S. Fire Statistics." U.S. Fire Administration. https://www.usfa.fema.gov/data/statistics/#tab-2.

14. Wright, David, Clayton Sandell, and Christina Ng. "Lone Survivor of Arizona Wildfire Was Lookout Who Warned Colleagues to Get Out." ABC News. July 2, 2013. http://abcnews.go.com/US/lone-survivor-arizona-wildfire-lookout-warned-colleagues/story?id=19550986.

15. Abdollah, Tami, and Felicia Fonseca. "Coroner: Firefighters Died from Burns, Oxygen Deprivation." *Las Vegas Review-Journal*. July 4, 2013. http://www.reviewjournal.com/news/nevada-and-west/coroner-arizona-firefighters-died-burns-oxygen-deprivation.

16. Summaries of survivor accounts cited in online search.

17. Crowley, C. F. "A Survivor's Story: Saved by a Pileup." *Providence Journal*. March 10, 2003.

18. "Carbon Monoxide–Related Deaths: United States, 1999–2004." *MMWR* 56, no. 50 (December 21, 2007): 1309–12. http://www.cdc.gov/mmwr/preview/mmwrhtml/mm5650a1.htm.

19. "QuickStats: Average Annual Number of Deaths and Death Rates from Unintentional, Non-Fire-Related Carbon Monoxide Poisoning, by Sex and Age Group: United States, 1999–2010." *MMWR* 63, no. 3 (January 24, 2014): 49–68. https://www.cdc.gov/mmwr/preview/mmwrhtml/mm6303a6.htm?s_cid=mm6303a6_w.

CHAPTER 10: CLEOPATRA REINCARNATE

1. Bean, Robert Bennett, comp., and William Bennett Bean, ed. *Sir William Osler: Aphorisms from His Bedside Teachings and Writings*. 2nd ed. Springfield, IL: Charles C. Thomas, 1961, aphorism 210, p. 105.

2. "Misuse of Prescription Drugs." National Institute on Drug Abuse. Last revised August 2016. https://www.drugabuse.gov/publications/research-reports/misuse-prescription-drugs/what-scope-prescription-drug-misuse.

3. Carollo, Kim. "Deaths from Painkiller Overdose on the Rise, Says CDC." ABC News. November 1, 2011. http://abcnews.go.com/health/prescription-painkiller-overdose-deaths-rise/story?id=14858375.

4. "John Fox Jr." The Literature Network. http://www.online-literature.com/john-fox.

5. Rosenberg, D. "How One Town Got Hooked." *Newsweek*. April 8, 2001.

6. "Stop Rx Abuse before It Starts." Kentucky Attorney General Andy Beshear. 2016. http://ag.ky.gov/rxabuse/Pages/default.aspx.

7. Childress, Sarah. "Veterans Face Greater Risks amid Opioid Crisis." *Frontline*. March 28, 2016. http://www.pbs.org/wgbh/frontline/article/veterans-face-greater-risks-amid-opioid-crisis; Miller, Matthew, Catherine W. Barber, Sarah

Leatherman, Jennifer Fonda, John A. Hermos, Kelly Cho, and David R. Gagnon. "Prescription Opioid Duration of Action and the Risk of Unintentional Overdose among Patients Receiving Opioid Therapy." *Journal of the American Medical Association Internal Medicine* 175, no. 4 (April 2015): 60815.

8. "Scores of Texas War Veterans Have Died of Overdoses, Suicide, and Vehicle Crashes, Investigation Finds." *Statesman*, September 29, 2012. http://www.statesman.com/news/news/local-military/texas-war-veteran-deaths-studied/nSPJs.

9. "Press Release: Opioids Drive Continued Increase in Drug Overdose Deaths." Centers for Disease Control and Prevention. February 20, 2013. http://www.cdc.gov/media/releases/2013/p0220_drug_overdose_deaths.html.

10. Roberts, Joel. "Bill Clinton: I Never Denied Smoking Marijuana." Yahoo News. December 4, 2013. http://news.yahoo.com/bill-clinton--i-never-denied-smoking-marijuana-092753311.html;_ylt=AwrTceHa3PRUXTcAjD0lnIlQ;_ylu=X3oDMTEzbmdoYXFmBHNlYwNzcgRwb3MDMDMgRjb2xvA2dxMQR2dGlkAllI UzAwNF8x.

11. "Youth Risk Behavior Surveillance: United States, 1991–2011." *MMWR* 61, no. 4 (June 8, 2012). http://www.cdc.gov/mmwr/pdf/ss/ss6104.pdf.

12. "The Surgeon General's Warning on Marijuana." *MMWR* 31, no. 31 (August 13, 1982): 428–29. https://www.cdc.gov/mmwr/preview/mmwrhtml/00001143.htm.

13. Wilkinson, Samuel T., and Deepak Cyril D'Souza. "Problems with the Medicalization of Marijuana." *Journal of the American Medical Association* 311, no. 23 (June 18, 2014): 2377–78.

14. "Surgeon General's Warning."

15. Wang, George S., Genie Roosevelt, Marie-Claire Le Lait, Erin M. Martinez, Becki Bucher-Bartleson, Alvin C. Bronstein, and Kennon Heard. "Association of Unintentional Pediatric Exposures with Decriminalization of Marijuana in the United States." *Annals of Emergency Medicine* 63, no. 6 (June 2014): 684–89.

16. Tashkin, Donald P. "Effects of Marijuana Smoking on the Lung." *Annals of the American Thoracic Society* 10, no. 3 (June 1, 2013): 239–47.

17. Zhang, Li Rita, et al. "Cannabis Smoking and Lung Cancer Risk." *International Journal of Cancer* 136, no. 4 (February 15, 2015): 894–903.

18. Berzon, Alexandra. "Why Did These Oil Workers Die?" *Wall Street Journal*. April 21, 2015.

19. Saloner, Brendan, and Joshua Sharfstein. "A Stronger Treatment System for Opioid Use Disorders." *Journal of the American Medical Association* 315, no. 20 (May 24/31, 2016): 2165–66.

20. Quinones, Sam. *Dreamland: The True Tale of America's Opiate Epidemic*. New York: Bloomsbury Press, 2015.

CHAPTER 11: SMOKING BEAGLES

1. "Vintage Tobacco Advertising: How Cigarette Adverts Have Changed over the Years." Telegraph. http://www.telegraph.co.uk/news/health/pictures/8620411/

Vintage-tobacco-advertising-how-cigarette-adverts-have-changed-over-the-years
.html?image=3.

2. Auerbach, Oscar, E. Cuyler Hammond, David Kirman, Lawrence Garfinkel, and Arthur Purdy Stout. "Histologic Changes in Bronchial Tubes of Cigarette-Smoking Dogs." *Cancer* 20, no. 12 (December 1967): 2055–66.

3. Auerbach et al., "Histologic Changes," p. 2060.

4. Auerbach, Oscar, E. Cuyler Hammond, and David Kirman. "Emphysema Produced in Dogs by Cigarette Smoking." *Journal of the American Medical Association* 199, no. 4 (January 23, 1967): 241–46, p. 245.

5. Wynder, Ernest L., and Evarts A. Graham. "Tobacco Smoking as a Possible Etiologic Factor in Bronchiogenic Carcinoma: A Study of Six Hundred and Eighty-Four Proved Cases." *Journal of the American Medical Association* 143, no. 4 (May 27, 1950): 329–36.

6. Fletcher, C. M. "Chronic Bronchitis: Its Prevalence, Nature, and Pathogenesis." *American Review of Respiratory Diseases* 80, no. 4, pt. 1 (October 1959): 483–94, p. 490.

7. Burkhart, Ford. "Oscar Auerbach, 92, Dies: Linked Smoking to Cancer." *New York Times*, January 16, 1997.

8. Borio, Gene. "Tobacco Timeline." Tobacco.org. 2001. http://archive.tobacco .org/History/Tobacco_History.html.

9. Borio, "Tobacco Timeline."

10. "Cigarettes: Men." Coffin Nails. 2005. http://tobacco.harpweek.com/ HubPages/CommentaryPage.asp?Commentary=Men.

11. "Cigarettes: Men."

12. Borio, "Tobacco Timeline."

13. Alberg, A., and J. Samet. "Epidemiology of Lung Cancer." In *Murray and Nadel's Textbook of Respiratory Medicine.* 5th ed. Robert J. Mason, V. Courtney Broaddus, Thomas R. Martin, Talmedge E. King Jr., Dean E. Schraufnagel, John F. Murray, and Jay A. Nadel, eds. Philadelphia: Saunders Elsevier, 2010.

14. Burns, David M. Personal communication, February 2016.

15. "Tobacco Use: United States, 1900–1999." *Oncology* (November 30, 1999). http://www.cancernetwork.com/lung-cancer/tobacco-use-united-states-1900-1999.

16. Bach, Laura. "Tobacco Industry Targeting of Women and Girls." Campaign for Tobacco-Free Kids. November 21, 2016. https://www.tobaccofreekids.org/ research/factsheets/pdf/0138.pdf.

17. "Doctors Recommend Smoking Camels." OTR Commercials. http://www.old-time.com/commercials/1940's/More%20Doctors%20Smoke%20Camels.html.

18. "Before Becoming President, Ronald Reagan Was a Paid Cigarette Model." Forgotten History Blog. December 19, 2008. http://forgottenhistoryblog.com/before-becoming-president-ronald-reagan-was-a-paid-cigarette-model.

19. Mukherjee, Siddhartha. *The Emperor of All Maladies: A Biography of Cancer.* New York: Scribner, 2011, p. 252.

20. "Surgeon General's Warning." http://www.cigarettes.1emallway.com/ warning.htm.

21. "History of the Surgeon General's Reports on Smoking and Health." Centers for Disease Control and Prevention. Last updated December 2006. http://www.cdc.gov/tobacco/data_statistics/sgr/history/index.htm.

22. "History of the Surgeon General's Report."

23. Alberg and Samet, "Epidemiology of Lung Cancer," p. 1105.

24. Alberg and Samet, "Epidemiology of Lung Cancer," p. 1105.

25. Burns, personal communication 2016.

26. "History of the Surgeon General's Report."

27. "Prevalence of Tobacco Smoking." World Health Organization. http://www.who.int/gho/tobacco/use/en.

28. "Trends in Tobacco Use." American Lung Association. July 2011. http://www.lung.org/assets/documents/research/tobacco-trend-report.pdf.

29. "E-Cigarette Inventor Complains about Lack of Financial Rewards." Vape Ranks. October 14, 2013. http://vaperanks.com/e-cigarette-inventor-complains-about-lack-of-financial-rewards.

30. Gostin, Lawrence O., and Aliza Y. Glasner. "E Cigarettes, Vaping, and Youth." *Journal of the American Medical Association* 312, no. 6 (August 13, 2014): 595–96. http://jamanetwork.com/journals/jama/article-abstract/1886077.

31. O'Donnell, Jayne, and Laura Ungar. "Feds Announce Much Tougher E-Cigarette, Cigar Rule." *USA Today*. May 5, 2016. http://www.usatoday.com/story/news/politics/2016/05/05/feds-expected-announce-final-e-cigarette-rule-could-nearly-ban-them/83951786.

32. Szabo, Liz. "States Racing to Regulate E-Cigarettes." *USA Today*. February 7, 2015. http://www.usatoday.com/story/news/2015/02/07/state-e-cigarette-bills/22364765.

33. "Press Release: E-Cigarette Use More Than Doubles among U.S. Middle and High School Students from 2011–2012." Centers for Disease Control and Prevention. September 5, 2013. https://www.cdc.gov/media/releases/2013/p0905-ecigarette-use.html.

34. "Current Cigarette Smoking among Adults in the U.S." Centers for Disease Control and Prevention. Last updated December 1, 2016. http://www.cdc.gov/tobacco/data_statistics/fact_sheets/adult_data/cig_smoking.

35. Boseley, Sarah. "Hon Lik Invented the E-Cigarette to Quit Smoking—but Now He's a Dual User." *Guardian*. June 9, 2015. https://www.theguardian.com/society/2015/jun/09/hon-lik-e-cigarette-inventor-quit-smoking-dual-user.

CHAPTER 12: DAD, AND THE WEREWOLF

1. Zastrow, Sam. "25 Inspirational Cancer Quotes to Share with Your Friends and Family." *Exact Sciences*. March 20, 2014. http://www.beseengetscreened.com/blog/25-inspirational-cancer-quotes-to-share-with-your-friends-and-family.

2. Zastrow, "25 Inspirational Cancer Quotes."

3. "Lung Cancer Statistics." Centers for Disease Control and Prevention. Last reviewed August 20, 2015. http://www.cdc.gov/cancer/lung/statistics/index.htm.

4. "Common Cancer Types." National Cancer Institute. Last updated February 1, 2016. https://www.cancer.gov/types/common-cancers#1. Citing *American Cancer Society: Cancer Facts and Figures 2016*. Atlanta, GA: American Cancer Society, 2016.

5. Hensley, George T., and Kevin P. Glynn. "Hypertrichosis Lanuginosa as a Sign of Internal Malignancy." *Cancer* 24, no. 5 (November 1969): 1051–56.

6. Alberg, Anthony, and J. Samet. "Epidemiology of Lung Cancer." In *Murray and Nadel's Textbook of Respiratory Medicine*. 5th ed. Robert J. Mason, V. Courtney Broaddus, Thomas R. Martin, Talmedge E. King Jr., Dean E. Schraufnagel, John F. Murray, and Jay A. Nadel, eds. Philadelphia: Saunders Elsevier, 2010, pp. 1573ff.

7. American Thoracic Society. "Asbestos Exposure, Asbestosis, and Smoking Combined Greatly Increase Lung Cancer Risk." *Science Daily*. April 12, 2013. http://www.sciencedaily.com/releases/2013/04/130412084227.htm.

8. Goldsmith, David F., Tee L. Guidotti, and Donald R. Johnston. "Does Occupational Exposure to Silica Cause Lung Cancer?" *American Journal of Industrial Medicine* 3, no. 4 (1982): 423–40.

9. "Lung Cancer Prevention and Early Detection." American Cancer Society. Last updated February 22, 2016. http://www.cancer.org/cancer/lungcancer-non -smallcell/moreinformation/lungcancerpreventionandearlydetection.

10. Alberg and Samet, "Epidemiology of Lung Cancer," p. 1106.

11. Mulloy, Karen B., David S. James, Kim Mohs, and Mario Kornfeld. "Lung Cancer in a Nonsmoking Underground Uranium Miner." *Environmental Health Perspectives* 109, no. 3 (March 2001): 305–9.

12. "A Citizen's Guide to Radon: The Guide to Protecting Yourself and Your Family from Radon." United States Environmental Protection Agency. Last updated December 2016. http://www.epa.gov/radon/pubs/citguide.html.

13. "NIOSH Worker Health Study Summaries: Research on Long-Term Exposure: Uranium Miners (1)." Centers for Disease Control and Prevention. Last reviewed October 1, 2015. https://www.cdc.gov/niosh/pgms/worknotify/uranium .html.

14. Brugge, Doug, and Rob Goble. "The History of Uranium Mining and the Navajo People." *American Journal of Public Health* 92, no. 2 (September 2002): 1410–19.

15. Moran, Kristen. "Uranium Mining in the United States." Uranium Investing News. September 13, 2016. http://uraniuminvestingnews.com/7680/uranium -mining-in-the-united-states.html.

16. "Domestic Uranium Production Report: Annual." U.S. Energy Information Administration. May 5, 2016. http://www.eia.gov/uranium/production/annual.

17. "Lung Cancer Fact Sheet." American Lung Association. Last reviewed November 3, 2016. http://www.lung.org/lung-disease/lung-cancer/resources/ facts-figures/lung-cancer-fact-sheet.html.

18. Homicides account for 16,000 deaths annually; suicides account for 41,000 deaths; and motor vehicle accidents account for 35,000 deaths.

19. "Lung Cancer (Non-Small Cell)." American Cancer Society. Last updated May 16, 2016. www.cancer.org/cancer/lungcancer-non-smallcell/detailedguide/non-small-cell-lung-cancer-survival-rates.

20. "The Health Consequences of Smoking—50 Years of Progress: A Report of the Surgeon General: Executive Summary." U.S. Department of Health and Human Services. 2014. http://www.surgeongeneral.gov/library/reports/50-years-of progress/exec-summary.pdf.

21. Glynn, Kevin P. "Piano Lessons." *Journal of the American Medical Association* 306, no. 10 (September 14, 2011): 1063–64.

CHAPTER 13: THE LETHAL BROWN CLOUD

1. "Quotes about Pollution." Goodreads. http://www.goodreads.com/quotes/tag/pollution.

2. Murray, Ann. "Smog Deaths in 1948 Led to Clean Air Laws." *All Things Considered*, NPR. April 22, 2009. http://www.npr.org/templates/story/story.php?storyId=103359330.

3. Kiester, Edwin, Jr. "A Darkness in Donora." *Smithsonian Magazine* (November 1999).

4. Kiester, "Darkness in Donora."

5. Williams, Jack. "U.S. Once Had Air Pollution to Match China's Today." *Washington Post*, October 25, 2013.

6. "1948 Donora Smog." Wikipedia. https://en.wikipedia.org/wiki/1948_Donora_smog.

7. Kiester, "Darkness in Donora."

8. Kiester, "Darkness in Donora."

9. Hamill, Sean. "Unveiling a Museum: Pennsylvania Town Remembers the Smog That Killed 20." *New York Times*, November 1, 2008.

10. Davis, Devra Lee. *When Smoke Ran Like Water: Tales of Environmental Deception and the Battle against Pollution*. New York: Basic Books, 2002, p. 29.

11. Mooney, Chris, and Brady Dennis. "WHO: Global Air Pollution Is Worsening, and Poor Countries Are Being Hit the Hardest." *Washington Post*, May 12, 2016.

12. Eisner, M. D., and J. R. Balmes. "Indoor and Outdoor Air Pollution." In *Murray and Nadel's Textbook of Respiratory Medicine*. 5th ed. Robert J. Mason, V. Courtney Broaddus, Thomas R. Martin, Talmedge E. King Jr., Dean E. Schraufnagel, John F. Murray, and Jay A. Nadel, eds. Philadelphia: Saunders Elsevier, 2010, pp. 1601–18.

13. "State of the Air 2013." American Lung Association. 2013. http://www.stateoftheair.org/2013.

14. Marcum, Diana. "A Menacing Air in the Central Valley." *Los Angeles Times*, January 24, 2014.

15. Jacobs, Chip, and William J. Kelly. *Smogtown: The Lung-Burning History of Pollution in Los Angeles*. Woodstock, NY: Overlook Press, 2008, p. 10.

16. Ritz, Beate, Michelle Wilhelm, and Yingxu Zhao. "Air Pollution and Infant Death in Southern California, 1989–2000." *Pediatrics* 118, no. 2 (August 2006): 493–502.

17. Weber, Rodney. "Air Pollution: History." Georgia Tech: Earth and Atmospheric Sciences, College of Sciences. 2005. http://www.aerosols.eas.gatech.edu /EAS%20Air%20Pollution%20Phys%20Chem/Intro1%20AP%20History.pdf.

18. Dickens, Charles, quoted in Metcalfe, John. "December 2, 1952: Killer Fog Smothers Up to 12,000 Londoners." WJLA.com. December 9, 2011. http://wjla .com/weather/dec-9-1952-killer-fog-smothers-4-000-people-in-london-13893.

19. Joesten, Melvin, Mary E. Castellion, and John L. Hogg. *The World of Chemistry: Essentials*. 4th ed. Belmont, CA: Thomson Brooks/Cole, 2007.

20. "The Southland's War on Smog: Fifty Years of Progress toward Clean Air (through May 1997)." South Coast AQMD. 2014. http://www.aqmd.gov/home/library/ public-information/publications/50-years-of-progress.

21. Dockery, Douglas. "Health Effects of Particulate Air Pollution." *Annals of Epidemiology* 19 (2009): 257–63.

22. Pope, C. Arden, III. "Respiratory Disease Associated with Community Air Pollution and a Steel Mill, Utah Valley." *American Journal of Public Health* 79, no. 5 (May 1989): 623–28.

23. Pope, C. Arden, III, Michael J. Thun, Mohan M. Namboodiri, Douglas W. Dockery, John S. Evans, Frank E. Speizer, and Clark W. Heath. "Particulate Air Pollution as a Predictor of Mortality in a Prospective Study of U.S. Adults." *American Journal of Respiratory and Critical Care Medicine* 151, no. 3, pt. 1 (March 1, 1995): 669–74.

24. Dockery, Douglas W., C. Arden Pope III, Xiping Xu, John D. Spengler, James H. Ware, Martha E. Fay, Benjamin G. Ferris Jr., and Frank E. Speizer. "An Association between Air Pollution and Mortality in Six U.S. Cities." *New England Journal of Medicine* 329, no. 24 (December 9, 1993): 1753–59.

25. Wong, Edward. "Pollution Leads to Drop in Life Span in Northern China, Research Finds." *New York Times*, July 8, 2013.

26. Wong, Edward. "Air Pollution Linked to 1.2 Million Premature Deaths in China." *New York Times*, April 1, 2013.

27. Wong, Edward. "Urbanites Flee China's Smog for Blue Skies." *New York Times*, November 22, 2013.

28. Harris, Gardener. "Beijing's Bad Air Would Be Step Up for Smoggy Delhi." *New York Times*, January 26, 2014.

29. Busch, Simon. "And the World's Most Polluted City Is . . ." CNN Travel. January 31, 2014. http://www.cnn.com/2014/01/30/travel/most-polluted-city.

30. Yee, Amy. "The Air That Kills in India." *New York Times: Green*. February 14, 2013. http://green.blogs.nytimes.com/2013/02/14/the-air-that-kills-in-india/ ?_r=0.

31. Taylor, David A. "The ABCs of Haze." *Environmental Health Perspectives* 111, no. 1 (January 2003): A21.

32. Taylor, "ABCs of Haze," p. A21.

33. Pope, C. Arden, III, Richard T. Burnett, George D. Thurston, Michael J. Thun, Eugenia E. Calle, Daniel Krewski, and John J. Godleski. "Cardiovascular Mortality and Long-Term Exposure to Particulate Air Pollution: Epidemiological Evidence of General Pathophysiological Pathways of Disease." *Circulation* 109, no. 1 (January 6, 2004): 71–77.

34. Pope, C. Arden, III, Joseph B. Muhlestein, Heidi T. May, Dale G. Renlund, Jeffrey L. Anderson, and Benjamin D. Horne. "Ischemic Heart Disease Events Triggered by Short-Term Exposure to Fine Particulate Air Pollution." *Circulation* 114, no. 23 (December 5, 2006): 2443–48.

35. Kuehn, Bridget M. "WHO: More Than 7 Million Air Pollution Deaths Each Year." *Journal of the American Medical Association* 311, no. 15 (April 16, 2014): 1486. See also Jacobs, Andrew, and Ian Johnson. "Pollution Killed 7 Million People Worldwide in 2012, Report Finds." *New York Times*, March 25, 2014; "Public Health, Environmental and Social Determinants of Health (PHE)." World Health Organization. http://www.who.int/phe/health_topics/outdoorair/databases/en; Poon, Linda. "Pollution from Home Stoves Kills Millions of People Worldwide." NPR. March 25, 2014. http://www.npr.org/blogs/health/2014/03/25/294339956.

36. Brennan, Deborah Sullivan. "Highest Praise from U.N. Goes to Scripps Professor: Climate Expert Receives Award for Discoveries Tied to Soot as Pollutant." *San Diego Union-Tribune*, September 23, 2013.

37. Victor, David G., Charles F. Kennel, and Veerabhadran Ramanathan. "The Climate Threat We Can Beat: What It Is and How to Deal with It." *Foreign Affairs* (May/June 2012).

38. Roger Haines, a fellow Rotary Club member interested in reducing air pollution, gave me the solar cooker to try.

39. Victor, Kennel, and Ramanathan, "Climate Threat."

40. Brennan, Deborah Sullivan. "Scientist Hopes Pope Will Make Declaration." *San Diego Union-Tribune*, May 4, 2014.

41. Brennan, "Highest Praise," p. B3.

42. "Southland's War on Smog."

43. Berhane, Kiros, Chih-Chieh Chang, Rob McConnell, W. James Gauderman, Edward Avol, Ed Rapapport, Robert Urman, Fred Lurmann, and Frank Gilliland. "Association of Changes in Air Quality with Bronchitic Symptoms in Children in California, 1993–2012." *Journal of the American Medical Association* 315, no. 14 (April 12, 2016): 1491–1501.

44. "Report to the Community: 2015–2016." San Joaquin Valley Air Pollution Control District. http://www.valleyair.org/General_info/pubdocs/2015-Annual-Report-WEB.PDF.

45. Laden, Francine, Joel Schwartz, Frank E. Speizer, and Douglas W. Dockery. "Reduction in Fine Particulate Air Pollution and Mortality: Extended Follow-up of the Harvard Six Cities Study." *American Journal of Respiratory and Critical Care Medicine* 173, no. 6 (March 15, 2006): 667–72; Pope, C. Arden, III, Richard T. Burnett,

and Michael J. Thun. "Lung Cancer, Cardiopulmonary Mortality, and Long-Term Exposure to Fine Particulate Air Pollution." *Journal of the American Medical Association* 287, no. 9 (March 6, 2002): 1132–41, citing *Whitman vs. American Trucking Associations* 532 U.S. 457 (2001).

CHAPTER 14: PANTING FOR AIR

1. Osler, William. *The Principles and Practice of Medicine*. 3rd ed. New York: D. Appleton, 1899, p. 630.

2. McAlpine, Fraser. "Happy Birthday, T. S. Eliot: 20 of His Most Life-Affirming Quotes." Anglophenia. 2014. http://www.bbcamerica.com/anglophenia/2014/09/happy-birthday-t-s-eliot-20-quotes.

3. Sakula, Alex. "Henry Hyde Salter (1823–71): A Biographical Sketch." *Thorax* 40, no. 12 (December 1985): 887–88.

4. Holgate, Stephen T. "Brief History of Asthma and Its Mechanisms to Modern Concepts of Disease Pathogenesis." *Allergy, Asthma, and Immunology Research* 2, no. 3 (July 2010): 165–71.

5. "A History of Allergies, Part Three: The 16th Century to the 20th Century." Achoo Allergy. 2016. http://www.achooallergy.com/history-allergies-three.asp.

6. Glyn, John H. "The Discovery of Cortisone: A Personal Memory." *BMJ* 317, no. 7161 (September 19, 1998): 822. http://www.ncbi.nlm.nih.gov/pmc/articles/PMC1113923/

7. Holgate, "Brief History of Asthma."

8. Lugogo, Njira, Loretta G. Que, Daniel Fertel, and Monica Kraft. "Asthma." In *Murray and Nadel's Textbook of Respiratory Medicine*. 5th ed. Robert J. Mason, V. Courtney Broaddus, Thomas R. Martin, Talmedge E. King Jr., Dean E. Schraufnagel, John F. Murray, and Jay A. Nadel, eds. Philadelphia: Saunders Elsevier, 2010, p. 885.

9. Stein, Michelle M., et al. "Innate Immunity and Asthma Risk in Amish and Hutterite Farm Children." *New England Journal of Medicine* 375, no. 5 (August 4, 2016): 411–21.

10. Weiss, Scott T. "Genetics of Asthma." Medscape. August 5, 2015. http://emedicine.medscape.com/article/2068244-overview#a30.

11. Lugogo, et al., "Asthma."

12. Stevenson, Donald D. Personal communication, January, 27, 2016.

13. Holloway, John W., Tim P. Keith, Donna E. Davis, Robert Powell, Hans-Michael Haitchi, and Stephen T. Holgate. "The Discovery and Role of *ADAM33*, a New Candidate Gene for Asthma." *Expert Reviews in Molecular Medicine* 6, no. 17 (August 3, 2004): 1–12. http://www.ncbi.nlm.nih.gov/pubmed/15387895.

14. Holgate, "Brief History of Asthma."

15. Heron, Melonie, Donna L. Hoyert, Sherry L. Murphy, Jiaquan Xu, Kenneth D. Kochanek, and Betzaida Tejada-Vera. "Deaths: Final Data for 2006." *National*

Vital Statistics Reports 57, no. 14 (April 17, 2009); cited in "Asthma Facts and Figures." Asthma and Allergy Foundation of America. August 2015. http://www.aafa.org/page/asthma-facts.aspx.

16. "Asthma May Raise Risk of COPD, Emphysema." WebMD Health News. July 12, 2004. http://www.webmd.com/lung/copd/news/20040712/asthma-may-raise-risk-copd-emphysema.

CHAPTER 15: LUNGS THAT DO NOT COLLAPSE

1. Osler, William. *The Principles and Practice of Medicine*. 3rd Edition. New York: D. Appleton, 1899, p. 657.

2. Laennec, R. T. H. *A Treatise on Diseases of the Chest and on Mediate Auscultation*. 4th ed. John Forbes, trans. London: Henry Renshaw, 1834, p. 164. https://books.google.com/books?id=fSUbXEB8cS8C&pg=PA166&lpg=PA166&dq=lungs+that+do+not+collapse+%2B+rene+laennec&source=bl&ots=aD2RLxrz-0&sig=o79T2r68i-xCn9pFKMZLaU9vkL8&hl=en&sa=X&ved=0ahUKEwiK2sit8qXMAhVQ7WMKHZW_CMkQ6AEIJzAD#v=onepage&q=lungs%20that%20do%20not%20collapse%20%2B%20rene%20laennec&f=false.

3. Part of Ray's story was originally published in Glynn, Kevin, and Max Adler. "A Pro Made Me a Better Doctor." *Golf Digest* (November 12, 2012): 18. © 2012 Conde Nast/Golf Digest.

4. "Lung Health and Diseases: How Serious Is COPD?" American Lung Association. Last reviewed November 1, 2016. http://www.lung.org/lung-disease/copd/resources/facts-figures/COPD-Fact-Sheet.html.

5. "Statistics about Bronchiectasis." Right Diagnosis. 2014. http://www.rightdiagnosis.com/b/bronchiectasis/stats.htm.

6. Sadatsafavi, Mohsen, and Don D. Sin. "COPD Undefeated." *Chest* 147, no. 4 (April 2015): 868–69.

7. Taylor, Tim. "Lungs." Inner Body. 2016. http://www.innerbody.com/anatomy/respiratory/lungs.

8. Laennec, *A Treatise on Diseases of the Chest*. Translated from the French. London: T. and G. Underwood, 1821, p. 89; cited by Petty, Thomas L. "The History of COPD." *International Journal of Chronic Obstructive Pulmonary Disease* 1, no. 1 (March 15, 2006): 3–14.

9. "Chronic Obstructive Pulmonary Disease (COPD)." World Health Organization. November 2016. http://www.who.int/mediacentre/factsheets/fs315/en.

10. Recent reports suggest that medical errors may cause more deaths than COPD. However, if lung cancer and COPD are added together, then breathing disorders move back into third place in the ranks of major killers.

CHAPTER 16: THE GREAT MASQUERADER

1. "Herman Melville: Quotes: Quotable Quote." Goodreads. 2017. http://www.goodreads.com/quotes/302241-all-men-live-enveloped-in-whale-lines-all are-born-with.

2. Bělohlávek, Jan, Vladimír Dytrych, and Aleš Linhart. "Pulmonary Embolism, Part I: Epidemiology, Risk Factors and Risk Stratification, Pathophysiology, Clinical Presentation, Diagnosis and Nonthrombotic Pulmonary Embolism." *Experimental and Clinical Cardiology* 18, no. 2 (Spring 2013): 129–38. https://www.ncbi.nlm.nih.gov/pmc/articles/PMC3718593.

3. Bělohlávek, Dytrych, and Linhart, "Pulmonary Embolism, Part I."

4. Bělohlávek, Dytrych, and Linhart, "Pulmonary Embolism, Part I."

5. McFadden, P. Michael, and John L. Ochsner. "A History of the Diagnosis and Treatment of Venous Thrombosis and Pulmonary Embolism." *Ochsner Journal* 4, no. 1 (January 2002): 9–13.

6. Simpson, Keith. "Shelter Deaths from Pulmonary Embolism." *Lancet* 236, no. 6120 (December 14, 1940): 744; cited by Beasley, R., S. Hill, M. Nowitz, and R. Hughes. "eThrombosis: The 21st Century Variant of Venous Thromboembolism Associated with Immobility." *European Respiratory Journal* 21 (2003): 374–76.

7. Belcaro, G., G. Geroulakos, A. N. Nicolaides, K. A. Myers, and M. Winford. "Venous Thromboembolism from Air Travel: The LONFLIT Study." *Angiology* 52, no. 6 (June 2001): 369–74. Cited by Beasley et al., "eThrombosis."

8. Beasley et al., "eThrombosis."

9. Shirakawa, Toru, Hiroyasu Iso, Kazumasa Yamagishi, Hiroshi Yatsuya, Naohito Tanabe, Satoyo Ikehara, Shigekazu Ukawa, and Akiko Tamakoshi. "Watching Television and Risk of Mortality from Pulmonary Embolism among Japanese Men and Women: The JACC Study (Japan Collaborative Cohort." *Circulation* 134 (July 26, 2016): 355–57.

10. Moser, Kenneth M., and Nina S. Braunwald. "Successful Surgical Intervention in Severe Chronic Thromboembolic Pulmonary Hypertension." *Chest* 64, no. 1 (July 1973): 29–35.

CHAPTER 17: CELLS LIKE ELONGATED CRESCENTS

1. Shakespeare, William. *Julius Caesar*, act 1, sc. 2, ll. 140–41.

2. Roberson, Lynn. "Researcher Passes Away after Lifelong Battle with Cystic Fibrosis." Inside UNC Charlotte. June 12, 2015. http://inside.uncc.edu/news-features/2015-06-12/researcher-passes-away-after-lifelong-battle-cystic-fibrosis.

3. Savitt, Todd L., and Morton F. Goldberg. "Herrick's 1910 Case Report of Sickle Cell Anemia: The Rest of the Story." *Journal of the American Medical Association* 261, no. 2 (January 13, 1989): 266–71.

4. Herrick, James B. "Peculiar Elongated and Sickle-Shaped Red Blood Corpuscles in a Case of Severe Anemia." *Archives of Internal Medicine* (Chicago) 6, no. 5 (November 1910): 517–21.

5. Savitt and Morton, "Herrick's 1910 Case Report."

6. Herrick, "Peculiar Elongated and Sickle-Shaped."

7. Ross, Richard S. "A Parlous State of Storm and Stress: The Life and Times of James B. Herrick." *Circulation* 67, no. 5 (May 1983): 955–59.

8. Miller, Andrew C., and Mark T. Gladwin. "Pulmonary Complications of Sickle Cell Disease." *American Journal of Respiratory and Critical Care Medicine* 185, no. 11 (June 1, 2012): 1154–65.

9. Miller and Gladwin, "Pulmonary Complications."

10. "Sickle Cell Disease (SCD): Data and Statistics." Centers for Disease Control and Prevention. Last updated August 31, 2016. http://www.cdc.gov/ncbddd/sicklecell/data.html.

11. Winter, William P. "A Brief History of Sickle Cell Disease." Howard University Hospital. http://huhealthcare.com/healthcare/hospital/specialty-services/sickle -cell-disease-center/disease-information/breif-history.

12. "Sickle Cell Disease." Eight percent of 39 million African Americans have the trait. Siddiqui, A. K., and S. Ahmed. "Pulmonary Manifestations of Sickle Cell Disease." *Postgraduate Medical Journal* 79, no. 933 (2003): 384–90.

13. Savitt and Morton, "Herrick's 1910 Case Report."

14. Ernest Irons was James Herrick's partner; later, Frank Kelly became Irons's partner. Dr. Kelly was my parents' physician and one of my models of how my life would play out if I became a doctor. I was born at Presbyterian Hospital in 1936, thirty-two years after Walter Clement Noel first presented for care. Forty-two years after Noel's visit, I made my first emergency visit for asthma to that same hospital, recounted in the introduction.

15. Fitzgerald, F. T. "Curiosity." *Annals of Internal Medicine* 130, no. 1 (January 5, 1999): 70–72.

16. Creager, Reid. "Charlotte Cystic Fibrosis Patient Studies His Own Disease." *Charlotte Observer*, May 6, 2015.

17. These comments came from "Josh's Story," Children's Organ Transplant Association, which was part of the online plea for donations for Stokell's lung transplant. See also Creager, "Charlotte Cystic Fibrosis Patient"; and "Unraveling Cystic Fibrosis Puzzle, Taking It Personally Matters." UNC Charlotte, Office of Public Relations. March 26, 2015. http://publicrelations.uncc.edu/news-events/news-releases/unravel-ing-cystic-fibrosis-puzzle-taking-it-personally-matters.

18. Stokell, Joshua R., Raad Z. Gharaibeh, Timothy J. Hamp, Malcolm J. Zapata, Anthony A. Fodor, and Todd R. Streck. "Analysis of Changes in Diversity and Abundance of the Microbial Community in a Cystic Fibrosis Patient over a Multiyear Period." *Journal of Clinical Microbiology* 53, no. 1 (January 2015): 237–47.

19. From "Josh's Story." See also Creager, "Charlotte Cystic Fibrosis Patient"; and "Unraveling Cystic Fibrosis Puzzle."

20. Sharma, Girish D. "Cystic Fibrosis." Medscape. June 8, 2016. http://emedicine.medscape.com/article/1001602-overview?pa=nOW%2FKo%2BXJPjDA9S n8sWpKLJSD8eXUqN7eVvSpOrTqGmuhq1vniG8ik2yV4FxNRW056MI7dGTgNaw PfsOtJla9Q%3D%3D.

21. Sharma, "Cystic Fibrosis."

22. From "Josh's Story." See also Creager, "Charlotte Cystic Fibrosis Patient"; and "Unraveling Cystic Fibrosis Puzzle."

CHAPTER 18: THE PUMP AND THE BELLOWS

1. Barker, Kenneth, ed. *The New International Version Study Bible*. Grand Rapids, MI: Zondervan, 1995.

2. Jackson, Chevalier. "All That Wheezes Is Not Asthma." *BMQ* 16 (1865): 86; cited by Kaminsky, David A. "'All That Wheezes Is Not Asthma' (or COPD)!" *Chest* 147, no. 2 (February 2015): 284–86.

3. Mørch, E. T. "History of Mechanical Ventilation." In *Mechanical Ventilation*. Robert R. Kirby, Robert A. Smith, and David A. Desautels, eds. New York: Churchill Livingstone, 1985.

4. Colice, G. "Historical Perspective on the Development of Mechanical Ventilation." In *Principles and Practice of Mechanical Ventilation*. 3rd ed. Martin J. Tobin, ed. New York: McGraw-Hill Medical, 2013, p. 15.

5. Colice, "Historical Perspective."

6. Ribatti, Domenico. "William Harvey and the Discovery of Circulation of Blood." *Journal of Angiogenesis Research* 1 (2009): 3. http://www.ncbi .nlm.nih.gov/pmc/articles/PMC2776239;

7. Osler, William. *The Principles and Practice of Medicine*. 3rd ed. New York: 1899, p. 635.

CHAPTER 19: THAT SLEEP OF DEATH

1. "Mahatma Gandhi: Quotes: Quotable Quote." Goodreads. 2017. http://www .goodreads.com/quotes/1233102-each-night-when-i-go-to-sleep-i-die-and.

2. Shakespeare, William. *Hamlet*, act 3, sc. 1, ll. 71–75.

3. "Rising Prevalence of Sleep Apnea in U.S. Threatens Public Health." American Academy of Sleep Medicine. September 29, 2014. http://www.aasmnet.org/articles. aspx?id=5043.

4. Olson, Amy L., and Clifford Zwillich. "The Obesity Hypoventilation Syndrome." *American Journal of Medicine* 118, no. 9 (September 2005): 948–56.

5. Kryger, Meir H. "Sleep Apnea: From the Needles of Dionysius to Continuous Positive Airway Pressure." *Archives of Internal Medicine* 143, no. 12 (December 1983): 2301–3.

6. Kryger, "Sleep Apnea."

7. Dement, William C. "History of Sleep Physiology and Medicine." In *Principles and Practice of Sleep Medicine.* 4th ed. Meir H. Kryger, Thomas Roth, and William C. Dement, eds. Philadelphia: Elsevier Saunders, 2005.

8. Dement, "History of Sleep Physiology," p. 8.

9. Dement, "History of Sleep Physiology," p. 8.

10. Severinghaus, J. W., and R. A. Mitchell. "Ondine's Curse: Failure of Respiratory Center Automaticity." *Clinical Research* 10 (1962): 122.

11. Burnett, Lynn Barkley. "Sudden Infant Death Syndrome." Medscape. Last updated December 7, 2016. http://emedicine.medscape.com/article/804412 -overview.

12. I don't remember if the Stanford referral was before or after the failed trach. I called Stanford to see if they have records. Her name is listed, but records have been destroyed.

13. Psalm 146: 4. "English Standard Version." Bible Hub. http://biblehub.com/ psalms/146-4.htm.

CHAPTER 20: THE FIRST BREATHS

1. Shakespeare, William. *King Lear*, act 4, sc. 6, ll. 171–72. http://nfs.sparknotes. com/lear/page_246.html.

2. Pasteur, Louis. Lecture at the University of Lille, December 7, 1854. https:// en.wikiquote.org/wiki/Louis_Pasteur.

3. Calmes, Selma H. "Virginia Apgar: A Woman Physician's Career in a Developing Specialty." *Journal of the American Medical Women's Association* 39 (1984): 184–88.

4. "The Virginia Apgar Papers: Establishing a New Specialty, 1938–1949." *U.S. National Library of Medicine*. https://profiles.nlm.nih.gov/ps/retrieve/Narrative/CP/p-nid/180.

5. Greenough, Anne. "Respiratory Disorders in the Newborn." In *Kendig's Disorders of the Respiratory Tract in Children.* 7th ed. Victor Chernick, Thomas F. Boat, Robert W. Wilmott, and Andrew Bush, eds. Philadelphia: Saunders Elsevier, 2006, pp. 317ff.

6. Altman, Lawrence K. "A Kennedy Baby's Life and Death." *New York Times*, July 29, 2013.

7. Ryan, Michael S. *Patrick Bouvier Kennedy: A Brief Life That Changed the History of Newborn Care.* Minneapolis: MCP Books, 2015, p. 141.

8. Avery, Mary Ellen. "Surfactant Deficiency in Hyaline Membrane Disease." *American Journal of Respiratory and Critical Care Medicine* 161, no. 4 (April 1, 2000): 1074–75.

9. Wrobel, Sylvia. "Bubbles, Babies, and Biology: The Story of Surfactant." *FASEB Journal* 18, no. 13 (October 2004): 1–16.

10. Halliday, H. L. "Surfactants: Past, Present and Future." *Journal of Perinatology* 28, no. S1, "Evidence vs. Experience in Neonatal Practices: Proceedings from the 4th Annual Conference June, 2007" (May 2008): S47–S56.

11. Wrobel, "Bubbles."

12. Gregory, George A., Joseph A. Kitterman, Roderic H. Phibbs, William H. Tooley, and William K. Hamilton. "Treatment of the Idiopathic Respiratory-Distress Syndrome with Continuous Positive Airway Pressure." *New England Journal Medicine* 284, no. 24 (June 17, 1971): 1333–40.

13. In the 1970s, Gluck was at UC San Diego. He was a medical celebrity, and local pediatricians were enthusiastic about his research and felt it was an important advance in prenatal care.

14. Liggins G. C., and R. N. Howie. "A Controlled Trial of Antepartum Glucocorticoid Treatment for Prevention of the Respiratory Distress Syndrome in Premature Infants." *Pediatrics* 50, no. 4 (October 1972): 515–25.

15. Fujiwara, Tetsuro, Shoichi Chida, Yoshitane Watanabe, Haruo Maeta, Tomoaki Morita, and Tadaaki Abe. "Artificial Surfactant Therapy in Hyaline-Membrane Disease." *Lancet* 315, no. 8159 (January 12, 1980): 55–59.

16. Stoll, Barbara J., et al. "Trends in Care Practices, Morbidity, and Mortality of Extremely Preterm Neonates, 1993–2012." *Journal of the American Medical Association* 314, no. 10 (September 8, 2015): 1039–51. doi:10.1001/jama.2015.10244.

17. Pasteur, Lecture.

18. Wrobel, "Bubbles," p. 15.

CHAPTER 21: AROUND THE WORLD ON OXYGEN

1. "Allen Klein Quotes." Brainy Quote. https://www.brainyquote.com/quotes/quotes/a/allenklein285002.html.

2. "Anonymous Quote." Cool Funny Quotes. http://www.coolfunnyquotes.com/author/anonymous/live-without-love.

3. "A Taped Interview with Alvan L. Barach by Thomas L. Petty." Archive Sound Material. 1976. http://www.perf2ndwind.org/html/Alvan_Barach.html.

4. Petty, Thomas L., Robert W. McCoy, and Dennis E. Doherty. "Long Term Oxygen Therapy (LTOT)." *6th Oxygen Consensus Conference Recommendations, National Lung Health Education Program.* August 25–28, 2005. http://www.nlhep.org/Documents/lt_oxygen.pdf.

5. Barach, Alvan L. "A New Oxygen Tent." *Journal of the American Medical Association* 87, no. 15 (1926): 1213–14.

6. "Taped Interview."

7. Hollman, Gregory, Guanghong Shen, Lan Zeng, Rhonda Yngsdal-Krenz, William Perloff, Jerry Zimmerman, and Richard Strauss. "Helium-Oxygen Improves Clinical Asthma Scores in Children with Acute Bronchiolitis." *Critical Care Medicine* 26, no. 10 (October 1998): 1731–36. http://www.ncbi.nlm.nih.gov/pubmed/9781732.

8. Jones, Norman L. "E. J. Moran Campbell, 1925–2004." *American Journal of Respiratory and Critical Care Medicine* 170, no. 3 (August 1, 2004): 222.

9. Jones, "E. J. Moran Campbell."

10. Nikander, K., and M. Sanders. "The Early Evolution of Nebulizers." *Medica-Mundi* 54, no. 3 (2010): 47–53.

11. Kalei, Kalikiano. "A History of US Military Aviation Oxygen Systems to 1945 (Part 1 of 2)." Authors Den. Last updated February 6, 2008. http://www.authors den.com/visit/viewarticle.asp?id=36665.

12. I once met Bird at his corporate headquarters in Palm Springs. He was a big, ebullient fellow, quick to smile, full of energy, and a trove of technical information. I could see why he was a successful entrepreneur. Bird died in 2015 at the age of ninety-four.

13. "Timeline and History. AARC." American Association for Respiratory Care. 2017. https://www.aarc.org/aarc/timeline-history.

14. I refer to him either as Petty or Dr. Thomas Petty to avoid confusion with the singer Tom Petty.

15. Gellene, Denise. "Dr. Thomas L. Petty, 76; Researched Long-Term Oxygen Therapy." *New York Times*, January 17, 2010.

16. "Taped Interview."

17. Casaburi, Richard. "Dr. Alvan Barach: New York's Founder of Pulmonary Rehabilitation." Pulmonary Education and Research Foundation. 2013. http://perf2ndwind.org/messages-barach.html.

18. Because of gravity, more air flows to the upper region of the lungs and more blood to the lower portion, slightly mismatching airflow and blood flow.

19. Casaburi, "Dr. Alvan Barach."

CHAPTER 22: THANK YOU FOR MY LIFE

1. Macintyre, Neil R., and Richard D. Branson, eds. *Mechanical Ventilation.* 2nd ed. St. Louis, MO: Saunders Elsevier, 2008, p. xi.

2. Rosenberg, Henry, and Jean K. Axelrod. "Ernst Trier Mørch: Inventor, Medical Pioneer, Heroic Freedom Fighter." *Anesthesia and Analgesia* 90, no. 1 (January 2000): 218–21.

3. Rosenberg and Axelrod, "Ernst Trier Mørch," p. 218.

4. Rosenberg and Axelrod, "Ernst Trier Mørch," p. 220.

5. Colice, Gene L. "Historical Perspective on the Development of Mechanical Ventilation." In *Principles and Practice of Mechanical Ventilation.* 3rd ed. Martin J. Tobin, ed. New York: McGraw-Hill Medical, 2013, p. 15.

6. West, John B. "Galen and the Beginnings of Western Physiology." *American Journal of Physiology: Lung Cellular and Molecular Physiology* 307 (2014): L124.

7. Mørch, E. T. "History of Mechanical Ventilation." In *Mechanical Ventilation.* Robert R. Kirby, Robert A. Smith, and David A. Desautels, eds. New York: Churchill, Livingston, 1985, p. 1.

8. Mushin, W. W., and L. Rendell-Baker, eds. *The Principles and Practice of Thoracic Anesthesia: Past and Present*. Oxford, Blackwell Scientific, 1953, p. 39; cited in Colice, "Historical Perspective."

9. Bert, Paul. *Barometric Pressure: Researches in Experimental Physiology* (1878). Mary Alice Hitchcock and Fred Andrews Hitchcock, trans. Columbus, OH: College Books, 1943; cited in Colice, "Historical Perspective," p. 19.

10. Bowditch, H. P. "Physiological Apparatus in Use at the Harvard Medical School." *Journal of Physiology* 2, no. 3 (September 1, 1879): 202–5; cited in Colice, "Historical Perspective," p. 20.

11. Mørch, "History of Mechanical Ventilation," p. 20.

12. Mørch, "History of Mechanical Ventilation," p. 20.

13. Colice, "Historical Perspective," p. 27.

14. Trubuhovich, Ronald V. "History of Medicine: On the Very First, Successful, Long-Term, Large-Scale Use of IPPV: Albert Bower and V. Ray Bennett: Los Angeles, 1948–1949." *Critical Care and Resuscitation* 9, no. 1 (March 2007): 91–100.

15. Motley, H. L., L. Werko, and A. Cournand. "Observations on the Clinical Use of Intermittent Positive Pressure." *Journal of Aviation Medicine* 18, no. 5 (October 1947): 417–35; and Motley, H. L., A. Cournand, L. Werko, D. T. Dresdale, A. Himmelstein, and D. W. Richards Jr. "Intermittent Positive Pressure Breathing: A Means of Administering Artificial Respiration in Man." *Journal of the American Medical Association* 137, no. 4 (May 22, 1948): 370–83.

16. Colice, "Historical Perspective," p. 26. See also Mørch, "History of Mechanical Ventilation," p. 24.

17. West, John B. "The Physiological Challenges of the 1952 Copenhagen Poliomyelitis Epidemic and a Renaissance in Clinical Respiratory Physiology." *Journal of Applied Physiology* 99, no. 2 (August 2005): 424–32.

18. West, "Physiological Challenges."

19. Trubuhovich, "History of Medicine," p. 98.

20. Colice, "Historical Perspective," p. 26.

21. West, "Physiological Challenges," p. 426.

22. West, "Physiological Challenges," p. 427.

23. Colice, "Historical Perspective," p. 29.

24. Mørch, "History of Mechanical Ventilation," p. 33.

25. Ashbaugh, David G., D. Boyd Bigelow, Thomas L. Petty, and Bernard E. Levine. "Acute Respiratory Distress in Adults." *The Lancet* 290, no. 7511 (August 12, 1967): 319–23.

26. Kirby, R. "Is Intermittent Mandatory Ventilation a Satisfactory Alternative to Assisted and Controlled Ventilation." *American Society of Anesthesiology Refresher Course Lecture* (1975); cited in Mørch, "History of Mechanical Ventilation," p. 33.

27. Soo Hoo, GuyW. "Noninvasive Ventilation." Medscape. Last updated October 12, 2016. http://emedicine.medscape.com/article/304235-overview?pa=1Qwn61gn1E kEGrPcmuzCbokpdyqFY%2Fbu610qO56EbO0c36K9W35lxcfSKE7rpy6T43mU9jD %2B1DtnxY47OmyybA%3D%3D.

CHAPTER 23: I WOULDN'T WANT THAT FOR MYSELF

1. "Socrates: Quotes: Quotable Quote." Goodreads. 2017. www.goodreads.com/quotes/671772-when-you-want-wisdom-and-insight-as-badly-as-you.

2. Quoted in J. D. "Inspirational Quotes." Sources of Insight. http://sourcesof insight.com/inspirational-quotes.

3. McFadden, Robert D. "Karen Ann Quinlan, 31, Dies: Focus of '76 Right to Die Case." *New York Times*, June 12, 1986. http://www.nytimes.com/1985/06/12/nyregion/karen-ann-quinlan-31-dies-focus-of-76-right-to-die-case.html.

CHAPTER 24: A SCIENCE OF UNCERTAINTY

1. Bean, Robert Bennett, comp., and William Bennett Bean, ed. *Sir William Osler: Aphorisms from His Bedside Teachings and Writings*.2nd ed. Springfield, IL: Charles C. Thomas, 1961, epitome 265, p. 129.

2. Sontag, Susan. *Illness as Metaphor*. New York: Vintage Books, 1979, p. 3.

3. Osler, William. "Medicine in the Nineteenth Century." In *Aequanimitas: With Other Addresses to Medical Students, Nurses, and Practitioners of Medicine*. 3rd ed. Philadelphia: Blakiston's Son, 1932, pp. 219–62.

4. Osler, "Medicine," p. 257.

5. Osler, "Medicine," p. 259.

6. Luke, 4:23. In Barker, Kenneth, ed. *The New International Version Study Bible*. Grand Rapids, MI: Zondervan, 1995.

7. Glover, Anne. "The 21st Century: The Age of Biology." Organization for Economic Cooperation and Development, Forum on Global Biotechnology, Paris, November 12, 2012. https://www.google.com/url?sa=t&rct=j&q=&esrc=s&source=web&cd=1&ved=0ahUKEwitgPiKnObJAhUT02MKHRzqAeAQFggdMAA&url=http%3A%2F%2Fwww.oecd.org%2Fsti%2Fbiotech%2FA%2520Glover.pdf&usg=AFQjCNG2K83IctkCmFA_diBmvL9h_Y8fsw&sig2=CdAg44DvToWBjd9yjeWs2A.

8. Topol, Eric J. *The Patient Will See You Now: The Future of Medicine Is in Your Hands*. New York: Basic Books, 2015; Verghese, Abraham. *Cutting for Stone: A Novel*. New York: Alfred A. Knopf, 2009.

9. Farley, Thomas A. "Mass Diseases, Mass Exposures, and Mass Media." *Journal of the American Medical Association: Internal Medicine* 175, no. 11 (November 2015): 1743–44.

10. Pope Francis. *Encyclical Letter* Laudato Si' *of the Holy Father Francis on Care for Our Common Home*. Vatican Press, 2015, no. 89.

11. Sontag, *Illness as Metaphor*, p. 3.

SELECTED BIBLIOGRAPHY

Barry, John M. *The Great Influenza: The Epic Story of the Deadliest Plague in History*. New York: Viking, 2004.

Bates, Barbara. *Bargaining for Life: A Social History of Tuberculosis, 1876–1938*. Philadelphia: University of Pennsylvania Press, 1992.

Bean, Robert Bennett, comp., and William Bennett Bean, ed. *Sir William Osler: Aphorisms from His Bedside Teachings and Writings*. 2nd ed. Springfield, IL: Charles C. Thomas, 1961.

Cherniack, Martin. *The Hawk's Nest Incident: America's Worst Industrial Disaster*. New Haven, CT: Yale University Press, 1986.

Davis, Devra Lee. *When Smoke Ran Like Water: Tales of Environmental Deception and the Battle against Pollution*. New York: Basic Books, 2002.

Fishman, Alfred P., Jack A. Elias, Jay A. Fishman, Michael A. Grippi, Robert M. Senior, and Allan I. Pack, eds. *Fishman's Pulmonary Diseases and Disorders*. 4th ed. New York: McGraw-Hill Medical, 2008.

Garrison, Fielding H. *An Introduction to the History of Medicine: With Medical Chronology, Suggestions for Study and Bibliographic Data*. 4th ed. Philadelphia: W. B. Saunders, 1929.

Harrod, Kathryn E. *Man of Courage: The Story of Dr. Edward L. Trudeau*. New York: J. Messner, 1959.

Hawkins, Leonard C. *The Man in the Iron Lung: The Frederick B. Snite, Jr., Story*. Garden City, NY: Doubleday, 1956.

Jacobs, Chip, and William J. Kelly. *Smogtown: The Lung-Burning History of Pollution in Los Angeles*. Woodstock, NY: Overlook Press, 2008.

Jonsen, Albert R., Mark Siegler, and William J. Winslade. *Clinical Ethics: A Practical Approach to Ethical Decisions in Clinical Medicine*. 6th ed. New York: McGraw-Hill, 2006.

Kidder, Tracy. *Mountains beyond Mountains*. New York: Random House, 2003.

Mason, Robert J., V. Courtney Broaddus, Thomas R. Martin, Talmadge E. King Jr., Dean E. Schraufnagel, John E. Murray, and Jay A. Nadel, eds. *Murray and Nadel's Textbook of Respiratory Medicine*. 5th ed. Philadelphia: Saunders Elsevier, 2010.

Morgan, W. Keith C., and Anthony Seaton. *Occupational Lung Diseases*. 2nd ed. Philadelphia: W. B. Saunders, 1984.

Mukherjee, Siddhartha. *The Emperor of All Maladies: A Biography of Cancer*. New York: Scribner, 2010.

Osler, William. *Aequanimitas: With Other Addresses to Medical Students, Nurses, and Practitioners of Medicine*. 3rd ed. Philadelphia: Blakiston's Son, 1932.

———. *The Principles and Practice of Medicine*. 3rd ed. New York: D. Appleton, 1899.

Quinones, Sam. *Dreamland: The True Tale of America's Opiate Epidemic*. New York: Bloomsbury Press, 2015.

Ryan, Frank. *The Forgotten Plague: How the Battle against Tuberculosis Was Won—and Lost*. Boston: Little, Brown, 1993.

Sontag, Susan. *Illness as Metaphor*. New York: Vintage Books, 1979.

Topol, Eric. *The Patient Will See You Now: The Future of Medicine Is in Your Hands*. New York: Basic Books, 2015.

Trudeau, Edward Livingston. *An Autobiography*. New York: Doubleday, Doran, 1936.

Verghese, Abraham. *Cutting for Stone: A Novel*. New York: Alfred A. Knopf, 2009.

Wallace, Joseph. *Colleagues in Discovery: One Hundred Years of Improving Respiratory Health*. San Diego, CA: Tehabi Books, 2005.

ACKNOWLEDGMENTS

Since 2012, when I decided to write *Gasping for Air*, I had to make decisions about what to include, and left out some topics, such as altitude sickness, diving medicine, drowning, and strangulation. I wanted the book to be broad but not exhaustive. Along the way, I received encouragement and help from many people, and they deserve thanks. My wife, Patty, supported the project from start to finish and patiently listened to me read portions of the manuscript out loud week after week. She also gave me the perspective of "Everyreader," which was often sobering but always helpful. My children, Kevin, Mary Ellen, Kathleen, Patrick, and Terry Glynn, accomplished communicators in their own domains, encouraged me and spurred me on.

The Read and Critique Group, led by Rich Farrell and Sandra Younger, forced me to "think story." Rich also acted as content editor, which I value very much. Sandra was a wise cheerleader, a most helpful role. Jean Seager, Dave Knop, Amy Ohlson, Susan Gembrowski, Linda Salem, Jo-Anne Berelowitz, Carol Lail, Nancy Eisenberg, Leslie Ray, Sandy Robertson, and Stacey Riley were always constructive in their critiques, and I appreciate their support.

I am grateful to colleagues who reviewed sections of the manuscript and clarified my misstatements. From Scripps Health, these include Gonzalo Ballon-Landa, Tom Farrell, Herman Froeb, Jeff Sandler, Art Johnson, Don Stevenson, Bob Sarnoff, Larry Kline, and Dave Shaw. David Gambling from Sharp Mary Birch Hospital reviewed the chapter on infant respiratory distress.

From UC San Diego School of Medicine, John West, Tony Catanzaro, Bill Hughson, David Burns, Andy Ries, John Adamson, Peter Fedullo, Ted Vallejos, and Lynn Russell of the Scripps Institution of Oceanography graciously reviewed chapters related to their areas of expertise. Demo Pappagianis and Tim Albertson of UC Davis and Philip Hopewell of UC San Francisco reviewed specific chapters, as did Todd Steck of the University of North Carolina, Charlotte. Whitney Addington, my classmate from Northwestern Feinberg School of Medicine, reviewed sections on respiratory public health. Alon Winnie reviewed the chapter on ventilators. Al died while the manuscript was being revised. May he rest in peace. Gayle Hefner, my long-time medical assistant, recently deceased, assisted me in recalling details of patients' stories, which was a great help. May she rest in peace. Roger Haines from Rotary International reviewed the chapter on air pollution. I am grateful to all of you. Any errors that remain are solely my responsibility.

I am also grateful to the American Medical Association, American Cancer Society, American College of Chest Physicians, and Conde Nast. Part of Maude's story in chapter 10 is excerpted from "Exogenous Lipoid Pneumonia Due to Inhalation of Spray Lubricant (WD-40 Lung)," *Chest* 97 (1990): 1265–66. © American College of Chest Physicians. Part of Ozzie's story in chapter 12 is excerpted from "Hypertrichosis Lanuginosa as a Sign of Internal Malignancy," *Cancer* 24 (1969): 1051–56. © American Cancer Society. Part of Earl's story in chapter 12 is excerpted from "Piano Lessons," *Journal of the American Medical Association* 306, no. 10 (2011): 1063–64. © American Medical Association. Part of Ray's story in chapter 15 is excerpted from "A Golf Pro Made Me a Better Doctor," *Golf Digest* (November 2012). © Conde Nast.

In writing *Gasping for Air*, I learned how much book writing and publishing depend on teamwork. Chris Fortunato, my agent, saw a future for *Gasping*, worked untiringly to show the book proposal to the publishing industry, and taught me how the business works. Martha Murphy edited the book proposal, and Suzanne Staszak-Silva, acquisitions editor at Rowman & Littlefield, guided the manuscript as it emerged from my word processor, and nursed the book through the publishing process. Alden Perkins, production editor, and Niki Guinan, copy editor, also helped bring the manuscript to its final form. Sunny McGowan and Lee Luniewski of the McGuire Medical Library at Scripps Mercy Hospital helped me find important references, always with a "can do" attitude. I appreciate all of your help as well.

INDEX

jock itch, 50
Johansson, Gunnar, xiii
Jonsen, Albert, xiii, 220

Karolinska Institute, Stockholm,
    Sweden, 204
Keller, Helen, 63
Kelly, Frank, 248n14
Kelly, William, 125
Kendall, Edward, xii, 136
Kennedy, Patrick, 184, 187
Kentucky, 92–93
Kirby, Robert, 211
Klebs, Edwin, 23
Klein, Allen, 191
Koch, Robert, x, 13

Laennec, René, x, 12, 80, 141, 147, 153
large-cell carcinomas, 113
Lassen, Henry, 207–9
Leahy, Frank, 36
Legionnaires' disease, xiii, 55–62
leptin, 175
Levine, Edward, 198
Liggins, Graham, 186
Linde liquid oxygen reservoir, xiii
Linde walker, 195
Link, Karl, xi
lipoid pneumonia, 99
Lister, F. Spencer, 25
Loftus, Eileen, 122
London, England, xii, 126
Los Angeles, California, xii, 3, 126, 130
Los Angeles County Hospital, 207–8
Love Save Pneumoconiosis, 81
Lowell, A. Lawrence, 39
Lucky Strike, 105, 106
Luft, Benjamin, 85
lung cancer, 111–20; causes of, xii,
    102–3, 106, 112, 113, 115, 117–18;
    costs of, 118; deadliness of, 115,
    118; genetic factors in, 114; growth
    and spread of, 114–15; personal

account of, 111–13, 118–20;
    prevalence of, 3, 118; psychological
    effects of, 119; treatment of, xi, xv,
    3, 115; types of, 113–15
lung edema, 210–11
lung fibrosis, 170
lungs: heart working in tandem with,
    167–72; irritants of, 2; of newborns,
    183–86; physiology of, 2, 142, 147;
    respiratory process of, 205
lung surgery, 206, 209
lymphocytes, 52

MA-1 ventilator, xiii, 210
Macintosh, Robert, 204
Macintyre, Neil, 203
Maloney, Cynthia, 85
Malpighi, Marcello, 170
Manhattan Project, 118
Mann, Thomas, *The Magic Mountain*,
    12
March of Dimes, 41, 42, 188
marijuana, xiv, 94–96;
Massachusetts General Hospital, 39, 40
McDade, Joseph, 55, 57–59
McDonough, Brendan, 87–88
McKhann, Charles, 37
McMath, Jahi, xiv
Mead, Jere, xii, 184, 186
Medecins Sans Frontieres (Doctors
    without Borders), 64
Melville, Herman, 151
meningitis, 22
Merck, 16
MERS-CoV. *See* Middle East
    respiratory syndrome
mesothelioma, 79, 116
metastasis, 103, 113
methane, 129
methyl isocyanate (MIC), 86
Metropole Hotel, Hong Kong, 65
Middle East respiratory syndrome
    (MERS-CoV), xiv, 3, 66–69